T0263359

Pathology and Clinical Relevance of Neoplastic Precursor Lesions of the Tubal Gut, Liver, and Pancreaticobiliary System: A Contemporary Update

Editor

ROBERT D. ODZE

GASTROENTEROLOGY CLINICS OF NORTH AMERICA

www.gastro.theclinics.com

Consulting Editor
ALAN L. BUCHMAN

March 2024 • Volume 53 • Number 1

ELSEVIER

1600 John F. Kennedy Boulevard ● Suite 1800 ● Philadelphia, Pennsylvania, 19103-2899

http://www.theclinics.com

GASTROENTEROLOGY CLINICS OF NORTH AMERICA Volume 53, Number 1
March 2024 ISSN 0889-8553, ISBN-13: 978-0-443-13005-2

Editor: Kerry Holland
Developmental Editor: Isha Singh

Gastroenterology Clinics of North America (ISSN 0889-8553) is published quarterly by Elsevier Inc., 360 Park Avenue South, New York, NY 10010-1710. Months of issue are March, June, September, and December. Business and Editorial Offices: 1600 John F. Kennedy Blvd., Suite 1800, Philadelphia, PA 19103-2899. Customer Service Office: 6277 Sea Harbor Drive, Orlando, FL 32887-4800. Periodicals postage paid at New York, NY and additional mailing offices. Subscription prices are $387.00 per year (US individuals), $100.00 per year (US students), $407.00 per year (Canadian individuals), $100.00 per year (Canadian students), $496.00 per year (international individuals), $220.00 per year (international students). For institutional access pricing please contact Customer Service via the contact information below. Foreign air speed delivery is included in all *Clinics* subscription prices. All prices are subject to change without notice. **POSTMASTER**: Send address changes to *Gastroenterology Clinics of North America*, Elsevier Health Sciences Division, Subscription Customer Service, 3251 Riverport Lane, Maryland Heights, MO 63043. **Telephone: 1-800-654-2452 (U.S. and Canada); 314-447-8871 (outside U.S. and Canada). Fax: 314-447-8029. E-mail: journalscustomerservice-usa@elsevier.com (for print support); journalsonlinesupport-usa@elsevier.com (for online support).**

Reprints. For copies of 100 or more, of articles in this publication, please contact the Commercial Reprints Department, Elsevier Inc., 360 Part Avenue South, New York, New York 10010-1710. Tel. 212-633-3874, Fax: 212-633-3820, E-mail: reprints@elsevier.com.

Gastroenterology Clinics of North America is also published in Italian by Il Pensiero Scientifico Editore, Rome, Italy; and in Portuguese by Interlivros Edicoes Ltda., Rua Commandante Coelho 1085, 21250 Cordovil, Rio de Janeiro, Brazil.

Gastroenterology Clinics of North America is covered in *MEDLINE/PubMed (Index Medicus)*, *Excerpta Medica*, *Current Contents/Clinical Medicine*, *Science Citation Index*, *ISI/BIOMED*, and *BIOSIS*.

Contributors

CONSULTING EDITOR

ALAN L. BUCHMAN, MD, MSPH, FACP, FACN, FACG, AGAF
Professor of Clinical Surgery, Medical Director, Intestinal Rehabilitation and Transplant Center, The University of Illinois at Chicago, UI Health, Chicago, Illinois, USA

EDITOR

ROBERT D. ODZE, MD, FRCPc
Professor of Pathology, Tufts University Medical Center, Department of Pathology and Lab Medicine, Tufts University School of Medicine, President and Managing Partner, Dr Robert Odze Pathology LLC, Boston, Massachusetts, USA

AUTHORS

N. VOLKAN ADSAY, MD
Professor, Head of Pathology, Head of Surgical Sciences, Chair, Department of Pathology, Koç University School of Medicine, Zeytinburnu, Istanbul, Turkey

TOMIO ARAI, MD, PhD
Director, Department of Pathology, Tokyo Metropolitan Institute for Geriatrics and Gerontology, Itabashi-ku, Tokyo, Japan

OLCA BASTURK, MD
Attending Pathologist, Department of Pathology and Laboratory Medicine, Memorial Sloan Kettering Cancer Center, New York, New York, USA

MARK BETTINGTON, MBBS, PhD, FRCPA
Envoi Pathology, Faculty of Medicine, University of Queensland, Brisbane, Queensland, Australia; Queensland Institute of Medical Research, Brisbane, Queensland, Australia

LODEWIJK A. A. BROSENS, MD, PhD
Associate Professor, Department of Pathology, University Medical Center Utrecht, Utrecht University, GA Utrecht, Netherlands

IAN BROWN, MBBS, FRCPA
Faculty of Medicine, University of Queensland, Brisbane; Envoi Pathology, Pathology Queensland, Queensland, Australia

NOAM HARPAZ, MD, PhD
Professor, Department of Pathology, Molecular and Cell-Based Medicine, Department of Medicine, Icahn School of Medicine at Mount Sinai, New York, New York, USA

STEVEN H. ITZKOWITZ, MD
Professor, Department of Medicine, Division of Gastroenterology, Icahn School of Medicine at Mount Sinai, New York, New York, USA

SANJAY KAKAR, MD
Professor of Pathology; Director, GI-Hepatobiliary Pathology Fellowship Program; Chief, GI-Hepatobiliary Pathology Service, University of California, San Francisco, San Francisco, California, USA

GREGORY Y. LAUWERS, MD
Chief, Gastrointestinal Pathology Section, Senior Member, Department of Pathology, H. Lee Moffitt Cancer Center and Research Institute, Professor, Departments of Pathology and Oncologic Sciences, University of South Florida Morsani College of Medicine, Tampa, Florida, USA

MAURICE B. LOUGHREY, BSc, MB, MD, MRCP, FRCPath
Professor of Gastrointestinal Pathology, Department of Cellular Pathology, Royal Victoria Hospital, Belfast, Northern Ireland, United Kingdom

ROBERT D. ODZE, MD, FRCPc
Professor of Pathology, Tufts University Medical Center, Department of Pathology and Lab Medicine, Tufts University School of Medicine, President and Managing Partner, Dr Robert Odze Pathology LLC, Boston, Massachusetts, USA

SATOSHI ONO, MD, PhD
Department of Gastroenterology and Gastrointestinal Endoscopy, Tokyo Metropolitan Institute for Geriatrics and Gerontology, Itabashi-ku, Tokyo, Japan

DEEPA T. PATIL, MD
Associate Professor, Department of Pathology, Brigham and Women's Hospital, Boston, Massachusetts, USA

CHRISTOPHE ROSTY, MD, PhD
Envoi Specialist Pathologists, University of Queensland, Brisbane, Queensland; Colorectal Oncogenomics Group, Department of Clinical Pathology, Victorian Comprehensive Cancer Centre, The University of Melbourne, Victoria, Australia

NEIL A. SHEPHERD, DM, FRCPath
Professor of Gastrointestinal Pathology, Gloucestershire Cellular Pathology Laboratory, Cheltenham General Hospital, Cheltenham, United Kingdom

KAIYO TAKUBO, MD, PhD
Research Team for Geriatric Pathology, Tokyo Metropolitan Institute for Geriatrics and Gerontology, Itabashi-ku, Tokyo, Japan

TETSUO USHIKU, MD, PhD
Professor, Department of Pathology, The University of Tokyo, Bunkyoku, Tokyo, Japan

KWUN WAH WEN, MD, PhD
Associate Professor, Division of Surgical Pathology, Departments of Pathology and Laboratory Medicine, University of California, San Francisco, San Francisco, California, USA

Contents

> Early detection of dysplasia and effective management are critical steps in halting neoplastic progression in patients with Barrett's esophagus (BE). This review provides a contemporary overview of the BE-related dysplasia, its role in guiding surveillance and management, and discusses emerging diagnostic and therapeutic approaches that might further enhance patient management. Novel, noninvasive techniques for sampling and surveillance, adjunct biomarkers for risk assessment, and their limitations are also discussed.

> Clinicopathological and molecular studies have demonstrated that dysplasia is a precancerous and/or neoplastic lesion with malignant potential. Further, it is subclassified into two grades: high-grade and low-grade dysplasia. High-grade dysplasia is a clinically significant lesion requiring resection or ablation. Low-grade dysplasia has a much lower risk of carcinoma; thus, it should be followed by endoscopic surveillance. Because squamous dysplasia may progress to squamous cell carcinoma, periodic endoscopy is useful to detect the lesion in patients with risk factors. Squamous dysplasia is diagnosed histopathologically by evaluating both cytologic and structural changes.

> Gastric dysplasia is defined as an unequivocally neoplastic epithelium. Dysplastic lesions are characterized by cellular atypia reflective of abnormal differentiation and disorganized glandular architecture. The last few years have been marked by a refinement of the prognosis and risk of progression of gastric dysplasia and the recognition of novel morphologic patterns of dysplasia. Determination of the correct diagnosis and grade of dysplasia are critical steps since it will be predicting the risk of malignant transformation and help tailor appropriate surveillance strategy. This review describes the morphologic characteristics of conventional dysplasia and nonconventional gastric dysplasia that have been more recently characterized.

chronic inflammatory bowel disease. This review provides a contemporary overview of the pathologic and endoscopic classification of dysplasia in inflammatory bowel disease, their roles in determining surveillance and management algorithms, and emerging diagnostic and therapeutic approaches that might further enhance patient management.

Colorectal polyps are common, and their diagnosis and classification represent a major component of gastrointestinal pathology practice. The majority of colorectal polyps represent precursors of either the chromosomal instability or serrated neoplasia pathways to colorectal carcinoma. Accurate reporting of these polyps has major implications for surveillance and thus for cancer prevention. In this review, we discuss the key histologic features of the major colorectal polyps with a particular emphasis on diagnostic pitfalls and areas of contention.

Gastrointestinal polyposis disorders are a group of syndromes defined by clinicopathologic features that include the predominant histologic type of colorectal polyp and specific inherited gene mutations. Adenomatous polyposis syndromes comprise the prototypical familial adenomatous polyposis syndrome and other recently identified genetic conditions inherited in a dominant or recessive manner. Serrated polyposis syndrome is defined by arbitrary clinical criteria. The diagnosis of hamartomatous polyposis syndromes can be suggested from the histologic characteristics of colorectal polyps and the association with various extraintestinal manifestations. Proper identification of affected individuals is important due to an increased risk of gastrointestinal and extragastrointestinal cancers.

Anal cancer, mainly squamous cell carcinoma, is rare but increasing in prevalence, as is its precursor lesion, anal squamous dysplasia. They are both strongly associated with human papillomavirus infection. The 2-tiered Lower Anogenital Squamous Terminology classification, low-grade SIL and high-grade SIL, is preferred to the 3-tiered anal intraepithelial neoplasia classification because of better interobserver agreement and clearer management implications. Immunohistochemistry with p16 is helpful to corroborate the diagnosis of squamous dysplasia. Similarly, immunohistochemistry is helpful to differentiate primary Paget disease from secondary Paget disease, which is usually due to anal squamous mucosal/epidermal involvement by primary rectal adenocarcinoma.

GASTROENTEROLOGY CLINICS OF NORTH AMERICA

Foreword

Singing With or About Gastrointestinal Cancers

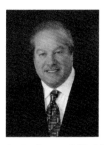

Alan L. Buchman, MD, MSPH
Consulting Editor

According to the World Cancer Research Fund International, the gastrointestinal (GI) tract is the organ system most affected by primary malignancies, with 30.7% of cancer cases originating in the GI tract. All areas of the GI tract, where food passes or are involved in the digestion or absorption of food, may be afflicted, from the mouth to the anus. Of these, colorectal cancers are the most common, with close to 2 million new cases annually worldwide.

Many songs have been written about GI cancers, including

- "Stronger Than That" by Craig Campbell, inspired by colorectal cancer survivor, Rose Hausmann, and Campbell's father, who died of colorectal cancer.
- "Hope's Alive" by Erin Willett, an anthem of hope for those impacted by pancreatic cancer
- "Liver Cancer" by the Piss Drinkers
- "Neoplasia" by the Argentinian brutal death metal band of the same name
- "Terminal Gastric Cancer" by the brutal death metal band Sakryn

While these artists may not be mainstream, GI cancers certainly are. A number of popular singers have also been stricken with GI tract malignancies, including

- Taylor Dane (colon cancer)
- Eddie Money (esophageal cancer)
- Aretha Franklin and Luciano Pavarotti (pancreatic cancer)
- David Bowie (liver cancer)

Many of these malignancies can be prevented by detection and proper treatment of precancerous neoplasia. Dr Odze has assembled a world-renowned group of experts

---

https://doi.org/10.1016/j.gtc.2023.11.001
0889-8553/24/© 2023 Published by Elsevier Inc.
gastro.theclinics.com

on the precursors of these various malignancies, their pathology, and their recognition. Best will be the day that artists no longer get GI cancers or need to write about them anymore, instead, write music about their prevention or recovery.

Alan L. Buchman, MD, MSPH
Intestinal Rehabilitation and Transplant Center
Department of Surgery/
UI Health University of Illinois at Chicago
840 South Wood Street, Suite 402 (MC958)
Chicago, IL 60612, USA

E-mail address:
buchman@uic.edu

Preface

Gastrointestinal Tract, Liver, and Pancreatic/Biliary Precursor Lesions

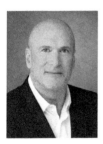

Robert D. Odze, MD, FRCPc
Editor

This issue of *Gastroenterology Clinics of North America* represents a contemporary clinical and pathology update of neoplastic precursors of the GI, liver, and pancreatic/biliary tract that was originally published in *Gastroenterology Clinics of North America* in 2007. Since the time of that publication, there have been many key developments in our understanding of the clinical and biological characteristics, pathogenesis, molecular features, and pathology of gastrointestinal (GI), liver, and pancreatic/biliary precursor lesions. For instance, regarding pathology specifically, there have been changes to the classification, terminology, and clinical relevance of neoplastic precursor lesions that clinicians should be aware of in order to provide appropriate and up-to-date care to their patients.

Similar to the original *Gastroenterology Clinics of North America* publication in 2007, in this issue, internationally recognized pathologists and clinicians have provided timely reviews on neoplastic precursor lesions but have also provided particular emphasis on the clinical relevance and associations of precursor lesions with molecular pathogenesis. For instance, due to recent advancements in molecular techniques and diagnostics, we have now been able to recognize the earliest forms of neoplasia, even prior to the morphologic expression of dysplasia, which until recently was considered by many to be the earliest manifestation of cancer risk identifiable in human tissue. Thus, the concept of "neoplasia without dysplasia" is now commonplace in pathology and now well accepted among GI pathologists worldwide. For instance, in the articles on Barrett's esophagus and gastric precursor lesions, entities now known as "crypt" and "pit" dysplasia, respectively, do not contain traditional morphologic features of "dysplasia" but are now recognized to be important early lesions associated with progression to cancer. In the colon, sessile serrate lesions are now

Gastroenterol Clin N Am 53 (2024) xi–xii
https://doi.org/10.1016/j.gtc.2023.11.006
0889-8553/24/© 2023 Published by Elsevier Inc.

recognized to have neoplastic potential, but most of these lesions do not show dysplasia morphologically. In the liver, we now recognize an elevated cancer risk associated with certain lesions never before thought to be cancer precursor lesions, such as in certain subtypes of hepatic adenomas. Parallel with the development of advanced and sophisticated molecular diagnostic techniques, scientists and pathologists alike have come to realize the importance of lesions that have previously been considered innocuous and have now been able to correlate molecularly abnormal signatures with the morphologic appearance of early changes in the progression to cancer. This information has been highlighted in this issue of *Gastroenterology Clinics of North America*.

Unfortunately, despite advancements in our diagnostic acumen, we still suffer from many limitations regarding our ability to recognize and predict cancer development at the histologic, and even the molecular, level, and as such, much important scientific work still needs to be performed. As I had mentioned in the first issue of *Gastroenterology Clinics of North America* in 2007, on precursor lesions, in some areas we have made few advancements. For instance, pathologists still suffer from high rates of interobserver error. Some of this error may be attributed to the relatively low prevalence rate of neoplastic precursor lesions in the general population and the relative inexperience with recognition of precursor lesions by most nontertiary care-affiliated general pathologists and the lack of access to advanced molecular diagnostic techniques that have yet to become mainstream in our medical societies. The problem associated with sampling error, unfortunately, still persists in diagnostics of many neoplastic entities in the GI tract, liver, and pancreatic/biliary tract, but most notably in conditions such as Barrett's esophagus, chronic gastritis, and inflammatory bowel disease. Thus, there is still a pressing need for more research in order to develop more sensitive and specific, reproducible, and accessible inexpensive biomarkers. Although we have made considerable gains in this area of cancer research in the last decade, much work remains to be done despite the challenges of doing large-scale population studies. Similar to our original report in 2007, although the medical and scientific community still feels that screening and surveillance for precursor lesions are both logical and scientifically valid, there is an ongoing need for more prospective controlled trials to determine the true costs and benefits of these programs.

Finally, I would like to thank all of the authors who have contributed reviews in this issue of *Gastroenterology Clinics of North America*, many of whom have spent a great portion of their medical careers exploring the science behind early cancer progression in the GI tract. As a result of the work of these dedicated individuals, considerable gains in patient care and longer survival rates have been achieved for patients at risk for cancer of the GI tract and associated organs.

Robert D. Odze, MD, FRCPc
Tufts University Medical Center
Boston, MA 02115, USA

Dr Robert Odze Pathology LLC
Boston, MA 02116, USA

E-mail address:
Rodze@tuftsmedicalcenter.org

Website:
http://Odzepathology.com

Barrett's Esophagus and Associated Dysplasia

Deepa T. Patil, MD[a],*, Robert D. Odze, MD[b]

KEYWORDS

- Barrett's esophagus • Endoscopy • Dysplasia • Surveillance

KEY POINTS

- The new definition of Barrett's esophagus includes endoscopic recognition of salmon-colored mucosa into the tubular esophagus, extending 1 cm or greater proximal to the gastroesophageal junction, which is confirmed pathologically to contain goblet cells.
- Pathologic diagnosis and grading of dysplasia in mucosal biopsies remain the best and most widely used methods of determining which patients are at highest risk for neoplastic progression, and for selecting patients who need a more intensive surveillance program or surgical intervention.
- Newer endoscopic and sampling techniques have the advantage of reducing sampling error.
- Use of standardized terminology for grading dysplasia is important for optimal and timely management.
- Recent advances in endoscopic resection techniques, such as endoscopic mucosal resection and endoscopic submucosal dissection, have the distinct advantage of improving the accuracy of grading dysplasia and staging early cancers.

INTRODUCTION

The incidence of esophageal and gastroesophageal junction (GEJ) adenocarcinoma has increased by approximately 600% in the United States during the past 30 years.[1,2] The precursor to esophageal adenocarcinoma (EAC) is Barrett's esophagus (BE), which is caused by chronic gastroesophageal reflux disease (GERD).[3] Histologic evaluation of dysplasia in esophageal mucosal biopsies is the mainstay of risk assessment in the surveillance and treatment of patients with BE. The current definition of dysplasia is "unequivocal" neoplastic epithelium confined to the basement membrane.[4,5] In most Western countries, including the United States, dysplasia in BE is classified as either negative, indefinite, or positive (low or high grade), based on a system initially developed

[a] Department of Pathology, Brigham and Women's Hospital, Boston, MA, USA; [b] Department of Pathology and Lab Medicine, Tufts University School of Medicine, Boston, MA, USA
* Corresponding author. Department of Pathology, Harvard Medical School, 75 Francis St. Cotran-3, Boston, MA 02115
E-mail address: deepa.patil@icloud.com

Gastroenterol Clin N Am 53 (2024) 1–23
https://doi.org/10.1016/j.gtc.2023.11.002
0889-8553/24/© 2023 Elsevier Inc. All rights reserved.

in 1983 for patients with inflammatory bowel disease.[4,5] This system has been applied to BE and to most, if not all, neoplastic precursor lesions of the tubal gut. However, many pathologists in Europe and Asia prefer the recently proposed Vienna classification system (**Table 1**),[6] which uses the term "noninvasive neoplasia" instead of "low-grade" or "high-grade" dysplasia, includes a category for "noninvasive" carcinoma (carcinoma in-situ) and also uses the term "suspicious for invasive carcinoma" for biopsies that show equivocal features of tissue invasion. This article focuses on dysplasia in BE in terms of its classification, risk factors and pathogenesis, pathologic diagnostic criteria, limitations, natural history, and treatment.

CLINICAL AND ENDOSCOPIC FEATURES

Although most cases of BE are acquired, a very small proportion of cases are congenital in origin. A familial predisposition for BE and EAC has been documented.[7] BE is found in approximately 5% to 15% of patients who undergo endoscopy for symptoms of GERD,[8] compared with 1.3% to 1.6% of the general population.[9]

Traditionally, BE is separated into long-segment (>3 cm), short-segment (1–3 cm), and ultrashort-segment (<1 cm) types, depending on the length of involved mucosa.[10,11] However, the biological significance of this classification is unclear. Sharma and colleagues[11] proposed an alternative consensus endoscopic classification system for BE, termed the Prague C&M criteria. This scoring system has been shown to be reliable in assessing the extent of endoscopic BE.[11,12]

Most experts use the "Seattle" protocol for surveillance of BE.[13,14] This includes 4-quadrant biopsies using jumbo biopsy forceps obtained from every 1 to 2 cm of BE mucosa, depending on the presence and degree of dysplasia, in addition to targeted biopsies of grossly apparent mucosal abnormalities.[13–15] The American College of Gastroenterology (ACG) and the American Gastroenterological Association (AGA) guidelines recommend that in patients with suspected BE, at least 8 random biopsies should be obtained to maximize the yield of intestinal metaplasia (IM) on histology. In those with shorter segments (1–2 cm), at least 4 biopsies per centimeter of circumferential BE, and 1 biopsy per centimeter in tongues of BE, should be obtained.[16]

Novel Tissue Acquisition Techniques for Screening and Surveillance

Nonendoscopic technologies for sampling BE have also gained significant interest because they are minimally invasive and have the potential for widespread

---

Table 1
Vienna classification and inflammatory bowel disease Dysplasia Morphology Study Group Classification of Neoplastic Precursor Lesions in Barrett's Esophagus

Vienna	IBD Study Group
Negative for neoplasia/dysplasia	Negative for dysplasia
Indefinite for neoplasia/dysplasia	Indefinite for dysplasia
Noninvasive low-grade neoplasia (low-grade adenoma/dysplasia)	Low-grade dysplasia
Noninvasive high-grade neoplasia	High-grade dysplasia
High-grade adenoma/dysplasia	
Noninvasive carcinoma (carcinoma in situ)	Suspicious for invasive carcinoma
Invasive neoplasia	Adenocarcinoma
Intramucosal adenocarcinoma	Intramucosal adenocarcinoma
Submucosal carcinoma or beyond	Invasive

applicability in the primary care setting. These technologies include Cytosponge™, which is an encapsulated sponge tethered to a string, which when swallowed and withdrawn out of the esophagus, collects cells from the esophageal lumen.[17] EsophaCap™, a sponge-on-string device, has been used in combination with methylated DNA biomarkers for diagnosing BE.[18] EsoCheck™ uses a swallowable encapsulated balloon device to sample the distal esophagus.[19] Wide area transepithelial sampling with computer-assisted 3-dimensional analysis of disaggregated tissue specimens, termed wide-area trans-epithelial sampling with 3 dimensional computer-assisted analysis (WATS^{3D}), is an approach that has shown enhanced detection rates of IM and dysplasia in BE.[20] Compared with forceps biopsies, WATS^{3D} samples a much broader area of mucosa, reducing sampling error. In addition, the procedure has been associated with good interobserver variability in pathology readings. WATS^{3D} has been shown to increase the diagnostic yield of IM and dysplasia in both screening and surveillance patients, in patients with BE postendoscopic ablation, and in patients with BE of all lengths of esophageal columnar mucosa equally.

Definition of Barrett's Esophagus

The ACG defines BE as endoscopically recognizable extension of salmon-colored mucosa into the tubular esophagus, extending 1 cm or greater proximal to the GEJ, which is confirmed pathologically to contain IM, the latter defined by the presence of goblet cells.[16] Both the endoscopic and the pathologic component must be present to establish a diagnosis of BE (**Fig. 1**A). By definition, this disease does not include patients who have IM (goblet cells) of the gastric cardia or when goblet cells are identified in patients who have a normal Z line or a Z line with less than 1 cm of variability. As much as one-third of patients with GERD who lack columnar mucosa within the distal esophagus show IM (goblet cells) in their otherwise anatomically normal GEJ, and these patients do not qualify as having BE based on the ACG definition.[16] This position is based on the assumption that the presence of a few intestinalized glands in the GEJ region of patients without endoscopically apparent columnar metaplasia of the distal esophagus does not confer the same increased risk of malignancy as endoscopically visible BE. Similarly, in large cohort studies with long-term follow-up, patients who demonstrate IM in segments less than 1 cm (referred to as specialized IM at GEJ)

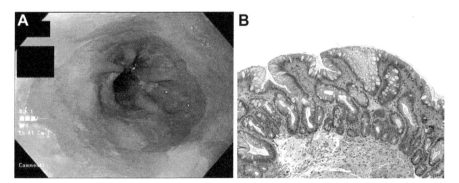

Fig. 1. (A) Endoscopic appearance of BE. Tongues of gastric-appearing columnar mucosa extend proximal to the GEJ in an irregular circumferential fashion. Notice the presence of squamous islands within the columnar mucosa. (B) BE, negative for dysplasia is characterized by the presence of incomplete IM, mucous columnar cells, scattered goblet cells, and reactive changes in the bases of the crypts. Nondysplastic BE shows mildly distorted crypt architecture characterized by mild crowding, branching, and budding.

have not shown an increase in the development of neoplasia compared to patients with segments of IM greater than 1 cm.[16] However, there is no worldwide agreement that IM (goblet cells) should be required for a diagnosis of BE. The British Society of Gastroenterology and the Japanese GERD Society Study Committee do not require IM to establish this diagnosis.[21,22]

Although histologic identification of intestinal (goblet) epithelium is required to establish a diagnosis of BE, the chance of detecting goblet cells is, essentially, proportional to the length of BE.[23–25] An increase in the number of biopsies also increases the likelihood of detecting goblet cells.[24]

PATHOGENESIS

The precise mechanism of development and the cell of origin of BE remain unknown but there has been much recent progress in this area. Chronic GERD leads to inflammation and ulceration of the esophageal squamous mucosa, which, if persistent and recurrent, ultimately leads to columnar metaplasia, usually with IM.[26–28] The proposed theories for pathogenesis of BE include the following: (1) conversion of squamous epithelium to gastric cardiac-type epithelium and to intestinal epithelium with ongoing injury and chronic inflammation, (2) exposure to bile acids,[29] and goblet cell development through a multistep process of transcommitment and transdifferentiation,[30] and (3) origin through progenitor stem cells including those residing in the basal layer of the esophageal squamous epithelium, mucosal and submucosal glands and their respective ducts.[31] In vitro experimental evidence supports the possibility that stem cells may be derived from undifferentiated mesenchymal cells, either in the lamina propria of the esophagus or in the bone marrow.[32] Using a rat model of reflux esophagitis via surgical esophagojejunostomy, Agoston and colleagues showed that metaplastic, columnar-lined esophagus develops via a wound healing process, and not via genetic reprogramming of progenitor cells.[33]

PATHOLOGY
Gross Features

Endoscopically, dysplasia may be undetectable or may seem as flat, irregular, plaque-like, nodular, polypoid, eroded, or ulcerated mucosa. Patients with one or more macroscopic lesions, especially nodules or ulcers are more likely to have and/or develop high-grade dysplasia (HGD) and cancer than patients without an endoscopically identifiable dysplastic lesion.

Microscopic Features

Dysplasia is defined as unequivocal neoplastic epithelium that remains confined within the basement membrane of the epithelium from which it develops.[34] In most Western countries, including the United States, specimens evaluated for dysplasia in BE are classified as negative, indefinite, or positive (either low grade or high grade).

Barrett's esophagus, negative for dysplasia
Because of persistent GERD, biopsies from patients with BE are often inflamed. Consequently, the epithelium normally shows a variable degree of regenerative change.[5] Biopsies with this type of morphology are categorized as "negative for dysplasia."[4] However, the spectrum of epithelial regeneration in BE is quite broad, so that at the severe end of the spectrum of regeneration, the degree of cytologic atypia may overlap with true dysplasia (see later discussion),[5,35] particularly in areas adjacent to ulcers. BE typically lacks evenly spaced test tube–like crypts characteristic of

the small and large bowel and also shows crypt budding, atrophy, branching, increased mitotic activity, hyperchromasia, dystrophic goblet cells, and mucin depletion (see **Fig. 1**). However, in contrast to well-developed dysplasia, the cells in nondysplastic BE maintain a low nuclear/cytoplasmic ratio, retain their polarity, and show progressive maturation (acquisition of cytoplasmic mucin) in epithelium at the mucosal surface. In fact, "surface maturation" is, in most instances, a helpful histologic sign of epithelial regeneration,[35] except in certain circumstances explained in later discussion.

Barrett's esophagus, indefinite for dysplasia

Pathologically, regenerating epithelium can, at times, be difficult to distinguish from true dysplasia. This is particularly apparent in instances where significant inflammation, or ulceration, is present in the biopsy specimen. In this context, the category "indefinite for dysplasia" is applied (**Fig. 2**).[4] Other reasons pathologists use the term "indefinite for dysplasia" include those related to technical issues, such as tangential or thick tissue sectioning, poor orientation, denuded surface epithelium, or marked cautery artifact. Finally, as explained in later discussion, some cases of dysplasia are limited to the crypt bases and, thus, mimic regeneration.[36] From a clinical perspective, "indefinite for dysplasia" should always be considered an interim diagnosis until mucosal biopsies can be processed better or until further biopsies can be evaluated after more aggressive treatment of the patient's reflux symptoms to decrease inflammation.

Barrett's esophagus, positive for dysplasia

In BE, 2 most common histologic types of dysplasia are intestinal (adenoma-like) and nonintestinal (foveolar or gastric type). A third type that has a serrated architecture (serrated dysplasia) may also show either intestinal or foveolar phenotype.[5] Intestinal dysplasia is much more common and is characterized by enlarged, elongated, and stratified nuclei (**Fig. 3**). The presence of (1) an abrupt transition between nondysplastic and dysplastic epithelium and (2) uniform nuclear changes extending evenly from the crypt base to the mucosal surface are helpful diagnostic features of low-grade dysplasia (LGD). Other features, including mitotic figures and pleomorphism, are typically only mild or absent.

In contrast to LGD, HGD shows increased crypt complexity, crowding, and branching, and cytologically, it shows more pronounced nuclear enlargement, loss of nuclear polarity, pleomorphism, nucleoli, and mitotic activity (**Fig. 4**). Two recent studies[37,38]

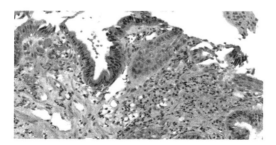

Fig. 2. BE, indefinite for dysplasia. The biopsy shows an area of atypical surface and crypt epithelium that is present adjacent to an area of erosion. The epithelium shows pseudostratification and loss of polarity. However, on the basis of its location adjacent to an ulcer, this specimen is best qualified as indefinite for dysplasia and would be best reevaluated after the ulcer has been treated.

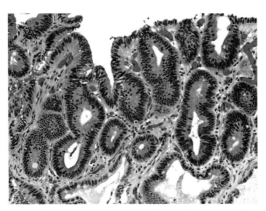

Fig. 3. Low-grade intestinal-type dysplasia in BE. The nuclei are stratified and pencil-shaped but are limited to the lower half of the cytoplasm. The architecture is similar to that of non-dysplastic epithelium.

have shown that solid (back to back glands) or cribriform architecture, ulcerated HGD, 3 or greater dilated dysplastic glands containing necrotic debris, prominent neutrophils within high-grade dysplastic epithelium, and dysplastic glands infiltrating the overlying squamous epithelium are significantly associated with the presence of EAC in corresponding surgical resection specimens.[37,38]

Foveolar dysplasia

Foveolar dysplasia is an uncommon form of dysplasia. Based on a series of 200 consecutive patients with BE dysplasia, the prevalence of foveolar-type dysplasia was found to be 15% at the patient level, and 20% at the biopsy level.[39] Foveolar-type dysplasia is more often high grade and occurs mostly in women, in patients who, on average, are a decade older than those with intestinal-type dysplasia. Low-grade foveolar dysplasia is characterized by cells that have a low nucleus to cytoplasmic ratio (N:C ratio) (far lower than intestinal type dysplasia; **Fig. 5** A). Thus, distinguishing reactive atypia from low-grade foveolar dysplasia can be quite challenging. A study by Patil and colleagues showed that surface nuclear stratification, "top-heavy" atypia, and noncrowded, villiform architecture were highly characteristic of reactive cardiac epithelium in patients with GERD (see **Fig. 5**B), in comparison to

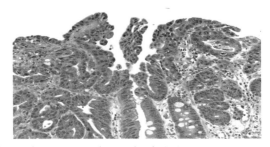

Fig. 4. High-grade dysplasia intestinal-type dysplasia in BE. In contrast to LGD (see **Fig. 3**), there is a greater degree of nuclear enlargement, pleomorphism, and loss of nuclear polarity. In this example, the glands show crowded architecture with focal cribriform arrangement (left lower aspect of image).

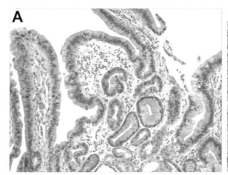
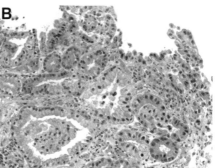

Fig. 5. Foveolar-type (gastric) dysplasia in BE. (*A*) In contrast to intestinal-type dysplasia, the cells have a more cuboidal or low columnar appearance, the nuclei are round or oval and irregular in shape, there is less nuclear stratification, and there is retention of the apical mucinous cytoplasm with a monolayer arrangement of cells. (*B*) High-grade foveolar dysplasia is characterized by a tight back-to-back crypt arrangement of atypical glands lined by cells with prominent nuclear atypia (nuclear size is usually greater than 3 to 4 times the size of an adjacent lymphocyte or plasma cell nucleus). The cells retain their monolayer arrangement of nuclei.

true dysplasia that more often revealed monolayered nuclei within crowded glands that occupied the full thickness of the mucosa.[40]

High-grade foveolar dysplasia often shows a monolayer of cells with markedly increased N:C ratio, with nuclei that often measure 3 to 4 times the size of lymphocytes or plasma cell nuclei. They may show an open chromatin pattern and often contain macronucleoli as well. With regard to the natural history, pure foveolar dysplasia is frequently high grade and associated with a higher risk of neoplastic progression compared with mixed gastric and intestinal-type dysplasia.[39]

Serrated dysplasia
Serrated dysplasia is the least common type. This type of dysplasia reveals a "hyperplastic" and/or "serrated" phenotype with a saw-toothed configuration of the epithelium and luminal infolding, similar to serrated polyps of the colon. The cells show small, oval-shaped nuclei with an open chromatin pattern, often with prominent nucleoli and less nuclear stratification. The cytoplasm is typically eosinophilic and wispy in appearance, especially at the surface. In HGD, the nuclei are more hyperchromatic and stratified and show an increased mitotic rate. In a study (published in abstract form) consisting of 214 patients with BE, the frequency of serrated dysplasia was found to be 2.8% (6 out of 214). Of these 6 patients, 3 progressed to cancer, suggesting a high potential for EAC.[41]

Intramucosal adenocarcinoma
Intramucosal adenocarcinoma is defined as neoplastic epithelium that has invaded beyond the basement membrane into the surrounding lamina propria or muscularis mucosae (**Fig. 6**). IMC is associated with an approximately 5% risk for lymph node metastases. Recommended criteria for the diagnosis of IMC include the following: (1) individual neoplastic cells that invade into the lamina propria and lack a connection to the crypts; (2) sheets of malignant cells without gland formation; (3) markedly angulated, infiltrative-appearing glands that reside in the lamina propria or muscularis mucosae; (4) a complex, anastomosing gland pattern within the lamina propria; and (5) neoplastic glands or cells arranged in a back-to-back or highly irregular

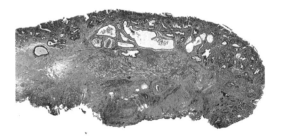

Fig. 6. EMR specimen with intramucosal adenocarcinoma in BE. Intramucosal adenocarcinoma is characterized by a proliferation of small, irregular glands with marked atypia infiltrating the lamina propria and muscularis mucosae.

architectural pattern that cannot be explained by the presence of preexisting Barrett's epithelium.

Crypt dysplasia

As mentioned above, lack of surface maturation is normally considered a cardinal feature of dysplasia.[35] However, in a study by Lomo and colleagues,[36] 15 cases of dysplasia-like atypia all showed basal crypt involvement only, with surface maturation, suggesting that in the early stages of progression, dysplasia involves only the crypt bases (**Fig. 7**). In their study, 47% of patients with basal crypt dysplasia also had conventional full-crypt dysplasia, or EAC, and a significantly higher incidence of 17p loss of heterozygosity (LOH) and flow cytometric abnormalities (see later discussion), compared with control patients without dysplasia. In another study, the bases of the crypts in foci of crypt dysplasia showed cellular DNA content abnormalities similar to those of basal crypt cells in foci of traditional full-crypt LGD but the surface epithelium in areas of basal crypt dysplasia was diploid.[42] A study by Coco and colleagues suggests that crypt dysplasia can be diagnosed reliably, with a moderate level of interobserver agreement.[43]

Recent data on the natural history of crypt dysplasia suggests that it progresses at a rate much higher than nondysplastic BE and even approaching that of traditional LGD.[44,45] In a large series of 4545 patients who had 2 sequential samples (separated by $\geq$ 12 months) obtained using the WATS[3D] technology, progression to HGD/EAC occurred in patients with baseline nondysplastic BE at a rate of 0.08%/patient-year. In contrast, the rate of progression was significantly higher (1.42%/patient-year) for patients with baseline crypt dysplasia and 5.79%/patient-year for those with baseline

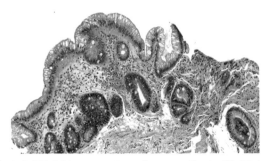

Fig. 7. Crypt dysplasia in BE. A biopsy specimen from a patient with BE shows LGD limited to the crypt bases but with evidence of surface maturation.

LGD.[46] These results indicate that patients with crypt dysplasia likely warrant close follow-up similar to those with LGD but this needs to be evaluated in further prospective studies.

Differential Diagnosis

Regenerative atypia versus dysplasia

Regenerative epithelial changes are always present in areas of neutrophilic inflammation and erosion/ulceration. There is a gradual transition between uninflamed mucosa and inflamed mucosa. However, the N:C ratio is usually preserved. In contrast, dysplastic changes often show an abrupt transition between normal and abnormal glands. Nuclear hyperchromasia, elongation, stratification, atypical mitotic activity, increased N:C ratio, without evidence of surface maturation are features that support a diagnosis of dysplasia (**Table 2**).

Low-grade dysplasia versus high-grade dysplasia

Because dysplasia progresses to cancer on a continuous (linear) scale, no well-defined cutoff points separate LGD from HGD. In general, the overall grade of dysplasia is determined by the most abnormal (highest grade) epithelium.

High-grade dysplasia versus intramucosal adenocarcinoma

At the high end of the spectrum of neoplasia, the degree of architectural distortion may reach a point at which a diagnosis of IMC is impossible to exclude with complete certainty. In a study performed at the Cleveland Clinic, overall agreement among several gastrointestinal (GI) pathologists for distinguishing HGD from IMC was only fair ($\kappa = 0.30$).[47] Because many institutions now consider endoscopic mucosal resection (EMR) followed by ablative therapy to be the main form of treatment of HGD or IMC and reserve esophagectomy for the treatment of submucosal EAC, the distinction between these 2 categories is less relevant.

Intramucosal versus submucosal adenocarcinoma

Dysplastic glands may be located between frayed fibers of muscularis mucosae, and differentiation of misplaced noninvasive dysplastic epithelium from truly invasive

Table 2
Reactive atypia vs dysplasia in Barrett's esophagus

Feature	Regeneration/ Reactive Atypia	Dysplasia
Inflammation	Very common	May be present
Ulceration	Common	May be present
Surface epithelial maturation	Present	Absent (except crypt dysplasia which is accompanied by surface maturation)
Pleomorphism	Absent	May be present
Loss of polarity	No	May be present (usually in HGD)
Atypical mitoses	Absent	May be present
Abrupt transition from normal to abnormal epithelium	No	Yes
Surface villiform change	May be present	May be present
Mucin depletion	May be present	Usually present
N:C ratio	Usually maintained	Increased

epithelium can be difficult. Given that most patients with BE have a duplicated muscularis mucosae, dysplastic glands that invade into, or even through, the new (superficial) muscularis mucosae are still considered "intramucosal" for management purposes.[48] However, in most superficial and even jumbo-forceps–derived mucosal biopsies, the deep (original) muscularis mucosae is not evident. Determination of true submucosal invasion is not possible in that circumstance.

Interobserver Variability

There is considerable interobserver variability among pathologists in the diagnosis of dysplasia in BE.[34,35,49] The highest degree of variability occurs at both the low end and the high end of the spectrum (ie, separating regenerative atypia from LGD and separating HGD from EAC). In a reproducibility study by Montgomery and colleagues[35] showed substantial agreement among pathologists for the diagnosis of HGD (k = 0.65) but only fair agreement for LGD (k = 0.32) and only slight agreement for indefinite cases (k = 0.15). As a result, the ACG and AGA have strongly recommended that all potential dysplasia diagnoses be confirmed by at least one experienced GI pathologist before embarking on a management plan.[16,50]

ADJUNCTIVE MARKERS OF DYSPLASIA

To improve the diagnostic accuracy of dysplasia by pathologists, many types of histochemical "'biomarkers'" have been evaluated, such as markers of cell proliferation (proliferating cell nuclear antigen and Ki-67), cyclin D1, and p53.[51–56] For example, studies have shown that the extent and distribution of Ki-67 staining correlates reasonably well with the grade of dysplasia.[51,54,55] Unfortunately, regenerating epithelium can also demonstrate increased cell proliferation,[54] which, in some instances, approaches that seen in HGD. Similarly, although the frequency of p53-positive staining has also been shown to be proportional to the grade of dysplasia and may have predictive value in assessing the risk of malignancy in patients with BE (discussed later), p53 may also be detected in as many as 10% of biopsy specimens that are histologically negative for dysplasia, and its staining results have high false-positive and false-negative rates. Regardless, in some parts of the world, p53 is used for the detection and confirmation of dysplasia. Kastelein and colleagues evaluated p53 immunohistochemical staining patterns in esophageal biopsy samples from 635 patients with BE with clinical follow-up. They found aberrant p53 staining in 11% of biopsy samples without dysplasia, 38% in LGD, 83% in HGD, and in 100% of EACs.[57] Kaye and colleagues found that adding p53 immunostain to histologic evaluation decreased interobserver variability with respect to dysplasia classification, and also increased the predictive value of the histologic diagnoses.[58] However, in the United States, none of these markers, including p53, are advocated for routine diagnostic use in patients with BE. Immunostaining for alpha-methylacyl-CoA racemase has shown promise as a marker for dysplasia.[59,60] In a more recent study by Rickelt and colleagues showed that the loss of basement membrane agrin (AGRN) expression was significantly higher in BE-related dysplasia and EAC compared with nondysplastic glands ($P<.001$; specificity = 82.2% and sensitivity = 96.4%). Thus, AGRN is another diagnostic marker that needs further validation.[61]

RISK ASSESSMENT IN BARRETT'S ESOPHAGUS

Patients with BE have a 10-fold to 55-fold increased risk of developing EAC.[62] Of those with nondysplastic BE, 0.33% per year show progression to EAC.[63] Presence of a hiatal hernia and length of the Barrett's segment[64–66] have been shown to be associated with an increased risk of progression to cancer in patients with BE.

Although many potential nonmorphology-based biomarkers have been studied, few, if any, have been validated as markers of risk of cancer in phase III or phase IV prospective trials. Immunostaining for p53 has been the most widely examined potential biomarker in BE.[53,56,67,68] For instance, previous studies have shown that mutations in TP53, or LOH of 17p, are present in up to 75% of patients with HGD or EAC.[68–71] In general, the frequency of positive immunostaining for p53 has been shown to be proportional to the grade of dysplasia.[53,56,68,70] Unfortunately, p53 may be detected in up to 10% of biopsies that are histologically negative for dysplasia. In addition, its immunostaining has a high rate of both false positives and false negatives.[5,70] Although p53 is not always helpful for diagnosing dysplasia, several studies have suggested that p53 immunostaining may have predictive value.[56,68] For instance, in an immunohistochemistry study by Younes and colleagues[68] of 21 patients with BE whose biopsy specimens were negative for p53, only 1 developed HGD on follow-up. In contrast, 2 patients with p53-positive biopsies showed progression. In a recent retrospective cohort analysis of 561 patients, abnormal p53 was associated with a hazard ratio of 5.27 (95% confidence interval, 3.93–7.07) for patients with exclusively nondysplastic disease before progression to HGD or EAC. When analyzed in a separate prospective validation cohort, the authors found that p53 immunohistochemistry (IHC) predicted progression among nondysplastic BE, indefinite for dysplasia, and LGD ($P<.001$).[72]

DNA content abnormalities, detected by flow cytometry (aneuploidy and tetraploidy),[73–76] and genetic alterations in TP53 and p16[71,77,78] are the most promising biomarkers studied to date. A variety of somatic mutations, aberrantly methylated genes, overexpressed microRNAs (miRNAs), as well as deregulated proteins have also been investigated as tools for patients with BE who are at a high-risk of progression to cancer.[19,79] Additional information on non–morphology-based biomarkers can be found in several articles.[80,81]

A recent study by the authors group characterized morphologic features of nondysplastic crypts in baseline biopsies from 212 patients with BE (2956 biopsies) and graded them histologically using a 4-point scale (crypt atypia levels 0–3). This study also analyzed DNA content abnormalities and found that in patients who had dysplasia in their baseline biopsies, dysplasia was significantly associated with increasing grades of crypt atypia in the background non-dysplastic Barrett's esophagus (NDBE) ($P < .001$). In a subset of patients without dysplasia at baseline (N = 149), a higher grade of crypt atypia was associated with longer BE segment length (5.5 vs 3.3 cm, $P = .0095$), and a higher percentage of cells with 4N DNA content (3.67 ± 1.27 vs 2.93 ± 1.22; $P = .018$). Although no significant association was noted between the grade of crypt atypia and increased 4N, aneuploidy or progression to HGD/EAC, only patients with grade 2 or 3 crypt atypia showed increased 4N, aneuploidy or progression to HGD/EAC. These results suggest that neoplastic progression in BE likely begins in the crypts at an early stage, before the onset of dysplasia, and that these changes may reflect a progressive accumulation of DNA abnormalities[82] and may be predictive of outcome.

RELEVANCE OF EXTENT OF DYSPLASIA

Several recent studies suggest that not only the presence of dysplasia but also the extent of dysplasia affects risk of EAC in BE.[83,84] For example, in a study by Buttar and colleagues[83] of 100 patients with BE with HGD, the risk of developing EAC was significantly higher (3.7-fold higher) in patients with "diffuse" HGD (defined as HGD involving either more than 5 crypts in a single biopsy specimen or more than 1 biopsy fragment) compared with those with "focal" HGD (defined as dysplasia involving a single focus of 5 or fewer crypts). However, in a subsequent study by Dar and colleagues,[85] no significant difference in the prevalence of EAC was detected in patients with "focal" versus "diffuse" HGD (48% vs 67%, respectively).

In contrast, a study by the authors' research group[84] did not reveal an association between risk of cancer and extent of HGD but instead detected an association between the extent of LGD and the development of EAC in a case-control study of 77 patients with BE, 44 of whom eventually developed EAC on endoscopic surveillance. Thus, it seems reasonable to attempt to define both the presence and grade of dysplasia and the extent of dysplasia when evaluating biopsy specimens from patients with BE.

NATURAL HISTORY OF DYSPLASIA

Combining the results of several prospective endoscopic surveillance studies of patients with BE, the absolute annual risk of cancer in patients without dysplasia, at baseline, is approximately 0.1% to 0.5% per year.[66,76,86,87] The reported risk of cancer for LGD is somewhat controversial with progression rates varying between 1% and 47%.[56,84,88,89] This uncertainty is in part due to low interobserver agreement for a diagnosis of LGD, even among expert GI pathologists.[35,90] Furthermore, many studies have used either HGD or EAC as an endpoint,[56,91] which also complicates interpretation of the results. However, several more recent studies suggest a higher risk of cancer progression in patients with "definite" LGD, particularly where there has been uniform consensus among at least 3 GI pathologists.[35,84,91]

In contrast, the risk of cancer in patients with HGD ranges from 16% to 59%.[66,76,92–94] In a recent meta-analysis, the weighted annual incidence rate of cancer for patients diagnosed with HGD was found to be 7% (95% CI 5–8).[95] However, the AIM-Dysplasia trial that randomized 127 patients with dysplasia to ablation therapy compared with surveillance reported a much higher yearly progression rate of 19% in the HGD surveillance arm.[96] The wide range in outcome is partially explained by the separation of patients into those with "prevalent" dysplasia (dysplasia detected either at initial screening endoscopy or during the first 12 months of surveillance)[66,76,94,97] versus incident dysplasia (dysplasia that develops during endoscopic surveillance).

SURVEILLANCE AND TREATMENT OF DYSPLASIA

It is recommended that patients with BE undergo periodic endoscopic surveillance to detect early neoplastic complications (dysplasia) and prevent the development of cancer.[16] The current guidelines recommend a follow-up surveillance interval of 3 years if 2 consecutive endoscopies with biopsy within 1 year show an absence of dysplasia (**Table 3**). Cases diagnosed as indefinite for dysplasia are usually treated more aggressively with antireflux medication to decrease the amount of inflammation, followed by rebiopsy after 3 to 6 months to reevaluate the indefinite focus. However, in some institutions, such cases are managed similarly to LGD. For cases of LGD, a repeat examination within 3 to 6 months with high-definition white-light endoscopy (HD-WLE), and preferably optical chromoendoscopy, should be performed to rule out the presence of a visible lesion, which should prompt endoscopic resection.

The management of HGD is more controversial and variable among different institutions. The finding of HGD in flat mucosa should lead to confirmation by an expert

Table 3
Recommendations for surveillance and management of Barrett's esophagus

Society (year)	Negative for Dysplasia	Indefinite for Dysplasia	Low-Grade Dysplasia	High-Grade Dysplasia
AGA (2011)	EGD every 3–5 y	Not specified	• EGD every 6–12 mo • Consider endoscopic eradication therapy	• EGD every 3 mo • Endoscopic eradication therapy rather than surveillance or surgery
ASGE (2012)	• EGD every 3–5 y • Consider no surveillance • Consider ablation in select cases	Repeat EGD with maximal acid suppression	• Repeat EGD in 6 mo to confirm LGD • EGD every year • Consider endoscopic therapy	• EGD every 3 mo (only patients who are not candidates for endoscopic or surgical treatment) • Consider endoscopic treatment • Consider surgical consultation
BSG (2014)	• Irregular Z-line: no surveillance • BE < 3 cm without IM: no surveillance • BE < 3 cm with IM: EGD every 3–5 y • BE ≥ 3 cm: EGD every 2–3 y • Consider no surveillance on the basis of patient's fitness and risk of progression	Repeat EGD at 6 mo with maximal acid suppression	• Surveillance: EGD every 6 mo • Ablation cannot be recommended routinely	• Mucosal irregularity: EMR • Endoscopic therapy is preferred over esophagectomy or surveillance
ACG (2016)	EGD every 3–5 y	• Repeat EGD at 3–6 mo after optimization of acid suppression • Persistent indefinite for dysplasia: EGD after 1 y	• Endoscopic treatment (patients without life-limiting comorbidity) • EGD every 12 mo	Endoscopic treatment (patients without life-limiting comorbidity)

(continued on next page)

Table 3
(continued)

Society (year)	Negative for Dysplasia	Indefinite for Dysplasia	Low-Grade Dysplasia	High-Grade Dysplasia
ESGE (2017)	• BE < 1 cm: no surveillance • BE 1–3 cm: EGD every 5 y • BE 3–10 cm: EGD every 3 y • BE ≥ 10 cm: referral to BE expert center • Consider discharge for patients with limited life expectancy and advanced age	Repeat EGD at 6 mo with optimization of antireflux medication	• Repeat EGD at 6 mo • If persistent LGD: endoscopic ablation	• Repeat EGD • Visible irregularity: EMR • Persistent HGD: ablation • No dysplasia: repeat EGD 3 mo

Abbreviations: ACG, American College of Gastroenterology; AGA, American Gastroenterological Association, ASGE; American Society for Gastrointestinal Endoscopy, BSG; British Society of Gastroenterology; EGD, esophagogastroduodenoscopy; EMR, endoscopic mucosal resection, ESGE; European Society of Gastrointestinal Endoscopy.

GI pathologist and a subsequent endoscopy using HD-WLE within 6 to 8 weeks months, with biopsies to rule out visible HGD. Continued surveillance or definitive intervention is typically determined on an individual basis. Patients who have HGD with mucosal irregularity should undergo EMR or endoscopic submucosal dissection (ESD).[16] Updated AGA guidelines recommend endoscopic ablation (eg, RFA) after EMR for visible lesions (see **Table 3**).

Radiofrequency ablation is now the standard of care therapy for eradicating dysplasia endoscopically. It has an acceptable safety profile, is durable, and is associated with a low risk of disease progression.[96] The success rates with radiofrequency ablation (RFA) are superior, with approximately 90% of patients showing no HGD after therapy.[98] However, its efficacy in eradicating IM varies based on factors such as severity of ongoing reflux, size of hiatal hernia, and length of BE.[99,100] The rate of recurrence of IM varies between 8% and 10% per patient-year of follow-up. Majority of recurrences are detected in the distal 2 cm of the esophagus, and thus, it is recommended that the entire neosquamous mucosa should be sampled starting immediately above the GEJ.[101]

Photodynamic therapy (PDT) destroys target tissue by sensitizing the neoplastic tissue by chemical agents known as photosensitizers followed by photoradiation. In a randomized trial by Overholt and colleagues[102] comparing PDT with the proton pump inhibitor omeprazole to omeprazole alone in patients with BE with HGD showed a higher rate of complete ablation of HGD in the PDT group (77% vs 39%). Following PDT, up to two-thirds of patients show complete squamous reepithelialization.[103] However, up to 50% of such patients show residual Barrett epithelium buried underneath islands of squamous epithelium.[104–106] This is clinically important because buried Barrett epithelium is endoscopically inapparent and thus may be missed during endoscopic surveillance and allowed to progress.[15,107,108] Recent studies by the authors' group have shown that buried Barrett epithelium, following either chronic proton pump inhibitor therapy[109] or PDT,[110] has a significantly lower crypt proliferation rate, compared with nonburied epithelium, and a significantly lower incidence of aneuploidy. These findings suggest that post-PDT buried (nondysplastic) Barrett epithelium may, in fact, have a lower neoplastic potential than nonburied Barrett epithelium. Prospective follow-up studies will be required to determine the natural history and the risk of malignancy of buried Barrett epithelium.

EMR and ESD are recommended for visible neoplastic lesions. These specimens enhance the ability of pathologists to establish an accurate diagnosis and provide an accurate stage of invasion (if any) when compared with the evaluation of mucosal biopsies (see **Fig. 6**). There is recent evidence to suggest that early stage, low-risk EAC defined as pT1sm1 cancers with submucosal invasion of 500 μm or lesser, without any other histologic risk factors for nodal metastasis may be managed by endoscopic therapy, followed by close endoscopic follow-up.[101] Esophagectomy still remains an important method of treatment of BE with HGD but it is usually reserved for treatment failures, for multifocal HGD not amenable to less-aggressive therapy, and for all patients with submucosally invasive and deep mural EACs.

SUMMARY

Although BE is a precursor to EAC, not all patients with this disorder require intensive surveillance. Pathologic diagnosis and grading of dysplasia in mucosal biopsies remain the best and most widely used methods of determining which patients are at highest risk for neoplastic progression and for selecting patients who need a more intensive surveillance program or surgical intervention. Diagnosing dysplasia suffers from considerable interobserver variability. Therefore, consultation with expert GI pathologists to confirm the diagnosis of dysplasia before definitive management is highly advisable. Detection of p16, p53, and DNA content abnormalities may help identify patients at particularly high risk for progression to cancer but these techniques are not yet widely available for routine clinical application. Newer cytology-based techniques that sample the esophageal mucosal lining and use computational techniques (eg, WATS[3D]) hold promise in not only reducing sampling variability but also providing noninvasive methods to triage and identify patients who are at a high risk for neoplastic progression.

CLINICS CARE POINTS

- Distinguishing reactive atypia from true dysplasia remains to be a problem area for pathologists, and therefore, it is helpful to confirm a diagnosis of dysplasia before initiating therapy.
- Advanced endoscopy using high-definition white light endoscopy and narrow band imaging is recommended for better visualization and sampling of BE segment.
- Proper orientation and fixation of endoscopically resected specimens is important for accurate grading and staging of BE-related neoplasia.
- Biopsy of normal Z-line, an irregular Z-line less than 1 cm in length or GE junction should be avoided because the presence of a few intestinalized glands in these situations does not confer the same increased risk of malignancy as true BE.

DISCLOSURE

The authors have no commercial or financial conflicts of interest, or any funding sources relevant to this article.

REFERENCES

1. Pohl H, Welch HG. The role of overdiagnosis and reclassification in the marked increase of esophageal adenocarcinoma incidence. J Natl Cancer Inst 2005; 97(2):142–6.
2. Souza RF, Spechler SJ. Concepts in the prevention of adenocarcinoma of the distal esophagus and proximal stomach. CA Cancer J Clin Nov-Dec 2005; 55(6):334–51.
3. Spechler SJ. Barrett's esophagus and esophageal adenocarcinoma: pathogenesis, diagnosis, and therapy. Med Clin North Am 2002;86(6):1423–45, vii.
4. Riddell RH, Goldman H, Ransohoff DF, et al. Dysplasia in inflammatory bowel disease: standardized classification with provisional clinical applications. Hum Pathol 1983/11//1983;14(11):931–68.
5. Odze RD. Diagnosis and grading of dysplasia in Barrett's oesophagus. J Clin Pathol 2006;59(10):1029–38.
6. Schlemper RJ, Riddell RH, Kato Y, et al. The Vienna classification of gastrointestinal epithelial neoplasia. Gut 2000;47(2):251–5.
7. Chak A, Faulx A, Kinnard M, et al. Identification of Barrett's esophagus in relatives by endoscopic screening. Am J Gastroenterol 2004;99(11):2107–14.
8. Westhoff B, Brotze S, Weston A, et al. The frequency of Barrett's esophagus in high-risk patients with chronic GERD. Gastrointest Endosc 2005;61(2):226–31.

9. Zagari RM, Fuccio L, Wallander MA, et al. Gastro-oesophageal reflux symptoms, oesophagitis and Barrett's oesophagus in the general population: the Loiano-Monghidoro study. Gut 2008;57(10):1354–9.

10. Sampliner RE, Practice Parameters Committee of the American College of Gastroenterology. Updated guidelines for the diagnosis, surveillance, and therapy of Barrett's esophagus. Guideline Practice Guideline. Am J Gastroenterol 2002;97(8):1888–95.

11. Sharma P, Dent J, Armstrong D, et al. The development and validation of an endoscopic grading system for Barrett's esophagus: the Prague C & M criteria. Gastroenterology 2006/11//2006;131(5):1392–9.

12. Vahabzadeh B, Seetharam AB, Cook MB, et al. Validation of the Prague C & M criteria for the endoscopic grading of Barrett's esophagus by gastroenterology trainees: a multicenter study. Gastrointest Endosc 2012;75(2):236–41.

13. Reid BJ, Weinstein WM, Lewin KJ, VanDeventer G, DenBesten L, Rubin CE. Endoscopic biopsy can detect high-grade dysplasia or early adenocarcinoma in Barrett's esophagus without grossly recognizable neoplastic lesions Comparative Study Research Support, U.S. Gov't, P.H.S. Gastroenterology 1988;94(1):81–90.

14. Levine DS, Haggitt RC, Blount PL, et al. An endoscopic biopsy protocol can differentiate high-grade dysplasia from early adenocarcinoma in Barrett's esophagus. Comparative Study. Gastroenterology 1993;105(1):40–50.

15. Reid BJ, Blount PL, Feng Z, et al. Optimizing endoscopic biopsy detection of early cancers in Barrett's high-grade dysplasia Comparative Study Research Support, U.S. Gov't, P.H.S. Am J Gastroenterol 2000;95(11):3089–96.

16. Shaheen NJ, Falk GW, Iyer PG, et al. ACG Clinical Guideline: Diagnosis and Management of Barrett's Esophagus. Am J Gastroenterol 2016/01//2016; 111(1):30–50, quiz 51.

17. Ross-Innes CS, Debiram-Beecham I, O'Donovan M, et al. Evaluation of a minimally invasive cell sampling device coupled with assessment of trefoil factor 3 expression for diagnosing Barrett's esophagus: a multi-center case-control study. PLoS Med 2015;12(1):e1001780.

18. Iyer PG, Taylor WR, Johnson ML, et al. Highly Discriminant Methylated DNA Markers for the Non-endoscopic Detection of Barrett's Esophagus. Am J Gastroenterol 2018;113(8):1156–66.

19. Moinova HR, LaFramboise T, Lutterbaugh JD, et al. Identifying DNA methylation biomarkers for non-endoscopic detection of Barrett's esophagus. Sci Transl Med 2018;10(424). https://doi.org/10.1126/scitranslmed.aao5848.

20. Gross SA, Smith MS, Kaul V, et al. Increased detection of Barrett's esophagus and esophageal dysplasia with adjunctive use of wide-area transepithelial sample with three-dimensional computer-assisted analysis (WATS). United European Gastroenterol J 2018;6(4):529–35.

21. Fitzgerald RC, di Pietro M, Ragunath K, et al. British Society of Gastroenterology guidelines on the diagnosis and management of Barrett's oesophagus. Gut 2014;63(1):7–42.

22. Ogiya K, Kawano T, Ito E, et al. Lower esophageal palisade vessels and the definition of Barrett's esophagus. Dis Esophagus 2008;21(7):645–9.

23. Jones TF, Sharma P, Daaboul B, et al. Yield of intestinal metaplasia in patients with suspected short-segment Barrett's esophagus (SSBE) on repeat endoscopy. Dig Dis Sci 2002;47(9):2108–11.

24. Harrison R, Perry I, Haddadin W, et al. Detection of intestinal metaplasia in Barrett's esophagus: an observational comparator study suggests the need for a

minimum of eight biopsies. Randomized Controlled Trial Research Support, Non-U.S. Gov't. Am J Gastroenterol 2007;102(6):1154–61.

25. Oberg S, Johansson J, Wenner J, et al. Endoscopic surveillance of columnar-lined esophagus: frequency of intestinal metaplasia detection and impact of antireflux surgery. Ann Surg 2001;234(5):619–26.

26. Hu Y, Williams VA, Gellersen O, et al. The pathogenesis of Barrett's esophagus: secondary bile acids upregulate intestinal differentiation factor CDX2 expression in esophageal cells. J Gastrointest Surg 2007;11(7):827–34.

27. Krishnadath KK. Novel findings in the pathogenesis of esophageal columnar metaplasia or Barrett's esophagus. Curr Opin Gastroenterol 2007;23(4):440–5.

28. Fitzgerald RC, Omary MB, Triadafilopoulos G. Dynamic effects of acid on Barrett's esophagus. An ex vivo proliferation and differentiation model. J Clin Invest 1996;98(9):2120–8.

29. Vaezi MF, Richter JE. Bile reflux in columnar-lined esophagus. Gastroenterol Clin N Am 1997;26(3):565–82.

30. Slack JM. Metaplasia and transdifferentiation: from pure biology to the clinic. Nat Rev Mol Cell Biol 2007;8(5):369–78.

31. Coad RA, Woodman AC, Warner PJ, et al. On the histogenesis of Barrett's oesophagus and its associated squamous islands: a three-dimensional study of their morphological relationship with native oesophageal gland ducts. J Pathol 2005;206(4):388–94.

32. Thiery JP. Epithelial-mesenchymal transitions in development and pathologies. Curr Opin Cell Biol 2003;15(6):740–6.

33. Agoston AT, Pham TH, Odze RD, et al. Columnar-Lined Esophagus Develops via Wound Repair in a Surgical Model of Reflux Esophagitis. Cell Mol Gastroenterol Hepatol 2018;6(4):389–404.

34. Reid BJ, Haggitt RC, Rubin CE, et al. Observer variation in the diagnosis of dysplasia in Barrett's esophagus. Research Support, U.S. Gov't, P.H.S. Hum Pathol 1988;19(2):166–78.

35. Montgomery E, Bronner MP, Goldblum JR, et al. Reproducibility of the diagnosis of dysplasia in Barrett esophagus: a reaffirmation. Hum Pathol 2001;32(4): 368–78.

36. Lomo LC, Blount PL, Sanchez CA, et al. Crypt dysplasia with surface maturation: a clinical, pathologic, and molecular study of a Barrett's esophagus cohort. Research Support, N.I.H., Extramural. Am J Surg Pathol 2006;30(4):423–35.

37. Zhu W, Appelman HD, Greenson JK, et al. A histologically defined subset of high-grade dysplasia in Barrett mucosa is predictive of associated carcinoma. Am J Clin Pathol 2009;132(1):94–100.

38. Patil DT, Goldblum JR, Rybicki L, et al. Prediction of adenocarcinoma in esophagectomy specimens based upon analysis of preresection biopsies of Barrett esophagus with at least high-grade dysplasia: a comparison of 2 systems. Comparative Study. Am J Surg Pathol 2012;36(1):134–41.

39. Mahajan D, Bennett AE, Liu X, et al. Grading of gastric foveolar-type dysplasia in Barrett's esophagus. Mod Pathol 2010;23(1):1–11.

40. Patil DT, Bennett AE, Mahajan D, et al. Distinguishing Barrett gastric foveolar dysplasia from reactive cardiac mucosa in gastroesophageal reflux disease. Hum Pathol 2013;44(6):1146–53.

41. Srivastava ACD, Odze RD. Foveolar and serrated dysplasia are rare high-risk lesions in Barrett's esophagus: a prospective outcome analysis of 214 patients. Mod Pathol 2010;23(1):742A.

42. Zhang X, Huang Q, Goyal RK, et al. DNA ploidy abnormalities in basal and superficial regions of the crypts in Barrett's esophagus and associated neoplastic lesions. Am J Surg Pathol 2008;32(9):1327–35.

43. Coco DP, Goldblum JR, Hornick JL, et al. Interobserver variability in the diagnosis of crypt dysplasia in Barrett esophagus. Am J Surg Pathol 2011;35(1): 45–54.

44. Srivastava A, Coco DP, Sanchez CA, et al. Risk of conventional dysplasia and adenocarcinoma in patients with Barrett's esophagus and crypt dysplasia: A prospective follow-up study of 214 patients. Mod Pathol 2010;23:168a–9a.

45. Askari SLBNG, Odze RD. Long-term outcome study of Barrett's esophagus with basal crypt dysplasia. Mod Pathol 2014;27(s2):163A.

46. Shaheen NJ, Smith MS, Odze RD. Progression of Barrett's esophagus, crypt dysplasia, and low-grade dysplasia diagnosed by wide-area transepithelial sampling with 3-dimensional computer-assisted analysis: a retrospective analysis. Gastrointest Endosc 2022;95(3):410–418 e1.

47. Downs-Kelly E, Mendelin JE, Bennett AE, et al. Poor interobserver agreement in the distinction of high-grade dysplasia and adenocarcinoma in pretreatment Barrett's esophagus biopsies. Am J Gastroenterol 2008;103(9):2333–40.

48. Abraham SC, Krasinskas AM, Correa AM, et al. Duplication of the muscularis mucosae in Barrett esophagus: an underrecognized feature and its implication for staging of adenocarcinoma. Am J Surg Pathol 2007;31(11):1719–25.

49. Kerkhof M, van Dekken H, Steyerberg EW, et al. Grading of dysplasia in Barrett's oesophagus: substantial interobserver variation between general and gastrointestinal pathologists. Histopathology 2007;50(7):920–7.

50. Spechler SJ, Sharma P, Souza RF, et al. American Gastroenterological Association medical position statement on the management of Barrett's esophagus. Practice Guideline Research Support, N.I.H., Extramural Research Support, U.S. Gov't, Non-P.H.S. Webcasts. Gastroenterology 2011;140(3):1084–91.

51. Feith M, Stein HJ, Mueller J, et al. Malignant degeneration of Barrett's esophagus: the role of the Ki-67 proliferation fraction, expression of E-cadherin and p53. Dis Esophagus 2004;17(4):322–7.

52. Bani-Hani K, Martin IG, Hardie LJ, et al. Prospective study of cyclin D1 overexpression in Barrett's esophagus: association with increased risk of adenocarcinoma. J Natl Cancer Inst 2000;92(16):1316–21.

53. Gimenez A, Minguela A, Parrilla P, et al. Flow cytometric DNA analysis and p53 protein expression show a good correlation with histologic findings in patients with Barrett's esophagus. Cancer 1998;83(4):641–51.

54. Hong MK, Laskin WB, Herman BE, et al. Expansion of the Ki-67 proliferative compartment correlates with degree of dysplasia in Barrett's esophagus. Cancer 1995;75(2):423–9.

55. Lorinc E, Jakobsson B, Landberg G, et al. Ki67 and p53 immunohistochemistry reduces interobserver variation in assessment of Barrett's oesophagus. Histopathology 2005;46(6):642–8.

56. Weston AP, Banerjee SK, Sharma P, et al. p53 protein overexpression in low grade dysplasia (LGD) in Barrett's esophagus: immunohistochemical marker predictive of progression. Am J Gastroenterol 2001;96(5):1355–62.

57. Kastelein F, Biermann K, Steyerberg EW, et al. Aberrant p53 protein expression is associated with an increased risk of neoplastic progression in patients with Barrett's oesophagus. Gut 2013;62(12):1676–83.

58. Kaye PV, Haider SA, Ilyas M, et al. Barrett's dysplasia and the Vienna classification: reproducibility, prediction of progression and impact of consensus reporting and p53 immunohistochemistry. Histopathology 2009;54(6):699–712.

59. Dorer R, Odze RD. AMACR immunostaining is useful in detecting dysplastic epithelium in Barrett's esophagus, ulcerative colitis, and Crohn's disease. Evaluation Studies. Am J Surg Pathol 2006;30(7):871–7.

60. Lisovsky M, Falkowski O, Bhuiya T. Expression of alpha-methylacyl-coenzyme A racemase in dysplastic Barrett's epithelium. Hum Pathol 2006;37(12):1601–6.

61. Rickelt S, Neyaz A, Condon C, et al. Agrin Loss in Barrett's Esophagus-Related Neoplasia and Its Utility as a Diagnostic and Predictive Biomarker. Clin Cancer Res 2022;28(6):1167–79.

62. Cook MB, Coburn SB, Lam JR, et al. Cancer incidence and mortality risks in a large US Barrett's oesophagus cohort. Gut 2018;67(3):418–529.

63. Desai TK, Krishnan K, Samala N, et al. The incidence of oesophageal adenocarcinoma in non-dysplastic Barrett's oesophagus: a meta-analysis. Gut 2012; 61(7):970–6.

64. Iftikhar SY, James PD, Steele RJ, et al. Length of Barrett's oesophagus: an important factor in the development of dysplasia and adenocarcinoma. Gut 1992;33(9):1155–8.

65. Menke-Pluymers MB, Hop WC, Dees J, et al. Risk factors for the development of an adenocarcinoma in columnar-lined (Barrett) esophagus. The Rotterdam Esophageal Tumor Study Group. Cancer 1993;72(4):1155–8.

66. Weston AP, Sharma P, Mathur S, et al. Risk stratification of Barrett's esophagus: updated prospective multivariate analysis. Am J Gastroenterol 2004;99(9): 1657–66.

67. Skacel M, Petras RE, Rybicki LA, et al. p53 expression in low grade dysplasia in Barrett's esophagus: correlation with interobserver agreement and disease progression. Am J Gastroenterol 2002;97(10):2508–13.

68. Younes M, Lebovitz RM, Lechago LV, et al. p53 protein accumulation in Barrett's metaplasia, dysplasia, and carcinoma: a follow-up study. Gastroenterology 1993;105(6):1637–42.

69. Paulson TG, Reid BJ. Focus on Barrett's esophagus and esophageal adenocarcinoma. Cancer Cell 2004;6(1):11–6.

70. Reid BJ. p53 and neoplastic progression in Barrett's esophagus. Am J Gastroenterol 2001;96(5):1321–3.

71. Reid BJ, Prevo LJ, Galipeau PC, et al. Predictors of progression in Barrett's esophagus II: baseline 17p (p53) loss of heterozygosity identifies a patient subset at increased risk for neoplastic progression. Am J Gastroenterol 2001; 96(10):2839–48.

72. Redston M, Noffsinger A, Kim A, et al. Abnormal TP53 predicts risk of progression in patients with barrett's esophagus regardless of a diagnosis of dysplasia. Gastroenterology 2022;162(2):468–81.

73. Menke-Pluymers MB, Mulder AH, Hop WC, et al. Dysplasia and aneuploidy as markers of malignant degeneration in Barrett's oesophagus. The Rotterdam Oesophageal Tumour Study Group. Gut 1994;35(10):1348–51.

74. Reid BJ, Blount PL, Rubin CE, et al. Flow-cytometric and histological progression to malignancy in Barrett's esophagus: prospective endoscopic surveillance of a cohort. Research Support, Non-U.S. Gov't Research Support, U.S. Gov't, P.H.S. Gastroenterology 1992;102(4 Pt 1):1212–9.

75. Rabinovitch PS, Longton G, Blount PL, et al. Predictors of progression in Barrett's esophagus III: baseline flow cytometric variables. Am J Gastroenterol 2001;96(11):3071–83.
76. Reid BJ, Levine DS, Longton G, et al. Predictors of progression to cancer in Barrett's esophagus: baseline histology and flow cytometry identify low- and high-risk patient subsets. Research Support, U.S. Gov't, P.H.S. Am J Gastroenterol 2000;95(7):1669–76.
77. Galipeau PC, Prevo LJ, Sanchez CA, et al. Clonal expansion and loss of heterozygosity at chromosomes 9p and 17p in premalignant esophageal (Barrett's) tissue. Research Support, U.S. Gov't, P.H.S. J Natl Cancer Inst 1999;91(24):2087–95.
78. Galipeau PC, Cowan DS, Sanchez CA, et al. 17p (p53) allelic losses, 4N (G2/tetraploid) populations, and progression to aneuploidy in Barrett's esophagus. Proc Natl Acad Sci U S A 1996;93(14):7081–4.
79. Paulson TG, Maley CC, Li X, Sanchez CA, Chao DL, Odze RD, Vaughan TL, Blount PL, Reid BJ. Chromosomal instability and copy number alterations in Barrett's esophagus and esophageal adenocarcinoma Research Support, N.I.H., Extramural Research Support, Non-U.S. Gov't. Clin Cancer Res 2009;15(10):3305–14.
80. Ong CA, Lao-Sirieix P, Fitzgerald RC. Biomarkers in Barrett's esophagus and esophageal adenocarcinoma: predictors of progression and prognosis. World J Gastroenterol 2010;16(45):5669–81.
81. Grady WM, Yu M, Markowitz SD, et al. Barrett's Esophagus and Esophageal Adenocarcinoma Biomarkers. Cancer Epidemiol Biomarkers Prev 2020;29(12):2486–94.
82. Wang HH, Patil DT, Paulson TG, et al. Significance of Crypt Atypia in Barrett's Esophagus: A Clinical, Molecular, and Outcome Study. Clin Gastroenterol Hepatol 2023;S1542-3565(23)00849-2.
83. Buttar NS, Wang KK, Sebo TJ, et al. Extent of high-grade dysplasia in Barrett's esophagus correlates with risk of adenocarcinoma. Comment Research Support, Non-U.S. Gov't Research Support, U.S. Gov't, P.H.S. Gastroenterology 2001;120(7):1630–9.
84. Srivastava A, Hornick JL, Li X, et al. Extent of low-grade dysplasia is a risk factor for the development of esophageal adenocarcinoma in Barrett's esophagus. Am J Gastroenterol 2007;102(3):483–93, quiz 694.
85. Dar MS, Goldblum JR, Rice TW, et al. Can extent of high grade dysplasia in Barrett's oesophagus predict the presence of adenocarcinoma at oesophagectomy? Gut 2003;52(4):486–9.
86. Hvid-Jensen F, Pedersen L, Drewes AM, et al. Incidence of adenocarcinoma among patients with Barrett's esophagus. N Engl J Med 2011;365(15):1375–83.
87. Wani S, Falk G, Hall M, et al. Patients with nondysplastic Barrett's esophagus have low risks for developing dysplasia or esophageal adenocarcinoma. Multicenter Study Research Support, Non-U.S. Gov't. Clin Gastroenterol Hepatol 2011;9(3):220–7, quiz e26.
88. Montgomery E, Goldblum JR, Greenson JK, et al. Dysplasia as a predictive marker for invasive carcinoma in Barrett esophagus: a follow-up study based on 138 cases from a diagnostic variability study. Hum Pathol 2001;32(4):379–88.
89. Curvers WL, ten Kate FJ, Krishnadath KK, et al. Low-grade dysplasia in Barrett's esophagus: overdiagnosed and underestimated. Multicenter Study Research Support, Non-U.S. Gov't. Am J Gastroenterol 2010;105(7):1523–30.

90. Haggitt RC. Barrett's esophagus, dysplasia, and adenocarcinoma Research Support, U.S. Gov't, P.H.S. Review. Hum Pathol 1994;25(10):982–93.
91. Skacel M, Petras RE, Gramlich TL, et al. The diagnosis of low-grade dysplasia in Barrett's esophagus and its implications for disease progression. Am J Gastroenterol 2000;95(12):3383–7.
92. Miros M, Kerlin P, Walker N. Only patients with dysplasia progress to adenocarcinoma in Barrett's oesophagus. Gut 1991;32(12):1441–6.
93. Robertson CS, Mayberry JF, Nicholson DA, et al. Value of endoscopic surveillance in the detection of neoplastic change in Barrett's oesophagus. Br J Surg 1988;75(8):760–3.
94. Schnell TG, Sontag SJ, Chejfec G, et al. Long-term nonsurgical management of Barrett's esophagus with high-grade dysplasia. Research Support, U.S. Gov't, Non-P.H.S. Gastroenterology 2001;120(7):1607–19.
95. Rastogi A, Puli S, El-Serag HB, et al. Incidence of esophageal adenocarcinoma in patients with Barrett's esophagus and high-grade dysplasia: a meta-analysis. Gastrointest Endosc 2008;67(3):394–8.
96. Shaheen NJ, Sharma P, Overholt BF, et al. Radiofrequency ablation in Barrett's esophagus with dysplasia. N Engl J Med 2009;360(22):2277–88.
97. Shaheen NJ, Falk GW, Iyer PG, et al. Diagnosis and management of barrett's esophagus: an updated ACG GUIDELINE. Am J Gastroenterol 2022;117(4):559–87.
98. Semlitsch T, Jeitler K, Schoefl R, et al. A systematic review of the evidence for radiofrequency ablation for Barrett's esophagus. Surg Endosc 2010;24(12):2935–43.
99. Krishnan K, Pandolfino JE, Kahrilas PJ, et al. Increased risk for persistent intestinal metaplasia in patients with Barrett's esophagus and uncontrolled reflux exposure before radiofrequency ablation. Gastroenterology 2012;143(3):576–81.
100. Tan MC, Kanthasamy KA, Yeh AG, et al. Factors Associated With Recurrence of Barrett's Esophagus After Radiofrequency Ablation. Clin Gastroenterol Hepatol 2019;17(1):65–72 e5.
101. Sharma P, Shaheen NJ, Katzka D, et al. AGA clinical practice update on endoscopic treatment of barrett's esophagus with dysplasia and/or early cancer: expert review. Gastroenterology 2020;158(3):760–9.
102. Overholt BF, Lightdale CJ, Wang KK, et al. Photodynamic therapy with porfimer sodium for ablation of high-grade dysplasia in Barrett's esophagus: international, partially blinded, randomized phase III trial. Gastrointest Endosc 2005;62(4):488–98.
103. Hage M, Siersema PD, van Dekken H, et al. 5-aminolevulinic acid photodynamic therapy versus argon plasma coagulation for ablation of Barrett's oesophagus: a randomised trial. Gut 2004;53(6):785–90.
104. Biddlestone LR, Barham CP, Wilkinson SP, et al. The histopathology of treated Barrett's esophagus: squamous reepithelialization after acid suppression and laser and photodynamic therapy. Am J Surg Pathol 1998;22(2):239–45.
105. Gore S, Healey CJ, Sutton R, et al. Regression of columnar lined (Barrett's) oesophagus with continuous omeprazole therapy. Aliment Pharmacol Ther 1993;7(6):623–8.
106. Mino-Kenudson M, Hull MJ, Brown I, et al. EMR for Barrett's esophagus-related superficial neoplasms offers better diagnostic reproducibility than mucosal biopsy. Gastrointest Endosc 2007;66(4):660–6, quiz 767, 769.

107. Overholt BF, Panjehpour M, Halberg DL. Photodynamic therapy for Barrett's esophagus with dysplasia and/or early stage carcinoma: long-term results. Gastrointest Endosc 2003;58(2):183–8.
108. Sampliner RE, Fass R. Partial regression of Barrett's esophagus–an inadequate endpoint. Am J Gastroenterol 1993;88(12):2092–4.
109. Hornick JL, Blount PL, Sanchez CA, et al. Biologic properties of columnar epithelium underneath reepithelialized squamous mucosa in Barrett's esophagus. Am J Surg Pathol 2005;29(3):372–80.
110. Hornick JL, Mino-Kenudson M, Lauwers GY, et al. Buried Barrett's epithelium following photodynamic therapy shows reduced crypt proliferation and absence of DNA content abnormalities. Am J Gastroenterol 2008;103(1):38–47.

Squamous Neoplastic Precursor Lesions of the Esophagus

Tomio Arai, MD, PhD[a],*, Satoshi Ono, MD, PhD[b],
Kaiyo Takubo, MD, PhD[c]

KEYWORDS

- Squamous dysplasia • Squamous intraepithelial neoplasia
- Squamous cell carcinoma in situ • Esophagus

KEY POINTS

- Squamous dysplasia is a neoplastic lesion that is recognized as a precursor to squamous cell carcinoma (SCC).
- This condition emerges from the accumulation of gene mutations and may progress to SCC.
- Alcohol and smoking are well-known risk factors but so are family history of cancer, oral hygiene, environment, aging, diet, and infectious agents.
- Early detection of squamous dysplasia is possible through periodic endoscopy in patients with risk factors.
- Low-grade dysplasia can be followed up endoscopically, whereas high-grade dysplasia should be treated by endoscopic resection.

INTRODUCTION

Clinical evidence has shown that squamous dysplasia is a precancerous lesion of esophageal squamous cell carcinoma (ESCC), especially in high-risk populations[1,2] and the relative risks for developing ESCC are much higher for high-grade dysplasia than for low-grade dysplasia.[2] Squamous cell carcinoma (SCC) is generally believed to develop through a sequence of such dysplastic precursor lesions, which can be detected endoscopically and microscopically. The term *dysplasia* is historical[3,4] but

[a] Department of Pathology, Tokyo Metropolitan Institute for Geriatrics and Gerontology, 35-2 Sakaecho, Itabashi-ku, Tokyo 173-0015, Japan; [b] Department of Gastroenterology and Gastrointestinal Endoscopy, Tokyo Metropolitan Institute for Geriatrics and Gerontology, 35-2 Sakaecho, Itabashi-ku, Tokyo 173-0015, Japan; [c] Research Team for Geriatric Pathology, Tokyo Metropolitan Institute for Geriatrics and Gerontology, 35-2 Sakaecho, Itabashi-ku, Tokyo 173-0015, Japan
* Corresponding author.
E-mail address: arai@tmig.or.jp

Gastroenterol Clin N Am 53 (2024) 25–38
https://doi.org/10.1016/j.gtc.2023.09.004
0889-8553/24/© 2023 Elsevier Inc. All rights reserved.
gastro.theclinics.com

is still in use.[5] On the other hand, the term *intraepithelial neoplasia* is still use by some pathologists in Europe and Asia.[5–7] This lesion is classified into two grades: low- and high-grade dysplasia. High-grade dysplasia is a key therapeutic target for endoscopic resection. This article focuses on squamous dysplasia of the esophagus and reviews the history of its concepts, definitions, pathologic findings, molecular biological features, and clinical management.

HISTORICAL PERSPECTIVE OF DYSPLASIA/INTRAEPITHELIAL NEOPLASIA

Mass cytologic screening began in the late 1950s in areas along the Yellow River in China, where the incidence of ESCC is very high.[8] This study revealed a close relationship between SCC and dysplasia and concluded that SCC develops from dysplasia. In the 1960s, Japanese researchers reported atypical proliferations of the esophageal epithelium in esophagi resected for SCC.[9] Other investigators reported multifocal epithelial dysplasia in males,[10] suggesting a possible relationship between varying degrees of dysplasia and invasive esophageal carcinoma. Several reports have examined the incidence of esophageal dysplasia using autopsy and esophagectomy series, either with or without esophageal carcinoma. The results demonstrated that the incidence was approximately 30%,[11,12] which was higher than expected. Since then, squamous dysplasia has been recognized worldwide as an important precursor lesion to carcinoma in the esophagus.

DEFINITION OF SQUAMOUS DYSPLASIA

Squamous dysplasia of the esophagus is defined as an unequivocal neoplastic alteration of the esophageal squamous epithelium, without invasion.[5] The lesion demonstrates structural and cytologic abnormalities.[7,13] Squamous dysplasia results from clonal genetic alterations and carries a predisposition for progression to invasive carcinoma and metastasis.

PREVALENCE/INCIDENCE

A few reports have investigated the incidence of esophageal dysplasia in Japan using autopsy and esophagectomy series, either with or without esophageal carcinoma. Of note, the incidence of dysplasia was reported to be 27%–37%,[11,12] and subclinical SCC was found in 2% of these autopsy series.[12] In contrast, in a high-risk population in China, endoscopic screening for healthy individuals revealed that the incidence of squamous dysplasia was 32%.[14] Tayler and colleagues reviewed the prevalence of ESCC precursor lesions in China and Iran and reported it to be 3% to 38%.[15] In Brazil, individuals who abuse alcohol, smoke, and consume "maté" had a high prevalence (approximately 7%) of dysplastic lesions.[16] Esophagi with unstained areas had an eightfold higher chance of revealing dysplasia than did the uniformly stained ones. Moreover, the prevalence of esophageal squamous dysplasia was 14.4% (11.5% in low-grade dysplasia and 2.9% in high-grade dysplasia) in Kenya.[17] The exact incidence of squamous dysplasia remains unclear, and the incidence trends vary across populations and regions.[18,19]

RISK FACTORS

Risk factors for dysplasia are similar to those previously identified for ESCC; alcohol intake and cigarette smoking are the two major risk factors.[14] Factors of alcohol metabolism, such as alcohol dehydrogenase (ADH1B) and aldehyde dehydrogenase (ALDH2), influence the risk of squamous neoplasia development in the esophagus.[20]

Hot beverages and dietary factors such as low intake of fresh fruits and vegetables, fresh or frozen meat or fish, barbecued meat, pickled vegetables, mycotoxins, or N-nitroso compounds are listed as risk factors for the development of ESCC.[7] These factors may also influence the development of esophageal squamous dysplasia. Family history of cancer, environment such as heating stove without chimney, oral hygiene including loss of teeth, serum Vitamin D, serum pepsinogens, aging, and low educational level are also listed as risk factors for dysplasia.[14,15,21–23]

A variety of organisms have been implicated in esophageal carcinogenesis, either directly or indirectly. The organisms with potential direct effects in ESCC include human papillomavirus (HPV), Epstein–Barr virus, and polyoma viruses.[24] HPV is a possible etiologic agent in esophageal carcinogenesis, most probably acting synergistically with physical, chemical, and/or nutritional factors that have previously been related to this malignancy in high-risk areas.[25] However, it was reported that HPV positivity was identified in 13% of subjects without squamous dysplasia, 8% to 16% with squamous dysplasia, and zero with invasive ESCC. Although HPV infection may be partly associated with squamous dysplasia, there is little association between HPV infection and the neoplastic progression of ESCC.[26]

ENDOSCOPIC CHARACTERISTICS

Esophageal squamous dysplasia is often discovered during routine screening for SCC. Although it is mostly located in the area adjacent to SCC, it can also be present in patients without carcinoma. Squamous dysplasia is usually difficult to detect using white light endoscopy (**Fig. 1**A); however, it can be detected by combining Lugol's chromoendoscopy (see **Fig. 1**B) and narrow band imaging (NBI) (see **Fig. 1**C).[27] With Lugol's iodine, low-grade dysplasia appears as unstained or weakly stained areas; in contrast, high-grade dysplasia shows a consistently unstained area. Overt neoplastic diseases are relatively large in size and have a non-flat appearance with irregular margins, positive pink color signs, and numerous distinct iodine-unstained lesions. In contrast, squamous dysplasia often shows flat, focal, regular margins, and normal color. Lugol's iodine chromoendoscopy is useful for screening squamous dysplasia and SCCs. NBI is also useful, and dysplastic lesions appear as brownish-discolored areas.[28,29] NBI, which focuses on changes in the intrapapillary capillary loops (IPCLs), shows that dysplasia can be recognized as a regional lesion with changes in the IPCL (see **Fig. 1**D). However, the degree of IPCL change is not as apparent as that in SCC.[30]

PATHOLOGY OF SQUAMOUS DYSPLASIA

Macroscopically, dysplasia is generally difficult to recognize because the lesion is usually flat and without color alteration. As a result of Lugol staining, it is possible to recognize it as a poorly stained or unstained area of mucosa. The lesion is usually small, measuring less than 10 mm and often has smooth margins in most instances.

Microscopically, squamous dysplasia is characterized by architectural and cytologic abnormalities that vary in extent and severity. Architectural abnormalities include loss of normal cell polarity, overlapping nuclei, and lack of surface maturation. Nuclear changes, such as enlargement, hyperchromasia, pleomorphism, increased nuclear/cytoplasmic ratio, and increased mitotic activity characterize cytologic abnormalities. World Health Organization (WHO) classification adopted a two-tiered system (low-grade and high-grade) for the grading of squamous dysplasia. In low-grade dysplasia, atypical cells are located only within the lower half of the epithelium and have only mild-to-moderate cytologic atypia (**Fig. 2**). In contrast, high-grade dysplasia is diagnosed when more than half of the epithelium is involved with dysplastic cells or

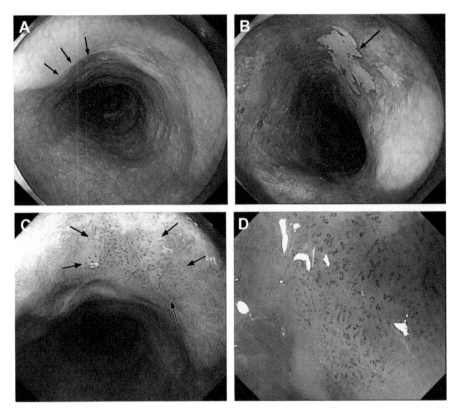

Fig. 1. Endoscopic findings of high-grade dysplasia/squamous cell carcinoma in situ. (*A*) White-light endoscopy. A flat and reddish lesion (*arrows*) is observed. (*B*) Lugol's chromoendoscopy shows the unstained area (*arrow*). (*C*) Narrow band image shows a greyish lesion with dilated intrapapillary capillary loops (*arrows*). (*D*) The high magnification image is shown in (*C*). Dilatation and irregularity of the intrapapillary capillary loops is observed.

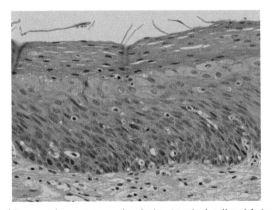

Fig. 2. Histology of low-grade squamous dysplasia. Atypical cells with increased cellularity are observed to be mainly located in the lower half of the epithelium. Hematoxylin and eosin staining.

when severe cytologic atypia is present (regardless of the extent of epithelial involvement) (**Fig. 3**). Thus, lesions with apparent severe cellular atypia are classified as high-grade dysplasia, even though atypical cells are located only within the lower half of the epithelium (**Fig. 4**). **Fig. 5** illustrates the histologic and cytologic characteristics of low-grade and high-grade dysplasia.

There exist differences in diagnostic criteria between Western countries and Japan. In Western countries, esophageal SCC is diagnosed when the neoplastic epithelium invades the lamina propria or beyond. In contrast, most Japanese pathologists regard high-grade dysplasia, sometimes even low-grade dysplasia, as "noninvasive squamous cell carcinoma." This is due to differences in the diagnostic criteria for carcinoma.[31,32] Japanese pathologists consider nuclear atypia to be more important, without considering the invasive growth of the tumor. However, although the concepts and terms differ, the clinical management is similar.[33]

DIFFERENTIAL DIAGNOSIS OF SQUAMOUS DYSPLASIA

The differential diagnoses include squamous cell papilloma, pseudoepitheliomatous hyperplasia, regenerative/reactive changes, radiation or chemotherapeutic effects, and verrucous carcinoma.[34,35] The differential diagnosis between reactive squamous epithelium and squamous dysplasia is of utmost importance in daily practice. **Table 1** summarizes the pathologic findings that can help distinguish reactive changes from dysplasia.[35,36] At the esophagogastric junctional area, it is also necessary to differentiate regenerative epithelium associated with reflux esophagitis from dysplasia, because the former can be quite marked.

On the other hand, the differential diagnosis between squamous dysplasia and SCC is also important. Squamous dysplasia and cancer are differentiated by the degree of nuclear atypia and more specifically, the presence or absence of invasion (**Fig. 6A–C**). The differential diagnosis between squamous dysplasia and SCC is easier when discontinuous infiltration is observed. However, it may be difficult to differentiate between high-grade dysplasia and SCC when the tumor proliferates downward expansively in a continuous fashion. When the lesion grows below the level of the basal layer of the surrounding nonneoplastic squamous epithelium, some pathologists consider this sufficient evidence of invasion, especially those from Asia; however, other

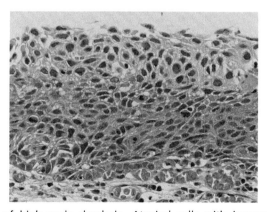

Fig. 3. Histology of high-grade dysplasia. Atypical cells with increased cellularity are observed to be distributed within the entire thickness of the epithelium. Hematoxylin and eosin staining.

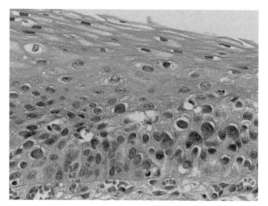

Fig. 4. Histology of high-grade dysplasia. Because high-grade cytologic atypia is observed in the neoplastic cells, this lesion is also diagnosed as high-grade dysplasia, even though the cells are limited to the basal half of the epithelium. Hematoxylin and eosin staining.

pathologists, such as those from western countries, require unequivocal evidence of tissue invasion in the form of discontinuous disease before true invasive carcinoma can be diagnosed confidentially (see **Fig. 6**D).

In addition, immunohistochemistry is occasionally useful for the differential diagnosis. Strong Ki-67 staining is extensively seen in high-grade dysplasia, and strong ProExC staining is also prevalent in the majority of high-grade dysplasia instances, but these can be positive in carcinoma and low-grade dysplasia as well.[37] Although the frequencies of intermediate/strong staining patterns of p53 increase with the severity of dysplasia, the sensitivity of p53 is considerably lower compared with that of Ki-67 and ProExC.[37] Because *TP53* gene mutation occurs frequently even in low-grade dysplasia,[38] p53 immunohistochemistry is not useful to differentiate

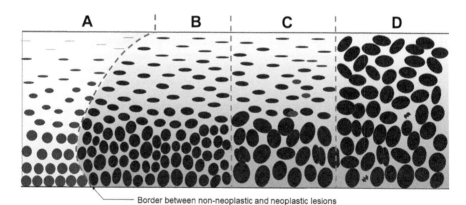

——— Border between non-neoplastic and neoplastic lesions

Fig. 5. Esophageal squamous dysplasia. This illustrates the concept of esophageal squamous dysplasia. The vague boundary is recognizable between nonneoplastic epithelium (*A*) and dysplasia (*B–D*). (*A*) Nonneoplastic epithelium. (*B*) Low-grade dysplasia is composed of mild atypical cells that show differentiation toward the surface. (*C*) This type of dysplasia, composed of severe atypical cells only within the lower half of the epithelium, can be also diagnosed as high-grade dysplasia. (*D*) High-grade dysplasia, composed of severe atypical cells distributed more than half of the epithelium, demonstrates apparent nuclear abnormalities.

Table 1
Clinical management of esophageal squamous epithelial neoplasia according to the modified Vienna classification[a]

Category	Diagnosis	Clinical Management
1	Negative for neoplasia/dysplasia	Optional follow-up
2	Indefinite for neoplasia/dysplasia	Follow-up
3	Low-grade dysplasia	Endoscopic resection or follow-up
4	High-grade dysplasia 4.1 High-grade dysplasia 4.2 Noninvasive carcinoma (CIS) 4.3 Suspicious for invasive carcinoma 4.4 Intramucosal carcinoma	Endoscopic or surgical local resection
5	Submucosal carcinoma or beyond	Surgical resection/chemo-radiotherapy/immune therapy

[a] This table was made with reference to the Vienna classification and modified Vienna classification (Dixon[33] and Shimizu et al[34]) for esophageal squamous epithelial neoplasia.

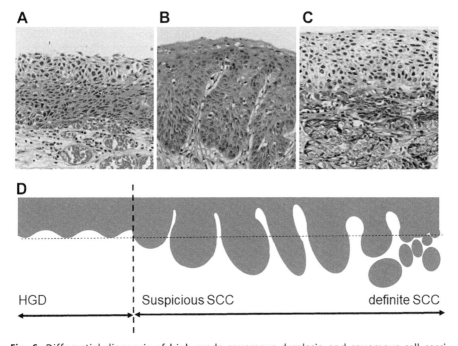

Fig. 6. Differential diagnosis of high-grade squamous dysplasia and squamous cell carcinoma. (*A*) High-grade dysplasia. Atypical cells proliferate within the entire epithelium but do not show invasion or extension into the lamina propria. (*B*) High-grade dysplasia considered suspicious for squamous cell carcinoma by some pathologists, particularly those from Asia. Tumor cells proliferate downward into the lamina propria, however, the cells are still continuous with the overlying epithelium. Thus, some pathologists consider this "pushing" invasion. (*C*) Definite squamous cell carcinoma. Small tumor cell nests are present in the lamina propria and they are separate from the overlying epithelium. (*D*) Progression from squamous dysplasia to invasive squamous cell carcinoma. Although determination of invasion is difficult at times, it is often helpful to assess the extent of downward growth from the level of the basal layer of the surrounding nonneoplastic epithelium (*dashed line*).

squamous dysplasia from high-grade dysplasia or SCC. However, p53 exhibits higher sensitivity and specificity for distinguishing normal/reactive hyperplasia from squamous dysplasia.[37] A few novel biomarkers were reported as potential candidates for the differential diagnosis of high-grade dysplasia that is likely to progress to carcinoma. Oral cancer overexpressed 1 (ORAOV1) overexpression seems to be significantly higher in ESCC, high- and low-grade squamous dysplasia than in the controls.[39] Increased expression of γ-glutamylcyclotransferase (GGCT) was common in invasive ESCC and high-grade dysplasia but was much less frequently observed in low-grade dysplasia.[40] In the differential diagnosis of low-grade dysplasia and high-grade dysplasia, GGCT possessed both high sensitivity and high specificity, whereas Ki-67 and p53 only possessed either high sensitivity or high specificity. Both ORAOV1 and GGCT expression correlated with the presence of lymph node metastasis and the degree of differentiation or advanced TNM stage.

GENETIC ALTERATIONS AND PATHOGENESIS

Cancer is a disease that develops due to the accumulation of gene mutations. ESCC is believed to progress from normal mucosa through dysplasia to invasive carcinoma by the influence of various risk factors. PT53 mutation is the most common gene mutation in ESCC and occurs in approximately 90% of all the cases.[41,42] PT53 mutation is also observed in high- and low-grade dysplasia with a rate of approximately 70%–80%,[38] suggesting that TP53 mutations occur early stage in the development of carcinogenesis. Recent molecular studies of ESCC have found an average of 83 gene mutations in an individual tumor.[41] In addition to TP53 mutation, the accumulation of gene mutations such as CCND1 amplification, TP63/SOX amplification, KDM6A deletion, and NOTCH1/3 mutations are observed in ESCC.[41,42]

Another study using next-generation sequence analysis reports that squamous dysplasia and ESCCs have similar mutations and markers of genomic instability at similar frequencies; these alterations differ from mutations in esophageal tissues with simple hyperplasia.[43] In addition, this study indicates that most ESCCs are formed from early-stage squamous dysplasia clones. Truncated mutations shared by squamous dysplasia and ESCC tissues are in genes that regulate DNA repair and cell apoptosis, proliferation, and adhesion. Mutations in TP53 and CDKN2A and copy number alterations in 11q (contains CCND1), 3q (contains SOX2), 2q (contains NFE2L2), and 9p (contains CDKN2A) are considered to be truncated variants; these were dominant mutations detected at high frequencies in clones of paired squamous dysplasia and ESCC tissues.[43] Thus, various gene mutations may occur in the early stage of carcinogenesis including squamous dysplasia.

Squamous dysplasia in cancerous and noncancerous esophagi demonstrated a non-diploid DNA histogram in 67.9% and 43.3% of cases, respectively.[44,45] Moreover, squamous dysplasia in cancerous esophagus shows more diverse non-diploid patterns than cancer-free esophagus.[44] This evidence suggests a higher degree of copy number alterations in squamous dysplasia in high-risk patients. Genomic changes observed in precancerous lesions may be used to identify patients at risk for ESCC.

NATURAL HISTORY

Several reports demonstrate the natural history of esophageal squamous dysplasia.[1,23,46–48] According to follow-up studies for esophageal squamous dysplasia, approximately two-thirds of cases of dysplasia have a regressive or stable status, and one-third have a progressive status.[23] In Linxian, China, which is a region with some of the highest incidence and mortality rates of ESCC in the world, the relative risks for developing ESCC over 13 years of follow-up were 2.9, 9.8, and 28.3 for individuals with mild, moderate, or severe dysplasia, respectively, compared with those of persons without histologic evidence of dysplasia or cancer.[1] Similarly, after 15 years of follow-up in asymptomatic subjects, one-third of patients with dysplasia, approximately 4% of subjects, developed SCC in the same area in China.[46] In addition, according to a recent nationwide study in the Netherlands, the annual risk of ESCC was 4.0% in patients with mild-to-moderate dysplasia and 8.5% in patients with high-grade dysplasia.[48] The rate of SCC development increased with the severity of dysplasia, and the prevalence of dysplasia increased significantly with age. These results suggest a close association between the histologic grading of squamous dysplasia and the risk of future ESCC; furthermore, a shift in the grade of dysplasia corresponds to a real change in cancer risk. One gene expression study demonstrated that local and systemic immune responses may influence the natural history of esophageal squamous dysplasia.[47]

RISK PREDICTION AND TREATMENT

Early detection for squamous dysplasia is possible through periodic endoscopy in subjects with various risk factors. In particular, individuals who consume alcohol and have a heterozygous single nucleotide variant of ALDH are at high risk of ESCC and squamous dysplasia.[20] Individuals possessing additional risk factors, such as a history of SCC or smoking, should be considered for regular screening. Because esophageal dysplasia is asymptomatic and difficult to detect by white-light endoscopy, Lugol chromoendoscopy and NBI are effective in high-risk populations. Endoscopic resection is considered for lesions diagnosed as high-grade dysplasia. Ablative methods, such as multipolar electrocoagulation, argon plasma coagulation, and radiofrequency ablation, may be adopted for patients who cannot undergo endoscopic resection.[7]

Several guidelines have been published for treating esophageal squamous dysplasia; however, the revised Vienna classification (**Table 2**) is recommended from a practical perspective.[33,49] This classification proves advantageous as it eliminates the diagnostic discrepancies between Japanese and Western pathologists, and each category is associated with different recommendations for further diagnostic and

Table 2
Useful pathologic findings distinguishing reactive change and intraepithelial neoplasia[a]

Reactive Change	Dysplasia
Basal cell hyperplasia	Highly atypical cells
Regular arrangement of basal layer	Irregular arrangement of basal layer
Nonkeratinizing epithelium	Increased cellularity
Glycogen depletion	Bizarre cell shapes
Fine and homogenous chromatin	Nuclear overlapping
Prominent hyperchromatic nucleoli	Nuclear hyperchromasia
Basophilic cytoplasm	Eosinophilic nucleoli (occasional)
Lack of irregular nuclear outline	Pleomorphism
Mucosal inflammation	Irregular nuclear outlines
Surface maturation	Increased nuclear/cytoplasmic ratio
Epithelial edema	Increased mitotic activity
Vascular congestion	Abnormal mitoses

[a] This table was made by modifying Dixon[33] and Shimizu et al.[34].

therapeutic measures. For cases of low-grade dysplasia, the recommendation includes either endoscopic resection or increased endoscopic surveillance with biopsy. Conversely, instances of high-grade squamous dysplasia mandate local endoscopic or surgical resection.

CLINICS CARE POINTS

The optimal management for distinct squamous dysplasia grades remains unclear due to the unknown associated risk of developing ESCC. Nevertheless, the diagnosis and treatment of esophageal squamous dysplasia revolves around essential clinical care points: chemoprevention, screening, endoscopic treatment, and follow-up strategy. In terms of chemoprevention, evidence for a beneficial effect on precancerous status was observed in the following agents: the combination of retinol, riboflavin and zinc,[50] multivitamins,[51] selenomethionine,[52] selenium,[52–54] and strawberries[55] improved cytologic or histologic features or reduced proliferation and expression of several cancer-related proteins. Recently, vitamin D has emerged as a promising anticancer agent. Although vitamin D dietary intake was associated with esophageal cancer, circulating 25-hydroxyvitamin D concentration showed inconsistent results.[56] Further investigations are imperative to substantiate its potential effects.

Screening holds paramount importance in the timely identification of esophageal squamous dysplasia, particularly among high-risk patients, as most of them remain asymptomatic. The ideal screening method should be cost-effective, well-tolerated, and suitable for primary care settings. Remarkable advancements in endoscopic imaging and optical enhancements have transpired over the past decade, revolutionizing the diagnosis of squamous dysplasia and early esophageal cancer. Alongside conventional white-light endoscopy and chromoendoscopy, innovative endoscopic techniques such as trans-nasal endoscopy, capsule endoscopy, electronic endoscopy, confocal laser endoscopy, and endocytoscopy have been introduced.[57,58] Despite existing challenges in endoscopic lesion diagnosis, artificial intelligence (AI) is rapidly evolving, and endoscopic systems integrated with AI display significant promise in the detection of squamous dysplasia and early SCC.[59,60] In addition, a recent study explored the feasibility of using circular miRNA-based blood tests to assist in the detection of squamous dysplasia and ESCC.[61]

Endoscopic follow-up or treatment should be considered in all patients with esophageal squamous dysplasia. For patients with low-grade dysplasia, endoscopic surveillance with careful inspection with NBI or dye-based chromoendoscopy of the esophageal mucosa is indicated, and for patients with high-grade dysplasia and in case of suspected SCC, endoscopic treatment should be performed.

SUMMARY

Clinicopathological and molecular studies have revealed the nature of squamous dysplasia as a precancerous and/or neoplastic lesion with malignant potential and genetic mutations. This condition holds the capacity to transition into ESCC, and its prevalence correlates with the extent of dysplasia. The risk factors associated with squamous dysplasia largely coincide with those linked to invasive ESCC. Identifying high-risk patients in their early stages, those with precursor lesions, is crucial for implementing therapeutic strategies such as chemoprevention and endoscopic therapy, leading to a reduction in ESCC-related mortality. Future research concerning squamous dysplasia and ESCC is expected to improve early detection methods through AI-assisted endoscopy. Furthermore, advancements in early detection via chemoprevention and biomarkers remain imperative for future endeavors.

CLINICS CARE POINTS

- Endoscopic screening is useful for patients who have risk factors for dysplasia.
- Increased endoscopic surveillance with biopsy is recommended for patients with low-grade dysplasia.
- High-grade squamous dysplasia requires local endoscopic or surgical resection.
- Ablative methods and radiofrequency ablation may be adopted for patients who cannot undergo endoscopic resection.

DISCLOSURE

The authors declare that they have no conflicts of interest.

REFERENCES

1. Dawsey SM, Lewin KJ, Wang GQ, et al. Squamous esophageal histology and subsequent risk of squamous cell carcinoma of the esophagus. A prospective follow-up study from Linxian, China. Cancer 1994;74:1686–92.
2. Wang GQ, Abnet CC, Shen Q, et al. Histological precursors of oesophageal squamous cell carcinoma: results from a 13 year prospective follow up study in a high risk population. Gut 2005;54:187–92.
3. Oota K, Sobin LH. Histological typeing of gastric and oesophageal tumours. 1st edition. Geneva: WHO; 1977.
4. Watanabe H, Jass JR, Sobin LH. Histological typing of oesophageal and gastric tumours. 2nd edition. Berlin: Springer-Verlag; 1990.
5. Takubo K, Fujii S. Oesophageal sqaumous dysplasia. In: Borad WCoTE, editor. WHO classification of tumours digestive system. 5th edition. Lyon: WHO Press; 2019.
6. Hamilton SR, Alaltonen LA. World Health Organization Classification of Tumours. Pathology and Genetics. In: Tumours of the digestive system. 3rd edition. Lyon: IARCPress; 2000.
7. Montgomery E, Field JK, Boffetta P, et al. Squamous cell carcinoma of the oesophagus. In: Bosman FT, Carneiro F, Hruban RH, et al, editors. WHO classification of tumours of the digestive system. 4th edition. Geneva: WHO Press; 2010. p. 18–24.
8. The Coordinating Groups for the Research of Esophageal Carcinoma, Honan Province and Chinese Academy of Medical Sciences. Studies on relationship between epithelial dysplasia and carcinoma of the esophagus. Chin Med J 1975;N1:110–6.
9. Takubo K. Squamous epithelial dysplasia and squamous cell carcinoma. Pathology of the esophagus. An Atlas and Textbook. 3rd edition. Tokyo: Wiley; 2015.
10. Ushigome S, Spjut HJ, Noon GP. Extensive dysplasia and carcinoma in situ of esophageal epithelium. Cancer 1967;20:1023–9.
11. Mukada T, Sato E, Sasano N. Comparative studies on dysplasia of esophageal epithelium in four prefectures of Japan (Miyagi, Nara, Wakayama and Aomori) with reference to risk of carcinoma. Tohoku J Exp Med 1976;119:51–63.
12. Takubo K, Tsuchiya S, Fukushi K, et al. Dysplasia and reserve cell hyperplasia-like change in human esophagus. Acta Pathol Jpn 1981;31:999–1013.
13. Japan Esophageal Society. Japanese Classification of Esophageal Cancer, 11th Edition: part II and III. Esophagus 2017;14:37–65.

14. Wei WQ, Abnet CC, Lu N, et al. Risk factors for oesophageal squamous dysplasia in adult inhabitants of a high risk region of China. Gut 2005;54:759–63.
15. Taylor PR, Abnet CC, Dawsey SM. Squamous dysplasia–the precursor lesion for esophageal squamous cell carcinoma. Cancer Epidemiol Biomarkers Prev 2013; 22:540–52.
16. Fagundes RB, de Barros SG, Putten AC, et al. Occult dysplasia is disclosed by Lugol chromoendoscopy in alcoholics at high risk for squamous cell carcinoma of the esophagus. Endoscopy 1999;31:281–5.
17. Mwachiro MM, Burgert SL, Lando J, et al. Esophageal Squamous Dysplasia is Common in Asymptomatic Kenyans: A Prospective, Community-Based, Cross-Sectional Study. Am J Gastroenterol 2016;111:500–7.
18. Abnet CC, Arnold M, Wei WQ. Epidemiology of Esophageal Squamous Cell Carcinoma. Gastroenterology 2018;154:360–73.
19. Wang QL, Xie SH, Wahlin K, et al. Global time trends in the incidence of esophageal squamous cell carcinoma. Clin Epidemiol 2018;10:717–28.
20. Yokoyama A, Hirota T, Omori T, et al. Development of squamous neoplasia in esophageal iodine-unstained lesions and the alcohol and aldehyde dehydrogenase genotypes of Japanese alcoholic men. Int J Cancer 2012;130:2949–60.
21. Abnet CC, Chen W, Dawsey SM, et al. Serum 25(OH)-vitamin D concentration and risk of esophageal squamous dysplasia. Cancer Epidemiol Biomarkers Prev 2007;16:1889–93.
22. Kamangar F, Diaw L, Wei WQ, et al. Serum pepsinogens and risk of esophageal squamous dysplasia. Int J Cancer 2009;124:456–60.
23. Su H, Liu K, Zhao Y, et al. High Serum Squamous Cell Carcinoma Antigen Level Associated with Remission of Mild/Moderate Dysplasia of the Esophagus: A Nested Case-Control Study. Gastroenterol Res Pract 2022;2022:2961337.
24. El-Zimaity H, Di Pilato V, Novella Ringressi M, et al. Risk factors for esophageal cancer: emphasis on infectious agents. Ann N Y Acad Sci 2018;1434:319–32.
25. Chang F, Shen Q, Zhou J, et al. Detection of human papillomavirus DNA in cytologic specimens derived from esophageal precancer lesions and cancer. Scand J Gastroenterol 1990;25:383–8.
26. Gao GF, Roth MJ, Wei WQ, et al. No association between HPV infection and the neoplastic progression of esophageal squamous cell carcinoma: result from a cross-sectional study in a high-risk region of China. Int J Cancer 2006;119: 1354–9.
27. Inoue H, Kaga M, Ikeda H, et al. Magnification endoscopy in esophageal squamous cell carcinoma: a review of the intrapapillary capillary loop classification. Ann Gastroenterol 2015;28:41–8.
28. Nagami Y, Tominaga K, Machida H, et al. Usefulness of non-magnifying narrow-band imaging in screening of early esophageal squamous cell carcinoma: a prospective comparative study using propensity score matching. Am J Gastroenterol 2014;109:845–54.
29. Morita FH, Bernardo WM, Ide E, et al. Narrow band imaging versus lugol chromoendoscopy to diagnose squamous cell carcinoma of the esophagus: a systematic review and meta-analysis. BMC Cancer 2017;17:54.
30. Oyama T, Inoue H, Arima M, et al. Prediction of the invasion depth of superficial squamous cell carcinoma based on microvessel morphology: magnifying endoscopic classification of the Japan Esophageal Society. Esophagus 2017;14: 105–12.

31. Schlemper RJ, Dawsey SM, Itabashi M, et al. Differences in diagnostic criteria for esophageal squamous cell carcinoma between Japanese and Western pathologists. Cancer 2000;88:996–1006.
32. Takubo K. Pathology of teh esophagus. An atlas and textbook. 2nd edition. Tokyo: Springer; 2007.
33. Dixon MF. Gastrointestinal epithelial neoplasia: Vienna revisited. Gut 2002;51: 130–1.
34. Shimizu M, Ban S, Odze RD. Squamous dysplasia and other precursor lesions related to esophageal squamous cell carcinoma. Gastroenterol Clin North Am 2007;36:797–811, v-vi.
35. Shimizu M, Nagata K, Yamaguchi H, et al. Squamous intraepithelial neoplasia of the esophagus: past, present, and future. J Gastroenterol 2009;44:103–12.
36. Fenoglio-Preiser CM, Noffsinger AE, Stermmermann GN. Gastrointestinal pathology. An atlas and text. 3rd edition. Philadelphia: Lippincott Williams & Wilkins; 2008.
37. Wang WC, Wu TT, Chandan VS, et al. Ki-67 and ProExC are useful immunohistochemical markers in esophageal squamous intraepithelial neoplasia. Hum Pathol 2011;42:1430–7.
38. Kobayashi M, Kawachi H, Takizawa T, et al. p53 Mutation analysis of low-grade dysplasia and high-grade dysplasia/carcinoma in situ of the esophagus using laser capture microdissection. Oncology 2006;71:237–45.
39. Li M, Cui X, Shen Y, et al. ORAOV1 overexpression in esophageal squamous cell carcinoma and esophageal dysplasia: a possible biomarker of progression and poor prognosis in esophageal carcinoma. Hum Pathol 2015;46:707–15.
40. Takemura K, Kawachi H, Eishi Y, et al. gamma-Glutamylcyclotransferase as a novel immunohistochemical biomarker for the malignancy of esophageal squamous tumors. Hum Pathol 2014;45:331–41.
41. Agrawal N, Jiao Y, Bettegowda C, et al. Comparative genomic analysis of esophageal adenocarcinoma and squamous cell carcinoma. Cancer Discov 2012;2: 899–905.
42. Cancer Genome Atlas Research Network. Integrated genomic characterization of oesophageal carcinoma. Nature 2017;541:169–75.
43. Liu X, Zhang M, Ying S, et al. Genetic Alterations in Esophageal Tissues From Squamous Dysplasia to Carcinoma. Gastroenterology 2017;153:166–77.
44. Itakura Y, Sasano H, Mori S, et al. DNA ploidy in human esophageal squamous dysplasias and squamous cell carcinomas as determined by image analysis. Mod Pathol 1994;7:867–73.
45. Itakura Y, Sasano F, Date F, et al. DNA ploidy, P53 expression, and cellular proliferation in normal epithelium and squamous dysplasia of non-cancerous and cancerous human oesophagi. Anticancer Res 1996;16:201–8.
46. Wang LD, Yang HH, Fan ZM, et al. Cytological screening and 15 years' follow-up (1986-2001) for early esophageal squamous cell carcinoma and precancerous lesions in a high-risk population in Anyang County, Henan Province, Northern China. Cancer Detect Prev 2005;29:317–22.
47. Joshi N, Johnson LL, Wei WQ, et al. Gene expression differences in normal esophageal mucosa associated with regression and progression of mild and moderate squamous dysplasia in a high-risk Chinese population. Cancer Res 2006;66:6851–60.
48. van Tilburg L, Spaander MCW, Bruno MJ, et al. Increased risk of esophageal squamous cell carcinoma in patients with squamous dysplasia: a nationwide cohort study in the Netherlands. Dis Esophagus 2023.

49. Schlemper RJ, Riddell RH, Kato Y, et al. The Vienna classification of gastrointestinal epithelial neoplasia. Gut 2000;47:251–5.
50. Munoz N, Hayashi M, Bang LJ, et al. Effect of riboflavin, retinol, and zinc on micronuclei of buccal mucosa and of esophagus: a randomized double-blind intervention study in China. J Natl Cancer Inst 1987;79:687–91.
51. Mark SD, Liu SF, Li JY, et al. The effect of vitamin and mineral supplementation on esophageal cytology: results from the Linxian Dysplasia Trial. Int J Cancer 1994; 57:162–6.
52. Limburg PJ, Wei W, Ahnen DJ, et al. Randomized, placebo-controlled, esophageal squamous cell cancer chemoprevention trial of selenomethionine and celecoxib. Gastroenterology 2005;129:863–73.
53. Ahsan A, Liu Z, Su R, et al. Potential Chemotherapeutic Effect of Selenium for Improved Canceration of Esophageal Cancer. Int J Mol Sci 2022;23.
54. Roth MJ, Katki HA, Wei WQ, et al. Serum cytokine analysis in a positive chemoprevention trial: selenium, interleukin-2, and an association with squamous preneoplastic disease. Cancer Prev Res 2010;3:810–7.
55. Chen T, Yan F, Qian J, et al. Randomized phase II trial of lyophilized strawberries in patients with dysplastic precancerous lesions of the esophagus. Cancer Prev Res 2012;5:41–50.
56. Rouphael C, Kamal A, Sanaka MR, et al. Vitamin D in esophageal cancer: Is there a role for chemoprevention? World J Gastrointest Oncol 2018;10:23–30.
57. di Pietro M, Canto MI, Fitzgerald RC. Endoscopic Management of Early Adenocarcinoma and Squamous Cell Carcinoma of the Esophagus: Screening, Diagnosis, and Therapy. Gastroenterology 2018;154:421–36.
58. Kumagai Y, Takubo K, Kawada K, et al. Diagnosis using deep-learning artificial intelligence based on the endocytoscopic observation of the esophagus. Esophagus 2019;16:180–7.
59. Hussein M, Gonzalez-Bueno Puyal J, Mountney P, et al. Role of artificial intelligence in the diagnosis of oesophageal neoplasia: 2020 an endoscopic odyssey. World J Gastroenterol 2020;26:5784–96.
60. Hussein M, Everson M, Haidry R. Esophageal squamous dysplasia and cancer: Is artificial intelligence our best weapon? Best Pract Res Clin Gastroenterol 2021; 52-53:101723.
61. Shen Y, Ding Y, Ma Q, et al. Identification of Novel Circulating miRNA Biomarkers for the Diagnosis of Esophageal Squamous Cell Carcinoma and Squamous Dysplasia. Cancer Epidemiol Biomarkers Prev 2019;28:1212–20.

Pathology and Clinical Relevance of Gastric Epithelial Dysplasia

Tetsuo Ushiku, MD, PhD[a], Gregory Y. Lauwers, MD[b,c],*

KEYWORDS

• Gastric • Dysplasia • Oxyntic gland adenoma • Pyloric • Diagnosis

KEY POINTS

- Gastric dysplasia carries a definite but variable risk of malignant transformation based on the grade.
- Nonconventional morphologic subtypes of gastric dysplasia have been recently recognized, and an understanding of their biological potential is being evaluated.
- Tailored endoscopic therapy and adequate surveillance is necessary for all gastric epithelial dysplastic lesions, although the risk is variable for nonconventional lesions.

INTRODUCTION

Gastric dysplasia is defined as an unequivocally neoplastic epithelium that may be associated with or give rise to invasive adenocarcinoma.[1–6] Establishing an accurate diagnosis of gastric dysplasia and its grade is important not only for establishing the risk of malignant transformation but also for determining the potential of synchronous and metachronous gastric cancer. We will discuss here not only conventional gastric dysplasia but also elaborate on nonconventional dysplastic patterns that have been more recently characterized (**Table 1**).

In addition to a better understanding of the clinical behavior of dysplasia, the last 2 decades have witnessed a diversification and improvement in therapeutic strategies. To date, endoscopic excision and surveillance offer an effective therapeutic and preventive strategy to successfully treat dysplasia and control the development of adenocarcinoma.[7]

Differences in the interpretation of histologic features, nomenclature, and classification between Far Eastern and Western pathologists are well known.[8] However, this review will present only the Western perspective.

a Department of Pathology, The University of Tokyo, 7-3-1 Hongo, Bunkyo-ku, Tokyo 113-0033, Japan; b Department of Pathology, Gastrointestinal Pathology Section, H. Lee Moffitt Cancer Center and Research Institute, 12902 USF Magnolia Drive, Tampa, FL 33612, USA; c Departments of Pathology and Oncologic Sciences, Tampa, FL, USA
* Corresponding author.
E-mail address: Gregory.Lauwers@Moffitt.org

Gastroenterol Clin N Am 53 (2024) 39–55
https://doi.org/10.1016/j.gtc.2023.11.003
0889-8553/24/© 2023 Elsevier Inc. All rights reserved.

Table 1
Morphologic characteristics of dysplastic subtypes

Lesions	Morphologic Characteristics
Intestinal dysplasia	Crowded tubules ± irregularly shaped dilated glands lined by columnar cells. Overlapping, elongated pencil-shaped hyperchromatic nuclei.
Foveolar dysplasia	Elongated foveolas lined by cuboidal/low-columnar cells with apical mucin cap. Round-to-oval hyperchromatic nuclei.
Serrated dysplasia	Foveolar presenting epithelial infoldings lined by low-columnar cells with apical mucin cap. Round-to-oval hyperchromatic nuclei.
Pyloric type dysplasia	Packed tubules ± irregularly shaped dilated glands lined by a single layer of low-columnar to cuboidal cells with a pale eosinophilic cytoplasm. Basally located round nuclei.
Oxyntic gland adenoma	Tight tubules lined by chief cells or admixture of chief and parietal cells or prominent mucous neck cells.
Pit dysplasia	Crowded, irregular branched glands +/budding, lined by hyperchromatic and enlarged dysplastic nuclei. Round-to-oval hyperchromatic nuclei.

CONVENTIONAL DYSPLASTIC PATTERNS
Clinical Features

Most individuals diagnosed with gastric dysplasia are in the sixth to seventh decade of life,[9,10] and men are commonly affected more often than women (male/female ratios range from 2.4–3.9:1).[10,11]

Although gastric epithelial dysplasia can develop over the entire mucosa, it most commonly affects the lesser curvature, particularly the antrum or the incisura angulus, where it is frequently detected in association with intestinal metaplasia.[10,12]

Pathogenesis and Risk Factors

Similar to gastric adenocarcinoma, the prevalence of gastric dysplasia shows marked variation worldwide between high-risk area (eg, 9%–20%) and regions where gastric cancer is less prevalent (eg, 0.5%–3.75%).[13–17] The difference reflects variations in the prevalence of risk factors (eg, prevalence of *Helicobacter pylori* infection) and the genetic makeup of the populations.

Gastric dysplasia share similar pathogenetic risk factors with adenocarcinoma. These include chronic *H. pylori* infection, atrophic gastritis, and intestinal metaplasia.[18] An autoimmune process such as chronic autoimmune gastritis is also associated with an elevated risk of dysplasia[19–21] However, the increased risk of developing adenocarcinoma is relatively moderate in these patients compared with the general population.[22–24]

Gastric dysplasia also develops in polyps in patients with a variety of polyposis syndromes.[25–28] For instance, patients with familial adenomatous polyposis (FAP) are at higher risk of developing dysplasia. These are typically located in the antrum, frequently multiple, and are observed in 2% to 50% of patients.[29–41] Polyps detected in GAPPS (gastric adenocarcinoma and proximal polyposis of the stomach) are also frequently associated with dysplasia.[42–44] In juvenile polyposis syndrome, gastric dysplasia is not uncommon, noted in up to 14% of cases.[45]

From a genetic point of view, any of the molecular alterations observed in gastric adenocarcinoma are observed in dysplasia. A full review goes beyond the scope of this article, but principal alterations are presented in a table form (**Table 2**).

Table 2
Clinical associations, risk of progression, and suggested therapeutic approach

Lesions	Associated Conditions	Risks of Malignant Transformation and Suggested Therapeutic Principles
Intestinal dysplasia	*Helicobacter pylori*, Atrophic gastritis, Intestinal metaplasia	Low-grade dysplasia: low progression rate and annual endoscopic surveillance with re-biopsy. High-grade dysplasia: high progression rate. EMR and biannual surveillance with chromoendoscopy and EUS advisable
Foveolar dysplasia	Sporadic, fundic gland polyp, raspberry polyp.	Low progression rate in fundic gland polyp and raspberry polyp. Limited data suggestive of high progression rate when sporadic or serrated pattern to be taken into consideration
Pyloric gland adenoma	Autoimmune gastritis, Lynch syndrome, FAP	Low-grade lesions have<10% recurrence rate and can be managed conservatively after complete excision. Endoscopic resection for large or high-grade lesions advisable
Oxyntic gland adenoma		Most have a benign course. Cytoarchitectural atypia and submucosal invasion may herald a malignant potential, and endoscopic resection is advisable for superficial lesions
Pit dysplasia	*Helicobacter pylori*, Atrophic gastritis, Intestinal metaplasia	25% rate of progression to conventional low-grade dysplasia

Abbreviations: EMR, endoscopic mucosal resection; EUS, endoscopic ultrasound; FAP, familial adenomatous polyposis.

Gross Findings

In years past, many cases of dysplastic lesions were detected haphazardly on random mucosal biopsies, without grossly observed abnormalities.[10,11] Nowadays, following the improvement of endoscopic techniques, most dysplastic foci are detected either as flat or elevated lesion or even as a polypoid lesions. In practice, the term gastric "adenoma" is commonly used for well-circumscribed polyps, whereas the term "dysplasia" is reserved for either endoscopically undetectable (invisible) or non-adenomalike (ie, flat) lesions.[2,13,46,47]

Flat dysplasia is usually inconspicuous and sometimes detected as an ill-defined erythematous mucosal area. An ill-defined nodular gross pattern is usually associated with a diagnosis of low-grade dysplasia while a slightly depressed or eroded pattern is commonly associated with a diagnosis of high-grade dysplasia.[48–50]

Adenomas can be either sessile or pedunculated and are usually solitary (with the exception of FAP patients). Gastric adenomas usually measure less than 2 cm in maximum diameter.[34] Large adenomas can be ulcerated and show active bleeding.

Of note, the mucosa surrounding any gastric dysplastic lesions commonly shows evidence of chronic gastritis and atrophy.[51]

Pathologic Features

While the original description of dysplasia emphasized predominantly the intestinal morphotype, several additional patterns of nonconventional subtypes of gastric dysplasia have been observed. Those include either predominantly flat (foveolar, serrated, and pit dysplasia) or polypoid dysplasia (pyloric gland adenoma [PGA], oxyntic gland adenoma [OGA], and a few rarer patterns). However, it is noteworthy that despite an expanding body of literature mostly in anatomic pathology publications that evaluate their behavior and their morphologic and molecular characteristics, to this day published clinical guidelines ignore these subtypes. We will first discuss the conventional gastric dysplastic patterns.

Intestinal type (or type 1) dysplasia

The majority of gastric dysplastic lesions present as an "intestinal" phenotype resembling the morphology of colonic adenomas. This type is classically referred to as adenomatous dysplasia (or type I). The lesions are architecturally characterized by crowded tubular glands lined by columnar cells with overlapping, penicillate, and hyperchromatic nuclei. Variable degree of pseudostratification and more or less conspicuous nucleoli are also noted[52] (**Fig. 1**A and B).

Foveolar type (or type 2) dysplasia

This subtype is usually detected in non-metaplastic foveolar epithelium.[52] It may develop de novo or as a progression of a fundic gland polyp. De novo cases are composed of glands of variable size and shape, occasionally with cystic dilatation. Papillary infoldings and serration can be detected. In some cases, the serration is prominent and the term of serrated dysplasia has been proposed (see the following paragraphs).

In comparison to intestinal-type dysplasia, the cells of foveolar dysplasia tend to be more cuboidal or low-columnar in shape although not universally. Another characteristic is the clear or pale eosinophilic cytoplasm with distinctly rounder to oval and sometimes vesicular nuclei with variably sized nucleoli. Nuclear stratification is uncommon (**Fig. 2**A).

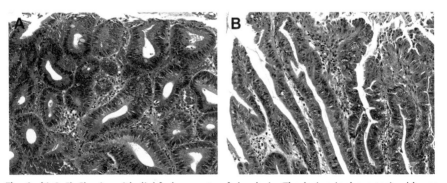

Fig. 1. (*A & B*) Classic epithelial [adenomatous] dysplasia. The lesion is characterized by an "intestinal" phenotype. **Fig. 1**A represents low-grade dysplasia displaying minimally crowded tubular glands and penicillate and hyperchromatic nuclei. High-grade dysplasia shows enlarged, rounded, and overlapping nuclei diagnostic of high-grade dysplasia (**Fig. 1**B).

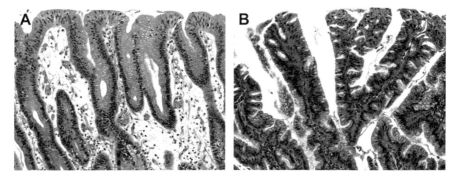

Fig. 2. (*A* & *B*) Foveolar (type II) dysplasia. **Fig. 2**A is a classic example of low-grade foveolar dysplasia displaying characteristic columnar-shaped cells with clear/pale eosinophilic cytoplasm with distinctly rounder-to-oval nuclei. **Fig. 2** B is an example of gastric serrated neoplasia with distinct lateral crenation.

Foveolar dysplasia can be detected in association with various processes. When sporadic, this type of dysplasia is more commonly associated with poorly differentiated adenocarcinoma.[52–54] Alternatively, it is the dysplastic subtype detected with fundic gland polyps when they develop dysplasia, either sporadic or in the setting of FAP. It is worth underscoring that dysplasia is seldom detected in sporadic fundic gland polyps but is much prevalent in polyps of FAP where it is observed in 25% to 42% of cases.[37,55]

In 2001, Rubio and colleagues[56] reported gastric serrated neoplasia as a new entity. Serrated dysplasia show elongated epithelial fronds with lateral crenation and sawtoothlike notches caused by scalloped epithelial indentations (see **Fig. 2**B).[56,57] Pure serrated dysplasia (>80% of the total tumor) and mixed serrated and conventional adenoma have been reported. Whereas conventional gastric adenoma has a low rate of malignant transformation, the limited data available report a higher propensity of serrated dysplasia to be associated of invasive carcinoma (to the rate of 74%).[58]

Recently, a new morphologic subtype of foveolar dysplasia characterized by a unique endoscopic appearance (ie, small raspberrylike polypoid lesion) has been described as "raspberrylike foveolar-type adenoma".[59] This lesion always arises in normal *H pylori*–naïve oxyntic mucosa and is often accompanied by fundic gland polyps. Morphologically, the adenoma shows papillary projections lined by foveolar-type epithelium with low-grade cytonuclear atypia (**Fig. 3**). This type of adenoma consistently harbors a unique *KLF4* c.A1322 C mutation that has never been detected in gastric carcinoma, a characteristic implying the benign nature of this neoplasm with virtually no malignant potential[60,61]

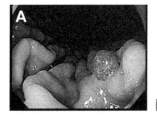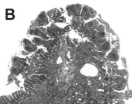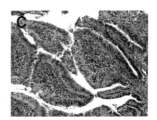

Fig. 3. (A–C) Raspberrylike polyps arising in an unremarkable gastric mucosa (see **Fig. 3**A). At low power (see **Fig. 3**B), epithelial papillary structures form the polyp. At higher magnification, the distinct low-grade foveolar-type epithelium is observed (see **Fig. 3**C).

The cells of foveolar-type dysplasia are predominantly immunoreactive for MUC5AC, and MUC6-positive cells may be seen at the bottoms of glands.[62] However, a pure immunophenotype is rare and a hybrid immunophenotype is common. In addition, rare MUC2-positive goblet cells can also be seen.[63] Thus, the histologic subtyping should primarily rely on hematoxylin rather than on immunophenotyping. Interestingly, despite clinical, morphologic, and immunophenotypic differences, the existence of cases with hybrid gastric and intestinal differentiation suggests the possibility of transdifferentiation between intestinal-type and foveolar-type dysplasia. The hybrid phenotype is just as likely to be due to clonal divergence of the same neoplastic process, leading to intralesional morphologic heterogeneity.[63]

Some authors suggest that foveolar lesions, which are more commonly diagnosed as high grade, may behave differently than adenomatous lesions.[64] However, the behavior of foveolar-type dysplasia is controversial, probably in part because of the low diagnostic reproducibility, particularly between low-grade foveolar dysplasia and regenerative foveolar epithelium.[65]

Grading of Gastric Dysplasia

The grading of gastric dysplasia is subject to interobserver variability. However, the challenges and clinical significance vary greatly for low-grade and high-grade dysplasia. Distinguishing between low-grade dysplasia and inflammatory cytoarchitectural atypia observed in the context of severe inflammation, or ulceration, can be difficult for pathologists with limited experience and even for gastrointestinal pathologists, particularly when evaluating small gastric biopsies.

Low-grade dysplasia displays minimal architectural disarray and[47,66,67] only mild-to-moderate cytologic atypia (see **Fig. 1**A).[46,66] Alternatively, reactive mucosal changes and regenerative epithelium associated with active inflammation may also display cytologic atypia, increased mitotic activity, and architectural disarray that may mimic dysplasia. In addition to taking into account the inflammatory and regenerative stromal background (maturing granulation tissue, vascular congestion), the recognition of subtle changes such as a gradual seamless transition between atypical cellular elements and surrounding normal epithelium rather than an abrupt transition and maturation of regenerative epithelium (from deeper glands as it reaches the luminal surface) are key in reaching a correct diagnosis.[46,47] However, in certain cases, it impossible to determine with certainty if the changes are nonneoplastic or dysplastic in nature, and a diagnosis of "indefinite for dysplasia" is appropriate. In this instance, clinical follow-up with repeated endoscopies and additional biopsies is the clinical norm.

A diagnosis of high-grade dysplasia is warranted when a lesion displays marked architectural disarray, such as glandular crowding and limited branching. Intraluminal necrotic debris is commonly present.[68] In addition, cytologic alterations are pronounced with cuboidal to low-columnar epithelial cells with a high nuclear-cytoplasmic (N/C) ratio rather than the columnar-shaped epithelium with lower N/C ratio commonly observed in low-grade dysplasia. Furthermore, high-grade dysplasia is characterized by usually round to oval, vesicular nuclei, with prominent nucleoli and loss of polarity (see **Fig. 1**B). Mitoses are also more common than in low-grade dysplasia and atypical mitoses figures may be detected.[46,47,67]

Natural History

A diagnosis of gastric dysplasia implies an increased risk of progression to gastric cancer. However, the risk is neither uniform nor certain. A large European study reported an annual incidence of gastric cancers within 5 years ranging from 0.6% to

6% after diagnoses of low-grade and high-grade dysplasia, respectively.[69] Modern publications show that high-grade dysplasia, for example, can rarely regress (6.25%).[70] Higher regression rates for high-grade dysplasia (57%) may be skewed by therapeutic intervention,[71] while most cases at least persist (25%–90%) or progress.[70,72]

Recent studies have confirmed the low risk of progression to cancer for patients with low-grade dysplasia (0%–17%) after at least 1 year of follow-up.[69,72] Notably, there is a substantial body of literature reporting that a fair number of cancer cases detected early after a diagnosis of gastric low-grade dysplasia made on endoscopic biopsy forceps may be related to inadequate sampling, particularly for larger lesions (>1 cm).[73,74] By the same token, a significant risk of malignant transformation is associated with high-grade dysplasia (10%–100%)[70,72] over an extended follow-up.[73 70] Similarly to the point made earlier, it is important to underscore that a high rate of progression observed in some studies with short follow-up (eg,<1 year) probably overestimates the risk due to undetected synchronous adenocarcinomas during the first endoscopy[72]

NONCONVENTIONAL GASTRIC DYSPLASIAS

Over the years, investigators have either refined or recognized uncommon dysplastic lesions, some presenting as flat lesions while others are characteristically polypoid. The cytomorphologic characteristics of these dysplastic lesions differ considerably from intestinal and foveolar dysplasias discussed earlier. Nevertheless, these unequivocal neoplastic lesions which present with variable risk of neoplastic progression deserve to be discussed.

Polypoid Nonconventional Gastric Dysplasias

Pyloric gland adenoma
Pyloric-type dysplasia almost exclusively presents as a polypoid lesion, and thus we will use the term PGAs going forward since it represents the term used in practice. Gastric PGAs make about 3% of gastric polypoid lesions when fundic gland polyps are excluded.[75]

Classically, most PGAs have been reported to develop in a background of autoimmune gastritis, mostly in older females and almost exclusively in the oxyntic mucosa.[75,76] Although still true, recent publications have noted the development of PGAs in the syndromic setting, including FAP, Lynch syndrome, and juvenile polyposis syndrome. These patients are also younger and equally distributed among males and females.[77,78]

PGAs are characteristically formed by packed tubules, although irregularly shaped cystically dilated glands can be seen (**Fig. 4**). Even less commonly broad villous projections can be detected. Irrespective of the low-power architecture, the glands are lined by a single layer of low-columnar to cuboidal cells with a distinctly pale eosinophilic cytoplasm with a ground glass quality as well as basally located round nuclei.[75,77] In contrast, high-grade lesions have the propensity of presenting varied cytoarchitectural anomalies. Commonly observed architectural alterations include back-to-back glands and cribriforming. Cytologic features of high-grade lesions include hyperchromasia, high N/C ratio, and loss of nuclear polarity, as well as enlarged nucleoli.

The immunophenotypic characteristics of PGA and most particularly MUC6 expression, a marker of pyloric gland differentiation, can be of importance in the differentiating PGA from polypoid foveolar dysplasia. However, the almost exclusive

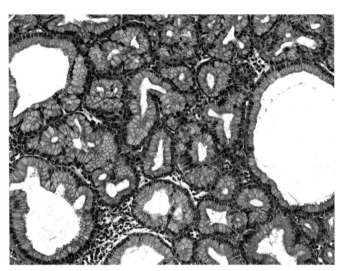

Fig. 4. Pyloric gland adenoma (low grade) with distinct clear ground glass eosinophilic cytoplasm and basal round nuclei.

expression of MUC6 has been reported in only about a quarter of the cases, while the others are decorated by mixed expression of MUC6 and MUC5, a marker of foveolar differentiation.[77]

A broader recognition of PGAs has also shed light on the prognosis of these lesions previously reported to have high malignant potential with high-grade dysplasia being present in 42% of cases[77] and a rate of association with adenocarcinoma ranging from 12% to 47%.[75,77,79,80] The risk of detecting high-grade dysplasia or adenocarcinoma is associated with large size, tubule-villous architecture, and a background of autoimmune gastritis.[77] In the background of Lynch syndrome, progression of PGA has been predominantly observed in males.[78]

Oxyntic gland adenoma

Neoplasm uniquely arising from the oxyntic mucosa and presenting with a multilineage phenotype with cells differentiating toward chief cells, parietal cells, and mucous neck cells. Tsukamoto and colleagues,[81] were the first to report on these unique gastric lesions.

It was recently recognized that these lesions present a diverse biological behavior ranging from benign (ie, OGA) to malignant (ie, gastric adenocarcinomas of the fundic gland type), and novel nomenclature has been proposed with the term oxyntic gland neoplasm encompassing the full histologic and biological characteristics of these neoplasms.[82–85]

OGAs are most frequently diagnosed in adult men (mean age 66 years and a male/female ratio of 2.2:1).[82] Most cases present in the upper third of the stomach and measure from 3 to 40 mm.

Cytologic heterogeneity is characteristic and the proportion of each cell subtype differs among cases. Some cases can show either a chief cell–predominant pattern or an admixture of chief and parietal cells, or they can show prominent mucous neck cells and even foveolar differentiation (**Fig. 5**).[82,85] In our experience, the chief cell–predominant pattern is the most common while the latter is rare. Cases with prominent mucous neck cells or foveolar differentiation are commonly associated with larger and

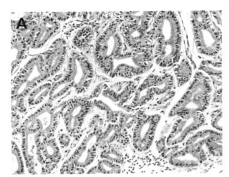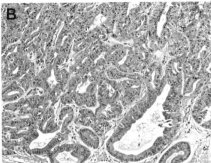

Fig. 5. Oxyntic gland adenoma (OGA). A illustrates a case of chief cell–predominant OGA, and **Fig. 5** B, an example of mixed **Fig.5** chief cell and parietal cells.

potentially more aggressive lesions.[85,86] Cytologic atypia is usually an inconspicuous feature of OGA with only mild-to-moderate nuclear enlargement and subtle nuclear irregularity. Architectural branching glands with pushing interface with surrounding mucosa and prolapse-type misplacement are characteristic of OGA. However, high-grade cytonuclear atypia, multilayering and nuclear stratification, and architectural complexity with cribriforming and glandular anastomosing can also be seen. Submucosal invasion with desmoplasia is limited to gastric adenocarcinomas of the fundic gland type.

Immunohistochemical evaluation can be helpful in underscoring the cellular heterogeneity. MUC6, a generic maker, highlights the entire lesion. More specifically, pepsinogen-I decorates the chief cells while parietal cells are highlighted by H+/K + -ATPase immunostaining.

Flat Nonconventional Gastric Dysplasias

Pit dysplasia

Atypical lesions limited to the basal aspects of the gastric mucosa and suspected to represent preneoplastic conditions have been reported. Pit dysplasia is a dysplastic lesion limited to the base of the pits.[87] Other terms have been used to report similar lesions such as **pit dysplasialike atypia**,[88] **intestinal metaplasia with basal gland atypia**,[89] and **immature proliferative lesions**.[90]

Pit dysplasia has been reported in 21% to 49% of patients who underwent gastric resection for adenocarcinoma but has been observed in only ~7% of gastric resections for nonneoplastic conditions.[87–89] On biopsy material, pit dysplasia has been detected in 2.8% of patients with chronic atrophic gastritis[89] and in 14% of those with intestinal metaplasia.[88] In 1 study, pit dysplasia was reported more commonly in association with incomplete metaplasia than in the background of complete intestinal metaplasia.[87] Data regarding the prevalence of pit dysplasia in the general population are lacking.

Morphologically, the anomalies observed in the basal parts of the gastric pits are similar to those present in traditional dysplasia but without surface involvement (**Fig. 6**). Architectural abnormalities, such as branching, crowding, budding, and irregularly shaped glands, can be seen. Stratification, an increased N/C ratio, hyperchromatic and enlarged nuclei, or nuclear clearing with prominent nucleoli are detected, as well as increased mitotic activity. Pit dysplasia can be classified as either low grade or high grade, depending on the severity of the morphologic anomalies.

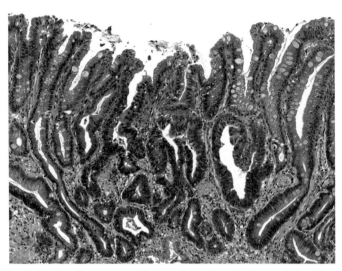

Fig. 6. Pit dysplasia with dysplastic epithelium limited to the base of the pits.

Metaplastic atypia, that is, the limited nuclear atypia uniquely detected in the proliferative zone of intestinal metaplasia represents the differential diagnosis of pit dysplasia, particularly of low-grade lesions.

In a retrospective study, it was shown that 38% of pit dysplasia persisted while 25% progressed to conventional low-grade dysplasia within a mean follow-up of 3.9 years.[88]

Tubule neck dysplasia

This exceedingly rare type of dysplasia is thought to be a unique precursor of diffuse-type gastric carcinoma and occurs more commonly in nonmetaplastic gastric epithelium.[91] Microscopically, it is characterized by the presence of atypical large cuboidal to polygonal clear cells confined to the basement membrane and occupying uniquely the neck region of gastric glands. Extension to deeper glands is less common while the mucosal surface is commonly spared. This unique dysplastic pattern has been defined on the basis of a large retrospective review of poorly cohesive adenocarcinomas. To date, no prospective evaluation of such lesion is available and management suggestions have not been established.[91,92]

MANAGEMENT OF DYSPLASIA

The therapeutic approach is dictated by the histologic grade and whether a lesion is endoscopically visible, that is, potentially amenable to endoscopic resection. To that end, high-definition endoscopy, narrow-band imaging, chromoendoscopy, and endoscopic ultrasound are crucial in evaluating the extent of dysplastic lesions. Complete excision is achievable in many cases by endoscopic mucosal resection or endoscopic submucosal dissection, obviating the need for surgical resection.[93]

In 2019, the British Society of Gastroenterology provided comprehensive therapeutic and surveillance recommendations after biopsy diagnoses of low-grade and high-grade dysplasia, based on an exhaustive review of the literature and very much in line with previously reported Japanese and European therapeutic guidelines (**Table 3**).[94–97]

Table 3
Molecular characteristics of dysplastic subtypes

Lesions	Major Molecular Alterations	Ref
Intestinal dysplasia	APC mutations (LGD and a subset of HGD), TP53 mutations (HGD)	Rokutan et al,[98] 2019; Lee et al,[99] 2002
Foveolar dysplasia	APC and KRAS mutations (sporadic and FAP-related), KLF4 (specific to raspberry-like)	Mishiro et al,[60] 2022; Naka et al,[62] 2023
Serrated dysplasia	KRAS mutations	Kwon et al,[57] 2013
Pyloric gland adenoma	GNAS, KRAS, APC mutations	Setia et al,[100] 2020; Matsubara et al,[101] 2013
Oxyntic gland adenoma	GNAS, KRAS mutations	Kushima et al,[102] 2013
Pit dysplasia	p53 overexpression	Shin et al,[87] 2011

Endoscopic Appearance	Histologic Diagnosis	Management	Surveillance
Invisible lesion	Low-grade dysplasia	Second enhanced endoscopy with biopsies to exclude a synchronous visible lesion	Every 3 y after 3 consecutive negative endoscopies Annual surveillance if persistent nonvisible low-grade dysplasia.
	High-grade dysplasia	Second enhanced endoscopy with biopsies to exclude a synchronous visible lesion	Biannual surveillance if persistent nonvisible high-grade dysplasia with careful follow-up.
Visible lesion	Low-grade dysplasia High-grade dysplasia	En bloc resection EMR: if ≤ 10 mm ESD: if >10 mm	Follow-up endoscopy at 6 mo after curative resection (ie, negative margins) followed by annual surveillance if negative.

Abbreviations: EMR, endoscopic mucosal resection; ESD, endoscopic submucosal dissection; HGD, high-grade dysplasia; LGD, low-grade dysplasia.

These guidelines relate essentially to conventional dysplastic lesions and do not address specifically the management for nonconventional dysplasias.

However, several investigators have underscored the biological behavior of some of these lesions and proposed some therapeutic approaches. A recent study by Baek and colleagues,[64] suggests a close surveillance after a diagnosis of foveolar dysplasia for which a biologically aggressive behavior is suspected but remains unproven. It has also been recommended that oxyntic gland neoplasms limited to the mucosa, that is, those likely to follow a benign course, be treated endoscopically based on the limited risk metastasis.[86] Alternatively, surgery is preferable to endoscopic resections for cases with atypical cytoarchitectural features and submucosal invasion which maintain a risk of lymphovascular invasion and subserosal intravenous spread.[85,86]

Finally, given the reportedly limited risk for local recurrence (<10% after endoscopic resection) and low-grade pyloric adenoma (<10% after endoscopic resection), watchful surveillance after complete excision has been suggested.[77] Alternatively, endoscopic resection appears advisable particularly for large or high-grade lesions, given a higher rate of recurrence.[77]

SUMMARY

The last few decades have been characterized by a better understanding of the risk of malignant transformation of dysplasia. Establishing accurately not only the diagnosis of gastric dysplasia but also its grade (as well as recently its subtype) is important to determine the risk of malignant transformation and the potential for synchronous and metachronous gastric cancer. Access to specialized endoscopic centers that offer high-quality endoscopic services is cardinal in the management of dysplastic gastric lesions before considering surgical options. Enhanced endoscopy in capable hands is important in considering the follow-up of invisible lesions. Alternatively, a large body of modern literature supports the role of endoscopic resection for visible low-grade and high-grade dysplasia.[94]

CLINICS CARE POINTS

- Diagnosis and grading of dysplasia are important indicators of the risk of malignant transformation and of synchronous and metachronous adenocarcinoma.
- Different subtypes of gastric dysplasia have varied risk of progression.
- High-quality endoscopic techniques are important when considering the follow-up of invisible lesions and endoscopic therapy for visible low-grade and high-grade dysplasia.

DISCLOSURE

The authors declare no conflicts of interest associated with this article.

REFERENCES

1. Riddell RH, Goldman H, Ransohoff DF, et al. Dysplasia in inflammatory bowel disease: standardized classification with provisional clinical applications. Hum Pathol 1983;14(11):931–68.
2. Ming SC, Bajtai A, Correa P, et al. Gastric dysplasia. Significance and pathologic criteria. Cancer 1984;54(9):1794–801.

3. Morson BC, Sobin LH, Grundmann E, et al. Precancerous conditions and epithelial dysplasia in the stomach. J Clin Pathol 1980;33(8):711–21.
4. Lauwers GY, Srivastava A. Gastric preneoplastic lesions and epithelial dysplasia. Gastroenterol Clin North Am 2007;36(4):813–29, vi.
5. Kushima RLG, Rugge M. Gastric dysplasia. WHO classification of tumours. digestive system tumours. Lyon (France): International Agency for Research on Cancer; 2019. p. 71–5.
6. Correa P. A human model of gastric carcinogenesis. Cancer Res 1988;48(13): 3554–60.
7. Kato M, Asaka M. Recent development of gastric cancer prevention. Jpn J Clin Oncol 2012;42(11):987–94.
8. Vieth M, Riddell RH, Montgomery EA. High-grade dysplasia versus carcinoma: east is east and west is west, but does it need to be that way? Am J Surg Pathol 2014;38(11):1453–6.
9. Lansdown M, Quirke P, Dixon MF, et al. High grade dysplasia of the gastric mucosa: a marker for gastric carcinoma. Gut 1990;31(9):977–83.
10. Di Gregorio C, Morandi P, Fante R, et al. Gastric dysplasia. a follow-up study. Am J Gastroenterol 1993;88(10):1714–9.
11. Rugge M, Farinati F, Di Mario F, et al. Gastric epithelial dysplasia: a prospective multicenter follow-up study from the Interdisciplinary group on gastric epithelial dysplasia. Hum Pathol 1991;22(10):1002–8.
12. You WC, Blot WJ, Li JY, et al. Precancerous gastric lesions in a population at high risk of stomach cancer. Cancer Res 1993;53(6):1317–21.
13. Zhang Y. Typing and grading of gastric dysplasia. In: Zhang Y, Kawai K, editors. Precancerous conditions and lesions of the stomach. Berlin: Springer-Verlag; 1993. p. 64–84.
14. Serck-Hanssen A. Precancerous lesions of the stomach. Scand J Gastroenterol Suppl 1979;54:104–5.
15. Farinati F, Rugge M, Di Mario F, et al. Early and advanced gastric cancer in the follow-up of moderate and severe gastric dysplasia patients. A prospective study. I.G.G.E.D.–Interdisciplinary Group on Gastric Epithelial Dysplasia. Endoscopy 1993;25(4):261–4.
16. Camilleri JP, Potet F, Amat C, et al. Gastric mucosal dysplasia: preliminary results of a prospective study of patients followed for periods of up to six years. In: Ming SC, editor. Precursors of gastric cancer. New York: Praeger; 1984. p. 83–92.
17. Bearzi I, Brancorsini D, Santinelli A, et al. Gastric dysplasia: a ten-year follow-up study. Pathol Res Pract 1994;190(1):61–8.
18. Dinis-Ribeiro M, Areia M, de Vries AC, et al. Management of precancerous conditions and lesions in the stomach (MAPS): guideline from the European Society of Gastrointestinal Endoscopy (ESGE), European Helicobacter Study Group (EHSG), European Society of Pathology (ESP), and the Sociedade Portuguesa de Endoscopia Digestiva (SPED). Endoscopy 2012;44(1):74–94.
19. Stockbrugger RW, Menon GG, Beilby JO, et al. Gastroscopic screening in 80 patients with pernicious anaemia. Gut 1983;24(12):1141–7.
20. Graem N, Fischer AB, Beck H. Dysplasia and carcinoma in the Billroth II resected stomach 27-35 years post-operatively. Acta Pathol Microbiol Immunol Scand [A] 1984;92(3):185–8.
21. Aste H, Sciallero S, Pugliese V, et al. The clinical significance of gastric epithelial dysplasia. Endoscopy 1986;18(5):174–6.

22. Ye W, Nyren O. Risk of cancers of the oesophagus and stomach by histology or subsite in patients hospitalised for pernicious anaemia. Gut 2003;52(7):938–41.
23. Song M, Camargo MC, Derkach A, et al. Associations between autoimmune conditions and gastric cancer risk among elderly adults in the United States. Am J Gastroenterol 2022;117(3):486–90.
24. Song M, Latorre G, Ivanovic-Zuvic D, et al. Autoimmune diseases and gastric cancer risk: a systematic review and meta-analysis. Cancer Res Treat 2019; 51(3):841–50.
25. Arnason T, Liang WY, Alfaro E, et al. Morphology and natural history of familial adenomatous polyposis-associated dysplastic fundic gland polyps. Histopathology 2014;65(3):353–62.
26. Stolte M, Vieth M, Ebert MP. High-grade dysplasia in sporadic fundic gland polyps: clinically relevant or not? Eur J Gastroenterol Hepatol 2003;15(11): 1153–6.
27. Bianchi LK, Burke CA, Bennett AE, et al. Fundic gland polyp dysplasia is common in familial adenomatous polyposis. Clin Gastroenterol Hepatol 2008;6(2): 180–5.
28. Garrean S, Hering J, Saied A, et al. Gastric adenocarcinoma arising from fundic gland polyps in a patient with familial adenomatous polyposis syndrome. Am Surg 2008;74(1):79–83.
29. Watanabe H, Enjoji M, Yao T, et al. Gastric lesions in familial adenomatosis coli: their incidence and histologic analysis. Hum Pathol 1978;9(3):269–83.
30. Bulow S, Lauritsen KB, Johansen A, et al. Gastroduodenal polyps in familial polyposis coli. Dis Colon Rectum 1985;28(2):90–3.
31. Burt RW, Berenson MM, Lee RG, et al. Upper gastrointestinal polyps in Gardner's syndrome. Gastroenterology 1984;86(2):295–301.
32. Shemesh E, Bat L. A prospective evaluation of the upper gastrointestinal tract and periampullary region in patients with Gardner syndrome. Am J Gastroenterol 1985;80(11):825–7.
33. Sarre RG, Frost AG, Jagelman DG, et al. Gastric and duodenal polyps in familial adenomatous polyposis: a prospective study of the nature and prevalence of upper gastrointestinal polyps. Gut 1987;28(3):306–14.
34. Domizio P, Talbot IC, Spigelman AD, et al. Upper gastrointestinal pathology in familial adenomatous polyposis: results from a prospective study of 102 patients. J Clin Pathol 1990;43(9):738–43.
35. Goedde TA, Rodriguez-Bigas MA, Herrera L, et al. Gastroduodenal polyps in familial adenomatous polyposis. Surg Oncol 1992;1(5):357–61.
36. Sawada T, Muto T. Familial adenomatous polyposis: should patients undergo surveillance of the upper gastrointestinal tract? Endoscopy 1995;27(1):6–11.
37. Bertoni G, Sassatelli R, Nigrisoli E, et al. Dysplastic changes in gastric fundic gland polyps of patients with familial adenomatous polyposis. Ital J Gastroenterol Hepatol 1999;31(3):192–7.
38. Iida M, Yao T, Itoh H, et al. Natural history of gastric adenomas in patients with familial adenomatosis coli/Gardner's syndrome. Cancer 1988;61(3):605–11.
39. Utsunomiya J, Maki T, Iwama T, et al. Gastric lesion of familial polyposis coli. Cancer 1974;34(3):745–54.
40. Spigelman AD, Williams CB, Talbot IC, et al. Upper gastrointestinal cancer in patients with familial adenomatous polyposis. Lancet 1989;2(8666):783–5.
41. Shimamoto Y, Ishiguro S, Takeuchi Y, et al. Gastric neoplasms in patients with familial adenomatous polyposis: endoscopic and clinicopathologic features. Gastrointest Endosc 2021;94(6):1030–1042 e1032.

42. Worthley DL, Phillips KD, Wayte N, et al. Gastric adenocarcinoma and proximal polyposis of the stomach (GAPPS): a new autosomal dominant syndrome. Gut 2012;61(5):774–9.
43. Shaib YH, Rugge M, Graham DY, et al. Management of gastric polyps: an endoscopy-based approach. Clin Gastroenterol Hepatol 2013;11(11):1374–84.
44. Alfaro EE, Lauwers GY. Early gastric neoplasia: diagnosis and implications. Adv Anat Pathol 2011;18(4):268–80.
45. Ma C, Giardiello FM, Montgomery EA. Upper tract juvenile polyps in juvenile polyposis patients: dysplasia and malignancy are associated with foveolar, intestinal, and pyloric differentiation. Am J Surg Pathol 2014;38(12):1618–26.
46. Lauwers GY, Riddell RH. Gastric epithelial dysplasia. Gut 1999;45(5):784–90.
47. Goldstein NS, Lewin KJ. Gastric epithelial dysplasia and adenoma: historical review and histological criteria for grading. Hum Pathol 1997;28(2):127–33.
48. Jeon SW. Endoscopic management of gastric dysplasia: cutting edge technology needs a new paradigm. World J Gastrointest Endosc 2010;2(9):301–4.
49. Ahn SY, Jang SI, Lee DW, et al. Gastric endoscopic submucosal dissection is safe for day patients. Clinical Endoscopy 2014;47(6):538–43.
50. Kang DH, Choi CW, Kim HW, et al. Predictors of upstage diagnosis after endoscopic resection of gastric low-grade dysplasia. Surg Endosc 2017;32(6):2732–8.
51. Oberhuber G, Stolte M. Gastric polyps: an update of their pathology and biological significance. Virchows Arch: An International Journal of Pathology 2000;437(6):581–90.
52. Jass JR. A classification of gastric dysplasia. Histopathology 1983;7(2):181–93.
53. Morson BC, Jass JR, Sobin LH. Precancerous lesions of the gastrointestinal tract: a histological classification. London: Bailliere Tindall; 1985.
54. Murayama H, Kikuchi M, Enjoji M, et al. Changes in gastric mucosa that antedate gastric carcinoma. Cancer 1990;66(9):2017–26.
55. Wu TT, Kornacki S, Rashid A, et al. Dysplasia and dysregulation of proliferation in foveolar and surface epithelia of fundic gland polyps from patients with familial adenomatous polyposis. Am J Surg Pathol 1998;22(3):293–8.
56. Rubio CA. Serrated neoplasia of the stomach: a new entity. J Clin Pathol 2001;54(11):849–53.
57. Kwon MJ, Min BH, Lee SM, et al. Serrated adenoma of the stomach: a clinicopathologic, immunohistochemical, and molecular study of nine cases. Histol Histopathol 2013;28(4):453–62.
58. Rubio CA. Traditional serrated adenomas of the upper digestive tract. J Clin Pathol 2016;69(1):1–5.
59. Shibagaki K, Mishiro T, Fukuyama C, et al. Sporadic foveolar-type gastric adenoma with a raspberry-like appearance in Helicobacter pylori-naive patients. Virchows Arch 2021;479(4):687–95.
60. Mishiro T, Shibagaki K, Fukuyama C, et al. KLF4 mutation shapes pathologic characteristics of foveolar-type gastric adenoma in helicobacter pylori-naive patients. Am J Pathol 2022;192(9):1250–8.
61. Naka T, Hashimoto T, Yoshida T, et al. A1322C mutation is a consistent and specific genetic feature of raspberry-like foveolar-type adenoma of the stomach. Am J Surg Pathol 2023;47(4):521–3.
62. Naka T, Hashimoto T, Cho H, et al. Sporadic and familial adenomatous polyposis-associated foveolar-type adenoma of the stomach. Am J Surg Pathol 2023;47(1):91–101.

63. Park DY, Srivastava A, Kim GH, et al. Adenomatous and foveolar gastric dysplasia: distinct patterns of mucin expression and background intestinal metaplasia. Am J Surg Pathol 2008;32(4):524–33.

64. Baek DH, Kim GH, Park DY, et al. Gastric epithelial dysplasia: characteristics and long-term follow-up results after endoscopic resection according to morphological categorization. BMC Gastroenterol 2015;15:17.

65. Serra S, Ali R, Bateman AC, et al. Gastric foveolar dysplasia: a survey of reporting habits and diagnostic criteria. Pathology 2017;49(4):391–6.

66. Misdraji J, Lauwers GY. Gastric epithelial dysplasia. Semin Diagn Pathol 2002; 19(1):20–30.

67. Rugge M, Correa P, Dixon MF, et al. Gastric dysplasia: the Padova international classification. Am J Surg Pathol 2000;24(2):167–76.

68. Watanabe Y, Shimizu M, Itoh T, et al. Intraglandular necrotic debris in gastric biopsy and surgical specimens. Ann Diagn Pathol 2001;5(3):141–7.

69. de Vries AC, van Grieken NC, Looman CW, et al. Gastric cancer risk in patients with premalignant gastric lesions: a nationwide cohort study in the Netherlands. Gastroenterology 2008;134(4):945–52.

70. Rugge M, Cassaro M, Di Mario F, et al. The long term outcome of gastric non-invasive neoplasia. Gut 2003;52(8):1111–6.

71. Kokkola A, Haapiainen R, Laxen F, et al. Risk of gastric carcinoma in patients with mucosal dysplasia associated with atrophic gastritis: a follow up study. J Clin Pathol 1996;49(12):979–84.

72. Yamada H, Ikegami M, Shimoda T, et al. Long-term follow-up study of gastric adenoma/dysplasia. Endoscopy 2004;36(5):390–6.

73. Choi CW, Kim HW, Shin DH, et al. The risk factors for discrepancy after endoscopic submucosal dissection of gastric category 3 lesion (low grade dysplasia). Dig Dis Sci 2014;59(2):421–7.

74. Lim H, Jung HY, Park YS, et al. Discrepancy between endoscopic forceps biopsy and endoscopic resection in gastric epithelial neoplasia. Surg Endosc 2014;28(4):1256–62.

75. Vieth M, Kushima R, Borchard F, et al. Pyloric gland adenoma: a clinicopathological analysis of 90 cases. Virchows Arch 2003;442(4):317–21.

76. Vieth M, Montgomery EA. Some observations on pyloric gland adenoma: an uncommon and long ignored entity. J Clin Pathol 2014;67(10):883–90.

77. Choi WT, Brown I, Ushiku T, et al. Gastric pyloric gland adenoma: a multicentre clinicopathological study of 67 cases. Histopathology 2018;72(6):1007–14.

78. Lee SE, Kang SY, Cho J, et al. Pyloric gland adenoma in Lynch syndrome. Am J Surg Pathol 2014;38(6):784–92.

79. Chen ZM, Scudiere JR, Abraham SC, et al. Pyloric gland adenoma: an entity distinct from gastric foveolar type adenoma. Am J Surg Pathol 2009;33(2): 186–93.

80. Vieth M, Kushima R, Mukaisho K, et al. Immunohistochemical analysis of pyloric gland adenomas using a series of Mucin 2, Mucin 5AC, Mucin 6, CD10, Ki67 and p53. Virchows Arch 2010;457(5):529–36.

81. Tsukamoto T, Yokoi T, Maruta S, et al. Gastric adenocarcinoma with chief cell differentiation. Pathol Int 2007;57(8):517–22.

82. Benedict MA, Lauwers GY, Jain D. Gastric adenocarcinoma of the fundic gland type: update and literature review. Am J Clin Pathol 2018;149(6):461–73.

83. Singhi AD, Lazenby AJ, Montgomery EA. Gastric adenocarcinoma with chief cell differentiation: a proposal for reclassification as oxyntic gland polyp/adenoma. Am J Surg Pathol 2012;36(7):1030–5.

84. Ueyama H, Yao T, Nakashima Y, et al. Gastric adenocarcinoma of fundic gland type (chief cell predominant type): proposal for a new entity of gastric adenocarcinoma. Am J Surg Pathol 2010;34(5):609–19.

85. Ushiku T, Kunita A, Kuroda R, et al. Oxyntic gland neoplasm of the stomach: expanding the spectrum and proposal of terminology. Mod Pathol 2020;33(2): 206–16.

86. Ueyama H, Yao T, Akazawa Y, et al. Gastric epithelial neoplasm of fundic-gland mucosa lineage: proposal for a new classification in association with gastric adenocarcinoma of fundic-gland type. J Gastroenterol 2021;56(9):814–28.

87. Shin N, Jo HJ, Kim WK, et al. Gastric pit dysplasia in adjacent gastric mucosa in 414 gastric cancers: prevalence and characteristics. Am J Surg Pathol 2011; 35(7):1021–9.

88. Agoston AT, Odze RD. Evidence that gastric pit dysplasia-like atypia is a neoplastic precursor lesion. Hum Pathol 2014;45(3):446–55.

89. Li Y, Chang X, Zhou W, et al. Gastric intestinal metaplasia with basal gland atypia: a morphological and biologic evaluation in a large Chinese cohort. Hum Pathol 2013;44(4):578–90.

90. Tava F, Luinetti O, Ghigna MR, et al. Type or extension of intestinal metaplasia and immature/atypical "indefinite-for-dysplasia" lesions as predictors of gastric neoplasia. Hum Pathol 2006;37(11):1489–97.

91. Ghandur-Mnaymneh L, Paz J, Roldan E, et al. Dysplasia of nonmetaplastic gastric mucosa. A proposal for its classification and its possible relationship to diffuse-type gastric carcinoma. Am J Surg Pathol 1988;12(2):96–114.

92. Grundmann E. Histologic types and possible initial stages in early gastric carcinoma. Beitr Pathol 1975;154(3):256–80.

93. Nakajima T. Gastric cancer treatment guidelines in Japan. Gastric Cancer 2002; 5(1):1–5.

94. Banks M, Graham D, Jansen M, et al. British society of gastroenterology guidelines on the diagnosis and management of patients at risk of gastric adenocarcinoma. Gut 2019;68(9):1545–75.

95. Japanese Gastric Cancer A. Japanese gastric cancer treatment guidelines 2010 (ver. 3). Gastric Cancer 2011;14(2):113–23.

96. Japanese Gastric Cancer A. Japanese gastric cancer treatment guidelines 2014 (ver. 4). Gastric Cancer 2017;20(1):1–19.

97. Pimentel-Nunes P, Dinis-Ribeiro M, Ponchon T, et al. Endoscopic submucosal dissection: European Society of Gastrointestinal Endoscopy (ESGE) Guideline. Endoscopy 2015;47(9):829–54.

98. Rokutan H, Abe H, Nakamura H, et al. Initial and crucial genetic events in intestinal-type gastric intramucosal neoplasia. J Pathol 2019;247(4):494–504.

99. Lee JH, Abraham SC, Kim HS, et al. Inverse relationship between APC gene mutation in gastric adenomas and development of adenocarcinoma. Am J Pathol 2002;161(2):611–8.

100. Setia N, Wanjari P, Yassan L, et al. Next-generation sequencing identifies 2 genomically distinct groups among pyloric gland adenomas. Hum Pathol 2020;97: 103–11.

101. Matsubara A, Sekine S, Kushima R, et al. Frequent GNAS and KRAS mutations in pyloric gland adenoma of the stomach and duodenum. J Pathol 2013;229(4): 579–87.

102. Kushima R, Sekine S, Matsubara A, et al. Gastric adenocarcinoma of the fundic gland type shares common genetic and phenotypic features with pyloric gland adenoma. Pathol Int 2013;63(6):318–25.

Early Cancerous Lesions of the Pancreas and Ampulla
Current Concepts and Challenges

Olca Basturk, MD[a], N. Volkan Adsay, MD[b],*

KEYWORDS

- Pancreas • Ampulla • PanIN • IPMN • ITPN • IOPN • MCN • IAPN

KEY POINTS

- Mass-forming preinvasive neoplasms (tumoral intraepithelial neoplasms) of pancreatobiliary tract (ie, intraductal neoplasms) represent adenoma-carcinoma sequence and comprise several entities including the intraductal papillary mucinous neoplasms (gastric, intestinal, and pancreatobiliary), intraductal oncocytic papillary neoplasm, intraductal tubulopapillary neoplasm, and those associated with ovarian-type stroma (mucinous cystic neoplasm), each with distinct clinicopathologic and molecular characteristics and cancer progression rates.

- Intra-ampullary papillary tubular neoplasms are distinct from the ampullary-duodenal surface adenomas. Instead, they are similar to pancreatic intraductal neoplasms, representing tumoral intraepithelial neoplasms, often with mixed cell lineages. They are proving to have high rate of invasive carcinoma that render them less amenable for ampullectomy.

- Both the conventional incidental/microscopic forms of dysplasia (<0.5 cm) as well as the mass-forming examples (intraductal or intra-ampullary neoplasms, typically > 1 cm) are now graded as low versus high grade, the latter encompassing the "in-situ"/"intramucosal" adenocarcinoma type lesions, which has very high association with (or progression into) invasive carcinoma.

- Invasive carcinoma types other than ordinary pancreatobiliary such as colloid (which has much better prognosis) as well as undifferentiated carcinoma with or without osteoclast like giant cells or poorly differentiated neuroendocrine carcinomas tend to occur more frequently in association with tumoral intraepithelial neoplasms. Therefore, the evaluation of invasive carcinomas in these neoplasms requires more nuanced documentation and classification.

[a] Department of Pathology and Laboratory Medicine, Memorial Sloan Kettering Cancer Center, 1275 York Avenue, New York, NY 10065, USA; [b] Department of Pathology, Koc University School of Medicine, Davutpaşa Cd. No:4, Zeytinburnu, Istanbul 34010, Turkey
* Corresponding author. Koç Üniversitesi Hastanesi, Davutpaşa Cd. No:4, Zeytinburnu, İstanbul 34010, Türkiye.
E-mail address: vadsay@kuh.ku.edu.tr

Gastroenterol Clin N Am 53 (2024) 57–84
https://doi.org/10.1016/j.gtc.2023.11.004
0889-8553/24/© 2023 Elsevier Inc. All rights reserved.

gastro.theclinics.com

PANCREAS

In the pancreas, preinvasive malignant neoplasia is currently viewed in two distinct categories.[1–4] One is the microscopic incidental forms of dysplasia (ie, intraepithelial neoplasia) termed pancreatic intraepithelial neoplasia (PanIN). The other is the mass-forming preinvasive neoplasia (ie, tumoral intraepithelial neoplasms, "adenoma-carcinoma sequence"), which by definition form clinically (radiologically) and grossly detectable lesions. The differential characteristics of this dichotomy are discussed in detail in the following section.

Pancreatic Intraepithelial Neoplasia

Definition

The spectrum included in the PanIN[5] category ranges from those that used to be called mucinous metaplasia (or mucinous hypertrophy), to all the way to those designated in situ carcinoma. Based on the degree of microscopic cytoarchitectural atypia, PanIN used to be graded using a three-tiered scale as PanIN1A, 1B, 2, and 3, but they are now graded as low-grade or high-grade PanIN (aka, carcinoma in situ [CIS]). Processes that used to be called mucinous metaplasia, which are essentially indistinguishable from normal gastric, ampullary or endocervical epithelium were included in this spectrum of "dysplasia" (intraepithelial neoplasia) in the pancreatic ducts because they are foreign to this area and can show mutations associated with neoplastic transformation such as clonality or KRAS mutations. As such they are believed to serve as the launching pad (previously called "1A") from which the true neoplastic transformation develops. Prior PanIN 1b and PanIN2 categories are also now regarded as "low-grade." These low-grade lesions are very common in general population and thus mostly believed to be clinically inconsequential aspect of the spectrum. In the other end of the spectrum is the full-blown carcinomatous transformation within the native duct epithelium, which can be indistinguishable from invasive carcinoma cells, in particular, from the intraductal spread from true invasive carcinomas ("colonization/cancerization"). This intraepithelial carcinomatous transformation is now classified as "high-grade" (designated "carcinoma in-situ" in some regions), which is the clinically significant aspect of the spectrum.[2]

Clinical features

More than 50% of older adults have foci of low-grade PanIN in their pancreas.[6] In contrast, high-grade PanIN is exceedingly uncommon to encounter in the absence of pancreatic invasive ductal adenocarcinoma (PDAC).[2,7,8]

Given their microscopic nature, PanIN lesions, when in isolation, are not symptomatic and typically cannot be detected on imaging studies. Thus, they virtually only come to clinical/diagnostic attention in pancreata resected for other lesions.

PanIN, similar to PDAC, has been found to be associated with advanced age, diabetes mellitus, and obesity.[5] Familial predisposition to PDAC is also a significant risk factor.[9]

Pathologic features

PanIN lesions are in general not visible on macroscopic examination. However, occasionally, in close inspection of resected pancreata, a focus of upstream atrophy pointing to a PanIN focus obstructing the region may be seen. Microscopically, low-grade PanIN are characterized by relatively bland mucinous columnar cells with either flat or papillary architecture. As mentioned previously, in the lowest end of the spectrum, the cells are indistinguishable from normal gastric or ampullary mucosa but are present in the pancreatic ducts where they do not belong. High-grade PanIN reveals all the attributes of cancerous transformation including significant cytoarchitectural atypia, increased mitotic figures, and even necrosis.

Special studies and molecular features
The immunohistochemical labeling pattern of PanIN parallels that of PDAC. Also, true to their nature as "mucinous" transformation, most express mucin-related glycoproteins/oncoproteins that are expressed in the upper GI tract including MUC1, MUC4, MUC5AC, and MUC6. They are, however, typically negative for MUC2, the intestinal mucin.[1] Not surprisingly, increasing Ki-67 labeling indices has been shown with increasing grades of "dysplasia" in PanINs[10]; however, it should be kept in mind that proliferation also increases, and in fact, often to a higher degree in foci of injury and regeneration.

Most of the molecular abnormalities identified PDACs have also been detected in PanIN, particularly in high-grade lesions. Some molecular changes occur early in the sequence (*KRAS* mutations), some in the middle stages (*CDKN2A* loss), and others only in the late stage (*DPC4* and *TP53* mutations).[11–13]

Differential diagnosis
PanIN should be distinguished from intraductal papillary mucinous neoplasms (IPMNs, see discussion on IPMNs section). As discussed previously, this is mostly definitional, with PanINs representing incidental/microscopic dysplasia, and the term IPMN preserved for those that form clinically detectable masses. However, at their earlier stages, there are naturally overlaps. Although most PanINs are smaller than IPMNs and involve ducts that usually measure less than 0.5 cm in diameter, distinction of these two types of intraductal neoplasms may be impossible in some cases as there are overlaps, especially at earlier stages of IPMNs. Furthermore, both PanIN and IPMN may be present within the same pancreas.[3,4,14,15] Of note, the overlap applies to the gastric- and pancreatobiliary-type IPMNs. Intestinal-type (MUC2/CDX2+) and oncocytic (MUC6+) dysplastic changes are not a feature of PanIN, and typically represent underrepresented (not properly sampled) tumoral intraepithelial neoplasm.

Biologic behavior and treatment
Low-grade PanINs are very common in general population and thus be clinically insignificant, with a very low risk for progression to carcinoma. In contrast, true foci of high-grade PanIN with the degree of atypia that is qualified as "carcinoma in-situ" is extremely uncommon to catch in the absence of invasive carcinoma. This highlights two important issues: (1) it is extremely difficult to distinguish high-grade PanIN from the cancerization/colonization phenomenon (ie, invasive cancer retrogradely invading into the duct epithelium). In other words, one cannot be sure whether one is studying true preinvasive cancer or invasive cancer. (2) Once the intraepithelial neoplastic cells become carcinomatous, they rapidly acquire invasive characteristics. This also goes along with the recent views challenging the concept of "pancreas cancer" remaining dormant for several years before it advances, something that had been advocated in some earlier studies.[16] Regardless, it is very clear that if high-grade PanIN (previous PanIN-3; CIS) is identified in pancreas resections that pancreas should be regarded highly suspicious for the presence of invasive adenocarcinoma, if not in that region, then somewhere else in the gland. In other words, for all practical purposes, high-grade PanIN should be regarded a surrogate marker for PDAC in the pancreas (**Table 1**).[17]

TUMORAL INTRAEPITHELIAL NEOPLASMS

There is a whole spectrum of preinvasive (premalignant) intraepithelial/intramucosal neoplasia that forms clinically (radiologically) detectable masses.[3,18] In essence, these represent adenoma-carcinoma sequence. It is believed that whatever leads these cells to keep growing within the epithelium and form masses before they become

Table 1 Pancreatic intraepithelial neoplasia	
Clinical features	• Asymptomatic and cannot be detected on imaging studies
Histopathologic features	• *Low grade:* Relatively bland mucinous columnar cells with either flat or papillary architecture; nuclear stratification and mild nuclear atypia can be seen • *High grade:* Significant loss of polarity, tufting of cells into the lumen, marked nuclear irregularity, frequent mitotic figures, and sometimes necrosis
IHC features	• Most expresses MUC1, MUC4, MUC5AC, and MUC6 • MUC2 is negative • Ki-67 labeling indices parallel to grades of dysplasia
Molecular features	• Most of the molecular abnormalities seen in PDACs have also been detected in PanIN • Some molecular changes (*KRAS* mutations) occur early, some (*CDKN2A* loss) in the middle, and others (*DPC4* and *TP53* mutations) in the late stages
Natural history	• *Low grade:* Very common in general population and clinically insignificant • *High grade:* Highly suspicious for the presence of PDAC, if not in that region, then somewhere else in the gland

Abbreviations: IHC, immunohistochemistry

invasive cancers confer a different biology to these tumors than the PanIN discussed above. The same concept has been well studied in the urothelium and biliary tract.[19-28] The entities that belong to this category are characterized by intraductal and cystic neoplasia that often have mucinous characteristics that overlap with PanIN. The tumors discussed under this heading are those in the "intraductal neoplasia" category: IPMNs, intraductal oncocytic papillary neoplasm (IOPN), and intraductal tubulo-papillary neoplasm (ITPN). Conceptually, mucinous cystic neoplasms (MCNs), which are associated with ovarian-type stroma, also belong to this group, but it is regarded as "de-novo" neoplasms without overt communication with the ductal system. The individual characteristics of these tumor types are discussed in detail as follows.

Intraductal Papillary Mucinous Neoplasms

Clinical features

IPMNs are now regarded as one of the most common neoplasms, not only in the pancreas but also in general. This is because a significant proportion of abdominal radiologic tests reveal incidental cysts in the pancreas, especially in the elderly population, which are qualified as IPMNs. IPMNs are defined as radiographically and macroscopically visible tumors characterized by an intraductal proliferation of mucin-producing cells, usually with a papillary architecture.[18,29-32]

Smaller IPMNs are asymptomatic and are often detected incidentally during abdominal imaging performed for other reasons. Larger and more papillary examples that manifest clinically are typically seen in the seventh to eighth decades. IPMNs occur more commonly (80%) in the pancreatic head.[33] Some IPMNs primarily involve the major pancreatic ducts (main-duct-type). However, others are limited to the secondary ducts (branch-duct-type). Preoperative separation of IPMNs into main duct and branch-duct types is important. Because the main duct type has a greater risk of having high-grade dysplasia or invasive carcinoma. In contrast, branch-duct IPMNs may not require surgical resection if they are small (<3 cm) and lack worrisome features such as mural nodules and growth during follow-up.[33-36] Cystic dilation of the ducts that form cyst-by-cyst appearance on imaging and, if present, mucin extrusion through the ampulla of Vater during endoscopy are diagnostic features.

Pathologic features

IPMNs may be localized, multicentric or, rarely, the entire ductal system may be involved. The extent of ductal dilation and the amount of gross papilla formation vary from case to case and even within an individual case (**Fig. 1**).[33] Moreover, high-grade dysplasia and invasive carcinoma may be focal, so it is vital to thorough sampling of the specimen to search for carcinoma is extremely important.[37]

Microscopically, mucinous cells with various degrees of atypia line the cystically dilated ducts. Three different papillary patterns have been described.[1,18,38,39] Considering that most incidentalomas prove to be gastric-type IPMNs, this is by far the most common in real life. Unfortunately, although the rate of invasion is rare, when they become invasive, the invasion is of the tubular type. In contrast, a significant proportion of the main duct-type IPMNs are of the intestinal type, also a substantial number of intestinal-type IPMNs have invasion, and thus, they are overrepresented in the resection cohorts (approximately, 35% of resected cases, **Fig. 2**), whereas the gastric type is about 50% (**Fig. 3**). The third subtype of IPMN, the pancreatobiliary type (15%, **Fig. 4**) is more difficult to define and it is believed to be a subset of transformed gastric-type IPMN.[18,33,40] It should be noted here that this classification pertains to the papillary proliferative components of IPMNs because gastric-type epithelium (also called "null" phenotype) is commonly encountered both in the background of intestinal- and pancreatobiliary-type IPMNs as well as any other pancreas with injury.

Like PanIN, the dysplasia in IPMNs is now graded as low or high grade. The prior low- and intermediate-grade dysplasia categories are regarded as low-grade dysplasia.[2] Grading is based on the most severely dysplastic region, emphasizing the need for extensive, if not complete, histologic sampling for accurate diagnosis.[3]

Invasive carcinoma is currently seen in about a third of resected cases in most institutions; however, this figure is bound to change with the changing criteria of resection as well as the quality of the detection methods. Invasion may be focal or multifocal or it may represent much of the tumor. There are two very distinct types of invasive cancer that develop from IPMNs.[41–43] More common is the tubular type, which is often indistinguishable from ordinary PDAC, although some has unusual characteristics.

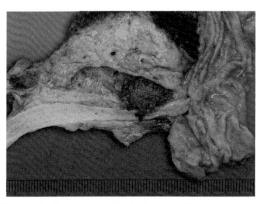

Fig. 1. Example of a main-duct-type intraductal papillary mucinous neoplasm (IPMN) involving the main pancreatic duct with friable papillary projections. Note that the duct is significantly dilated.

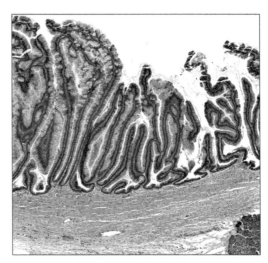

Fig. 2. Intestinal-type intraductal papillary mucinous neoplasm. Overall appearance is similar to that of colonic villous adenomas. The papillae are lined by pseudo-stratified columnar cells with cigar-shaped nuclei.

Tubular-type invasion may arise in association with any of the papilla types. The second type of invasion is colloid type, also called muconodular because it is characterized by gelatinous tumors composed of abundant mucin pools within which the carcinoma cells are suspended.[44] Colloid-type invasive carcinoma has been found to be incomparably more benevolent than PDAC, and this has been attributed to coupling of two factors observed at the histopathologic level.[1,44–46] The cells of colloid carcinoma have an inverse polarity in which they secrete their products to the stroma, and the mucin deposited, which is intestinal/goblet-type mucin with inhibitory properties, in turn serves as a containing factor. Colloid-type invasion invariably arises from intestinal-type IPMN.[33,44,45,47]

Special studies and molecular features
Immunohistochemically, IPMNs express keratins.[31,48] Most IPMNs also express mCEA, CA19 to 9, and MUC5AC.[48,49] Expression of MUC1 and MUC6 is more common in pancreatobiliary type. In contrast, expression of MUC2 and CDX2 is virtually

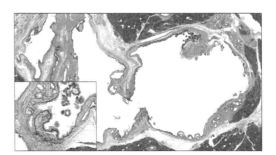

Fig. 3. Gastric-type intraductal papillary mucinous neoplasm. The cysts are lined by simple epithelium, composed of columnar cells with abundant mucin, resembling gastric foveolar epithelium (inset).

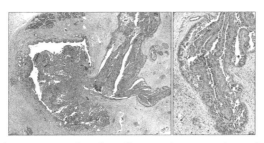

Fig. 4. Pancreatobiliary-type intraductal papillary mucinous neoplasm of with tall, thin complex papillae (left) lined by cuboidal cells that have little cytoplasmic mucin and severe cytologic atypia (right).

exclusive to the intestinal type and its invasive product, colloid carcinoma[50] rendering this group a distinct pathway of carcinogenesis in the pancreas.[1]

Many of the molecular alterations in IPMNs are similar to those of PDAC. However, mutations in *KRAS* and *TP53* are less frequent.[51] Also, no *DPC4* mutation is seen in IPMNs.[52] The Peutz–Jeghers gene (*STK11/LKB1*) inactivation as well as *APC* mutations are found in about 25% of IPMNs,[53] but not in PDACs. Two novel gene alterations have been described in IPMNs. *RNF43* is mutated in 75% of IPMNs, and *GNAS* is mutated in 60%.[54,55] The frequency of mutations varies according to the papilla type, with GNAS mutations being more frequent in IPMNs with intestinal-type papillae.[56] The detection of mutations in IPMNs can be used for preoperative diagnosis to help distinguish these neoplasms from other cystic lesions of the pancreas.[13,57]

Differential diagnosis

IPMNs should be distinguished from PanIN. As mentioned in the PanIN section, PanINs are by definition incidental, microscopic (not radiographically detectable) lesions that measure less than 0.5 cm in maximal diameter, whereas IPMNs are defined by radiographically or macroscopically detectable masses or cysts and are larger, typically more than 1.0 cm.[33] PanINs do not reveal intestinal-type lining. However, there are overlaps between small gastric-type IPMNs and larger PanINs.

Biologic behavior and treatment

IPMNs are very common "incidentalomas" and it is difficult to determine their relative risk for cancer formation. Therefore, their management is a nightmare. It is clear that the vast majority of these small cysts would remain clinically silent. However, the small percentage that advances to invasive carcinoma becomes detrimental because the carcinoma is practically a PDAC and mortal.[42] Although previous studies[58–60] states that 30% to 50% of resected IPMNs harbor invasive carcinoma, current series[61] report invasion in around 20% of resected IPMNs. From the PDAC perspective, an estimated 5% to 10% of PDACs arise from IPMNs.[62] This figure may be higher considering that once it forms, PDAC can destroy the IPMN rendering it unrecognizable at the time of diagnosis.

Various guidelines have been developed to determine which IPMN requires resection.[58,63–65] Some guidelines seem to be less applicable in capturing the true nature of these tumors.[66] In general, main duct-type IPMNs have a high risk and it is believed that they all warrant resection. For the more limited branch duct-type IPMNs, those with "worrisome features," such as large cyst size, presence of mural nodule(s), dilated main duct, and high CA-19 to 9 levels are also viewed as candidates for surgery.[65] Many patients managed by conservative resection of the highest risk areas and do not experience progression. However, for IPMNs that are main-duct type involving multiple segments of the organ or overtly multicentric at presentation, total pancreatectomy seems to be the best treatment.[67] Naturally, these all need to be evaluated in context.

Considering small incidentaloma-type IPMNs are common in general population, the overall prognosis of IPMNs is very good.[36,47,68] Resected noninvasive IPMNs have an almost excellent prognosis provided that invasion has been ruled out definitively both at the clinical and histopathologic levels. Few cases with progression are attributed to missed invasive cancers. At the same time, IPMNs are notorious for being multifocal, and some has been shown to "recur" (develop new tumors) in the remaining pancreas.[69–71] Accordingly, follow-up of the remaining pancreas is crucial. Pathologic factors that have been shown to be associated with higher rate of recurrence include multifocality and presence of margin positivity as well as high-grade dysplasia or invasive adenocarcinoma at the resection.[61] If there is invasion, the presence of poor differentiation, lymphovascular invasion, perineural invasion, and lymph node metastasis are also risk factors. The presence of poor differentiation has been reported to be associated with early recurrence (<12 months).[69,72,73] On the other hand, even patients with an associated invasive carcinoma have a better prognosis than those with an ordinary PDAC, particularly if the carcinoma is of the colloid type,[41,44–46] or the amount of invasive carcinoma is small. Invasive carcinomas measuring less than 0.5 cm (AJCC stage pT1a) have been designated "minimally invasive" and have an excellent prognosis.[74] It should be kept in mind that although overall tubular-type invasion may be less aggressive than classical PDAC, it is unclear whether this pattern of invasion is behaviorally and biologically better than PDAC when compared stage by stage.

In addition, IPMNs are seen in elderly who often have several comorbidities and patients with IPMNs seem to have a propensity to have other cancers. For this reason, management approach often needs to be individualized (**Table 2**).

Intraductal Oncocytic Papillary Neoplasm

IOPN of the pancreas was first recognized in 1996 as a distinct category.[75] However, for a while, it was regarded as a variant of IPMN including in World Health Organization (WHO) 2010[39,76] due to their clinicopathologic similarities.[77–80] Later on, various clinical, pathologic, behavioral, and genetic characteristics of this entity clearly distinguishing it from IPMNs have begun to be recognized, and since the WHO 2019 classification, it is recognized as a separate tumor type.[75,81–83]

Clinical features

IOPNs present as relatively large (often >5 cm) tumors, and radiologically, they are typically diagnosed as "complex cystadenocarcinomas with solid and cystic components."[33,40,81,84,85] Owing to their complex nature and formation of a large mass that pushes into the neighboring organs including the large vessels, they often give the erroneous impression of an unresectable mass, only to be found intraoperatively that they can be stripped of from the adjacent structures. Often their inflammatory companions also contribute to their "nasty" appearance at the radiologic level.

Pathologic features

IOPNs often form a multilocular cystic mass with fleshy papillary nodules filling some of the cysts. Owing to the large mass and inflammatory reaction, the intervening pancreatic parenchyma is atrophic and fibrotic. Microscopically, IOPNs are characterized by multilocular cystic dilatations of the ductal system with a florid intraductal

Table 2	
Intraductal papillary mucinous neoplasm of the pancreas	
Clinical features	• IPMNs in asymptomatic patients are often detected incidentally during abdominal imaging • Ectasia of the ducts on imaging and mucin spillage into the duodenum through the ampulla during endoscopy are diagnostic features

Histopathologic features	• Mucinous cells with various degrees of atypia line the cystically dilated pancreatic duct(s)
	• Three different papillary patterns with different degrees of dysplasia have been described:
	    Gastric type is characterized by cells that resemble the foveolar epithelium of the stomach, usually low grade
	    Intestinal type is morphologically similar to villous adenomas of the GI tract, more frequently high grade
	    Pancreatobiliary type has more complex papillae composed of cuboidal cells with significant atypia, by default high grade

IHC features	• *Gastric type:* Usually negative for MUC1 and CDX2; more papillary areas express MUC5AC, only small glandular elements at the base label with MUC6 • *Intestinal type:* Positive for MUC2, CDX2 and MUC5AC, while negative for MUC1 and MUC6 • *Pancreatobiliary type:* Labels with MUC1, MUC5AC, and to a lesser degree, with MUC6; does not express MUC2 and CDX2
Molecular features	• In contrast with PDACs, no *DPC4* mutation is seen in IPMNs and *KRAS* and *TP53* are less frequent • *STK11/LKB1* inactivation and *APC* mutations are found in about 25% of IPMNs but not in PDACs • IPMNs harbor two novel gene alterations: *RNF43* is mutated in 75%, and *GNAS* is mutated in 60% (*GNAS* mutations are more frequent in *intestinal type*)
Natural history	• 5-y survival rate of patients with IPMN is relatively good. • More than 75% of patients are free of disease 5 y after resection; however, recurrences can be seen even many years after surgery • Even patients with an associated invasive carcinoma have a good prognosis, especially if the carcinoma is of the colloid type, or invasive carcinoma component is small • Invasive carcinomas measuring <0.5 cm (AJCC stage pT1a) have been designated "minimally invasive" and have an excellent prognosis • Cases with a large invasive tubular-type adenocarcinoma component pursue an aggressive course, similar to that of conventional PDAC

Abbreviations: AJCC, American Joint Committee on Cancer; GI, gastrointestinal.

papillary growth pattern. Unlike the villous nature of the papillae in IPMN, the papillae of IOPNs are often very complex, delicate, and arborizing. This distinctive papillary architecture is combined with the oncocytic cytology that gives the entity its name (**Fig. 5**). Owing to their complex architecture, IOPNs are regarded as high-grade dysplastic (in situ carcinoma), justifying the clinical impression of "cystadenocarcinoma"; however, they are often curable even when invasive "Biologic behavior and treatment" section. Invasion is reported ranging from 15% to 60% of IOPNs. This is attributable to the fact that these tumors are highly complex with pagetoid extension into atrophic lobules, creating pseudo-invasive appearance, which could be indistinguishable from true invasion. In our experience, convincing invasion is seen in 30% or less. Most invasive carcinomas also reveal oncocytic features but some are characterized by abundant extracellular mucin.[84]

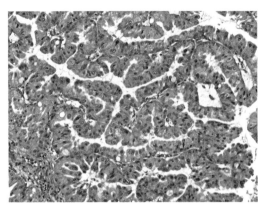

Fig. 5. Intraductal oncocytic papillary neoplasms (IOPNs) are characterized with arborizing papillae lined by oncocytic cells that have abundant granular cytoplasm.

Special studies and molecular features

Similar to pancreatobiliary-type IPMNs, IOPNs express MUC1 (usually focal) and MUC6.[50] Of note, most cases also express hepatocyte paraffin 1.[75,84,86] Recently, it has been shown that IOPNs have molecular profile very different than IPMNs. Most importantly, they reveal *DNAJB1-PRKACA* fusions, which had been thought specific for fibrolamellar hepatocellular carcinoma.[83] These fusions have not been detected in any other pancreatic tumors thus far. Moreover, IOPNs usually do not harbor mutations in *KRAS, TP53, SMAD4, GNAS,* and *CDKN2A,* and *RNF43* mutations that are commonly detected in IPMNs[80,82,87] Instead, recurrent mutations have been detected in *ARHGAP26, ASXL1, EPHA8,* and *ERBB4.*[82]

Biologic behavior and treatment

The prognosis of IOPNs is excellent, even the ones with an associated invasive carcinoma have a nearly 100% 5-year survival[84,88] and 10-year above 90%. Although recurrences after resection do occur, sometimes many years after the initial resection, reoperations often have excellent results in terms of survival.[88]

Intraductal Tubulopapillary Neoplasm

ITPN is a relatively new member of pancreatic intraductal neoplasms family. Initially, it was termed intraductal tubular neoplasms emphasizing the main feature that distinguish these tumors from other pancreatic tumors. However, later on formation of focal and abortive papillary units was also acknowledged in some publications and the term ITPN was adopted.[89-93]

Clinical features

The presentation of ITPNs is relatively similar to other intraductal neoplasms. They present as partially cystic and partially solid masses in elderly patients. However, they tend to form more solid and nodular architecture than IPMNs.

Pathologic features

ITPN exhibits a predominantly tubular architecture. Although the name bears the term "papillary," in most cases papilla formation is either focal or does not exist. The intraductal proliferation typically fills the entire duct, resulting in well-circumscribed nodules **(Fig. 6)** and may be difficult to recognize as intraductal unless continuity with the normal ductal epithelium can be identified.[91-93] ITPNs are regarded as high-grade dysplastic

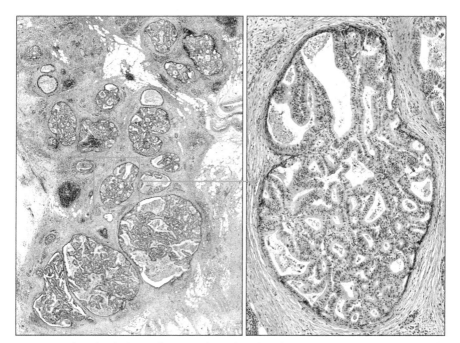

Fig. 6. Intraductal tubulopapillary neoplasm (ITPN) with a nodular growth pattern (left). The nodules are composed of back-to-back tubular glands lined by atypical cuboidal cells (right).

due to their significant architectural complexity and are frequently associated with invasive carcinoma. However, similar to IOPNs, ITPNs are also very prone to cause atrophy in the neighboring pancreas and show pagetoid extension to atrophic ducts, creating a pseudo-invasive appearance that is almost impossible to distinguish from true invasion. The fact that the reported rate of invasive carcinoma does not quite match the rate of metastatic carcinoma and the relatively indolent behavior suggests that overdiagnosis of invasion is common and that is what we observe in consultation practice. Invasive carcinoma is usually of the tubular type.[90]

Special studies and molecular features

ITPNs typically label with CK7 and CK19. MUC1 and MUC6 are also positive in most cases.[33] However, they are almost always negative for MUC5AC, an important difference from pancreatobiliary-type IPMNs.[90]

Molecular analysis of ITPNs reveals distinctive genetic characteristics compared with those of PDACs and other intraductal neoplasms of the pancreas. Mutations in *KRAS*, *GNAS*, and *RNF43* are not seen. However, certain chromatin remodeling genes (*MLL1*, *MLL2*, *MLL3*, *BAP1*, *PBRM1*, *EED*, and *ATRX*) as well as phosphatidylinositol 3-kinase (PI3K) pathway-related genes (*PIK3CA*, *PIK3CB*, *INPP4A*, and *PTEN*) have been found to be mutated in about one-third of ITPNs.[33,94] *FGFR2* fusions with various fusion partners are also observed in a subset of the cases.[91,95]

Differential diagnosis

ITPN histomorphology is highly similar to that of acinar cell carcinoma. In particular, intraductal and cystic variants of acinar cell carcinoma can be virtually indistinguishable from ITPNs. The presence of enzymatic concretions and crystals can be very helpful in this regard.[96] Another important differential diagnostic possibility is pancreatic neuro-endocrine neoplasms. Fortunately, immunohistochemical staining is very helpful for both differentials. ITPNs do not express acinar cell (trypsin, chymotrypsin, Bcl-10) or neuroendocrine (chromogranin and synaptophysin) differentiation markers.[40]

Biologic behavior
ITPNs appear to be less aggressive than PDACs, even when there is a component of invasive carcinoma.[96]

Mucinous Cystic Neoplasm

Defined by the presence of ovarian-type stroma as the pathognomonic characteristic, which for all practical purposes show all the characteristics of ovarian cortical stroma, MCN is a distinctive tumor type.[97] Similar to intraductal neoplasms discussed above, it represents an adenoma-carcinoma sequence, that is, tumoral intraepithelial neoplasm.

Clinical features
MCNs, defined by the ovarian-type stroma as a requirement, are seen almost exclusively (97%) in perimenopausal females and nearly always located in the pancreatic tail.[97] In fact, as a rule of thumb, studies on MCN encompassing less than 95% women are possibly using old criteria and are erroneously including non-MCN tumors like IPMNs. Presenting symptoms are nonspecific and reflect the effects of an enlarging mass. There is no mucin extrusion through the ampulla of Vater because MCNs do not communicate with the pancreatic ductal system unless there is a fistula formation. Radiologically, the lack of communication with the native ductal system is character-istic. As a result, although IPMNs form cyst-by-cyst appearance due to their intraduc-tal nature following the distribution of the involved ducts and their branches, the MCNs form a demarcated mass in which variable number of loculi and variably patterned septae can be seen. The arrangement is referred as "cyst-in-cyst" appearance.

It should be noted here that with the ovarian-type stroma requirement, which has been in place since WHO 2010, a definitive preoperative diagnosis of MCN is not possible. This is also true for fine needle aspiration (FNA) evaluation because ovarian-type stroma seldom, if ever, comes to the aspirates.

Pathologic features
Macroscopically, MCNs can become quite large (can be >10 cm) multilocular cysts surrounded by a thick fibrotic pseudocapsule (**Fig. 7**).[97] Soft friable polypoid projec-tions or solid nodules, which may harbor an invasive carcinoma component, can be seen within the cysts or within the peripheral capsule. Degenerative changes are also common.[97]

Microscopically, MCNs are usually lined by columnar cells with abundant cyto-plasmic mucin.[98] The epithelium may display a wide range of cytologic atypia. The de-gree of dysplasia should be graded (low or high grade) based on the most severely dysplastic region, which may be focal.

A prerequisite for the diagnosis of MCN is the presence of distinctive subepithelial hypercellular spindle cell stroma (**Fig. 8**). This stroma is not only morphologically but also immunohistochemically similar to ovarian-type stroma as it expresses estrogen and progesterone receptors as well as inhibin (ovarian-type stroma).[99–101] It may also have luteal cells. If a diagnosis of MCN is rendered that by default indicates that convincing ovarian-type stroma has been detected.

Fifteen percent of resected MCNs harbor invasive carcinoma component.[97,102,103] Just like high-grade dysplasia, the invasive carcinoma may also be focal and grossly invisible. Thus, it is very important to thoroughly examine any solid areas to properly

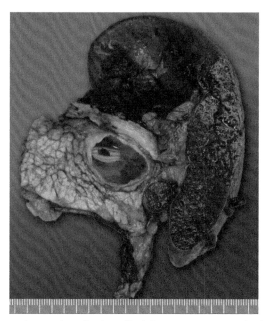

Fig. 7. A mucinous cystic neoplasm in the tail of the pancreas. Note the lack of communication with pancreatic duct system.

diagnose these neoplasms. Invasive carcinoma arising in MCNs is mostly (90%) of tubular type and resembles PDAC.[97] However, sarcomatoid carcinoma or undifferentiated carcinoma with osteoclast-like giant cells may also be seen.[97,104] In cases of MCN with an associated invasive carcinoma, the histologic type of invasive carcinoma as well as its size should be reported.

Differential diagnosis
Both clinically and microscopically in areas poor in ovarian-type stroma MCNs can closely resemble IPMNs. A cystic lesion in a male patient or a cyst located in the

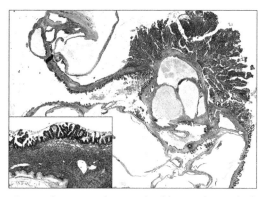

Fig. 8. Mucinous cystic neoplasms are characterized by mucin producing columnar epithelium surrounded by ovarian-type stroma (inset). A lesion with diffuse high-grade dysplasia is depicted here.

head of the pancreas, is exremely unlikely to be an MCN. The lack of communication with the ducts and formation of demarcated thick-walled cyst with cyst-in-cyst appearance are distinguishing features of MCNs. The cystic areas of MCNs are similar to gastric-type IPMN (except for ovarian-type stroma, of course) and the papillae in MCNs may have goblet cells but they do not have the characteristic villous pattern of intestinal-type IPMNs. In fact, the papillary elements in MCNs reveal pancreatobiliary pattern. Characteristic arborizing papillae and oncocytic cells of IOPNs are not seen in MCNs, either. Sometimes MCNs may develop extensive denudation of the lining epithelium, with the underlying stromal hemorrhage, fibrosis, and inflammation. Biopsies from these regions may resemble pseudocysts.[105] However, clinical setting (young female, usually without a history of pancreatitis and an otherwise normal-appearing pancreas) is a red flag to examine other regions of the cyst to find the characteristic mucinous lining or ovarian-type stroma. Simple mucinous cysts (see below) show various similarities to MCN at the clinical level but lack ovarian-type stroma.[106,107]

Special studies and molecular features
The epithelium of MCNs expresses keratin as well as glycoprotein markers, such as mCEA and CA19 to 9.[99,108,109] MUC1 is generally present only in the papillary high-grade dysplasia or in invasive carcinoma.

Molecular analysis of MCNs has disclosed alterations in many of the genes known to be abnormal in PDACs, including *KRAS*, *TP53*, *DPC4*, and *CDKN2A*. In addition, about half of MCNs have mutations in *RNF43*, which is also mutated in IPMNs.[54] However, *GNAS* mutations are not found in MCNs.[55]

Biologic behavior and treatment
Surgical resection is recommended for all patients with an MCN.[63,97] However, it is increasingly becoming recognized that invasion is extremely uncommon in MCNs that are less than 4 cm and noncomplex. As such, it is speculated that Sendai/Fukuoka criteria for IPMNs may in fact be also applicable to MCNs as well.[97] Invasion is typically seen in MCNs that are large (>5 cm) and complex with papillary nodules.[97] Although it has been suggested that invasive carcinomas arising in MCNs are less aggressive than PDACs, the difference may be stage-related. In some studies, even small invasive carcinomas have been found to behave aggressively[97]; however, other studies found microinvasive carcinomas to be more benevolent.[110] Undifferentiated carcinomas with osteoclast-like giant cells arising in MCNs appear to have a more protracted clinical course even when they are large. Of note, colloid-type invasive carcinoma, which constitutes a sizable percentage of invasion seen in IPMNs, typically in intestinal-type IPMNs, is virtually nonexistent in MCNs.

Simple Mucinous Cyst

The cyst type that is currently designated as "simple mucinous cyst" (previously also called mucinous non-neoplastic cyst) is also increasingly being recognized to harbor dysplastic changes and association with invasive carcinoma.[2,106,107,111] Before the recognition of this as a separate category in 2015 in the Baltimore International Consensus meeting, the cases currently included in this entity were previously diagnosed mostly as IPMNs or MCNs.

Clinical features
These present as cysts with an average size of 3 cm occurring in any region of the pancreas (equally distributed in the head vs corpus/tail) and in older ages (mean age 65 years).[106,107] Typically, they are unilocular. Recent studies show that they have radiologic findings distinct from IPMNs and retention cysts.[107] They do not exhibit overt

communication with the ductal system. The cyst contents commonly exhibit high CEA levels and *KRAS* mutations.

Pathologic features
Simple mucinous cysts tend to be unilocular and thick walled. They protrude to the peripancreatic soft tissues. The capsule-like wall may have hypercellular areas but not ovarian-type stroma. The cyst is lined by mucinous epithelium that is typically devoid of papilla and is often partially denuded. Atypia is common, with high-grade dysplasia detected in about 10%. Some simple mucinous cysts are associated with a PDAC. PDAC is often admixed with or is adjacent to the simple mucinous cyst. An analysis of PDACs reveals simple mucinous cyst in 1.5% of the cases.[107] These observations lead to the conclusion that simple mucinous cyst, like any mucin-epithelial lesions in the pancreas, is actually premalignant.

Differential diagnosis
Simple mucinous cysts mostly have flat lining. Papilla, if present, is stubby and not grossly visible. They do not have papillary nodules that characterize IPMNs. On the other hand, for practical purposes, simple mucinous cysts conceptually can be regarded as non-papillary ("1A") version of gastric/ branch-duct IPMNs. However, they do not show the radiologic characteristics and growth pattern of IPMNs. In addition, intestinal epithelium is not a feature of simple mucinous cysts. Especially in elderly female patients, simple mucinous cysts raise the differential of an MCN with postmenopausal burn out of ovarian-type stroma. Progesterone receptor (PR) immunohistochemistry may help in this distinction.

Special studies and molecular features
As expected, the lining of simple mucinous cysts is CK7 positive. The gastric-like and endocervical-like morphology of the lining epithelium is also supported by MUC5AC and to a lesser degree MUC6 expression. *KRAS* mutation is commonly detected. In one study,[112] *KMT2C (MLL3)* mutations was found in two-thirds of the cases, and other molecular alterations such as *BRAF, RNF3, CDKN2a,* and *TP53* mutations were also noted in a small percentage.

Biologic behavior and treatment
The presence of high-grade dysplasia as well as the molecular alterations otherwise characteristic of malignant transformation underscores the premalignant nature of simple mucinous cysts. In the papers published, the follow-up was relatively limited and because the tumors were resected, the natural course of the cases had been interfered. However, the occurrence of simple mucinous cysts in patients with PDACs suggests that if unresected, some simple mucinous cysts would progress to invasive carcinoma. Unfortunately, it is impossible to determine the risk and rate of such transformation.

AMPULLA

Similar to the pancreas, the flat type of dysplasia in the ampulla is seldom recognizable in daily practice outside the setting of invasive cancer. Therefore, most dysplastic lesions (intraepithelial neoplasms) that come to clinical attention are the "tumoral" examples. These occur in two distinct categories in this small site. One is the conventional intestinal-type adenomas that arise from the duodenal surface of the ampulla, which are similar to ordinary adenomas of tubular GI tract. These can occur in the setting of syndromes such as familial adenomatous polyposis (FAP) as well. The other group is intra-ampullary tumoral intraepithelial neoplasms, which are designated intra-ampullary papillary-tubular neoplasms (IAPNs).[113,114] In essence, this latter group is the intra-ampullary counterpart of the intraductal neoplasms discussed above in the pancreas as well as in the biliary tact section of this issue.

Adenomas of the Ampullary Duodenum

Clinical features

Intestinal-type adenomas, similar to the colorectal ones, may arise in the duodenal surface of the ampulla (ie, ampullary duodenum).[115] Although adenomas of the ampullary duodenum are usually sporadic; in patients with FAP, the duodenum including ampulla is the most common site of extracolonic adenomas.[116–120] About 90% of patients with FAP are found to have multiple adenomas in the duodenum, and one-fourth of these adenomas are located in the ampullary duodenum.

Sporadic adenomas of the ampullary duodenum are seen in patients in their 60s, usually in females. FAP patients are typically 20 years younger at the time of diagnosis and both sexes are affected equally.[116,117,119,121–126] Larger adenomas may cause bile duct obstruction with jaundice, pancreatitis, and abdominal pain.[125] The prevalence of carcinoma proportionately increases with the adenoma size.[116,117,119,126] Fortunately, due to FAP screening protocols, adenomas are increasingly detected, whereas they are still small and asymptomatic.[126]

Pathologic features

In order to be classified as an adenoma of the ampullary duodenum, more than 75% of the lesion should be located on the duodenal surface of the ampulla. If the lesion is predominantly or completely within the ampullary channel, it is classified as an IAPN.

Macroscopically, most villous adenomas have a feathery appearance, whereas most tubular ones are bosselated.[127,128] A firm texture is concerning for an invasive component.[116–120,126]

Microscopically, the adenomas are similar to those seen in colorectum. They are classified as tubular, tubulovillous, or villous, depending on the amount of glandular and papillary architecture.[116–120,126] It should be kept in mind that all adenomas are dysplastic. Dysplasia is graded as low or high grade, depending on the degree of cytoarchitectural atypia.

Differential diagnosis

Reactive changes resulting from inflammatory processes can closely mimic an adenoma. However, in addition to the presence of inflammatory cells, reactive changes usually do not reveal the degree of cytologic atypia seen in dysplasia. Moreover, there is no architectural complexity.

Intra-Ampullary Papillary-Tubular Neoplasms

Papillary/polypoid preinvasive lesions (ie, tumoral intraepithelial neoplasms) arising from and growing within the ampullary channel are designated IAPN.[113,114] Fundamentally, these are the intra-ampullary counterpart of pancreatic and biliary intraductal neoplasms.

Clinical features

Similar to sporadic adenomas of the ampullary duodenum, IAPNs are seen in patients in their 60s (mean age = 64 years) and they seem to be more common in man with a male-to-female ratio of about two. Most symptoms (eg, pruritus, jaundice, dark urine, light stool) are due to obstruction of the common bile duct, but nonspecific symptoms such as abdominal pain may also be present.

On radiologic examination, they often are described as filling defects or masses in the distal CBD or ampullary nodules. Some cases can be mistaken as stones impacted in the ampulla due to the dilatation they cause and the filling defect appearance. Double duct sign is not as striking as it is in ampullary-ductal (scirrhous) cancers due to the slow-growing nature of the adenomatous lesion.

From the endoscopic perspective, IAPNs typically present as bulging but mucosal covered masses. The duodenal surface of the ampulla is often smooth due to the compression from the underlying lesion, and the ampullary orifice is often patulous. Because they are not as exposed to the outside world, they do not show as much ulceration and bleeding as the duodenal surface adenomas do. Once the endoscopist punctures the mucosa, typically granular material from underneath readily bulges into the duodenal lumen.

Pathologic features

Macroscopic evaluation of the ampullary duodenum[129] typically reveals a hemispheric elevation of duodenal mucosa. The mucosa covering the duodenal surface of the ampulla is typically smooth and flattened due to the compression of the mass underneath. The ampullary orifice is typically dilated from within which granular material protruding into the duodenal lumen can be observed in some cases. Overt mucinous discharge, characteristic of pancreatic IPMN, is rare. Cut surface of the ampullary channel reveals an often large (mean diameter = 2.9 cm), exophytic lesion in the dilated distal bile and pancreatic ducts. Commonly, the lesion stops abruptly as it reaches to the duodenal mucosal segment of the ampulla.[113,114]

Microscopically, IAPNs usually show a mixture of papillary and tubular growth as well as a mixture of low- and high-grade dysplasia (**Fig. 9**). Unlike adenomas of the ampullary duodenum, approximately half of IAPNs reveal mixed intestinal and non-intestinal (pancreatobiliary or gastric) phenotype.[113] The cell typing used in IPMNs does not seem to be applicable much to IAPNs due to the frequent hybrid/mixed nature of the lesions. Most of the IAPNs (75–90+ %) are associated with invasive carcinoma but the invasive component is usually small (<1 cm in diameter). However, even when the invasion is small, they have lymph node metastasis in about a third of the cases. The histologic type of invasive carcinoma (intestinal vs pancreatobiliary) does not parallel that of the preinvasive component in all cases. Invasion is often focal and hidden at the base of

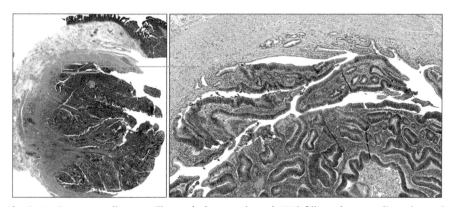

Fig. 9. An intra-ampullary papillary-tubular neoplasm (IAPN) filling the ampullary channel. The lesion is characterized by well-formed papillae projecting into the intra-ampullary ducts. The duodenal mucosa is spared (left). IAPNs display a spectrum of dysplasia. One with predominantly low-grade dysplasia is depicted here (right).

Table 3	
Intra-ampullary papillary-tubular neoplasm	
Clinical features	• Seen in patients in their 60s, more commonly in man • Present with obstruction-related symptoms (pruritus, jaundice, dark urine, light stool) • Imaging reveals filling defects or masses in the distal CBD or ampullary nodules • Endoscopist may detect a bulging mass covered with mucosa at the ampulla
Pathologic features	Gross • Granular material protruding from dilated ampullary orifice into the duodenal lumen can be seen • Sectioning reveals an exophytic lesion in the dilated distal bile and pancreatic ducts Microscopy • A papillary and tubular growth, usually with mixed intestinal and non-intestinal (gastric or pancreatobiliary) phenotype • Both low- and high-grade dysplasia can be seen in the same lesion • Most of the IAPNs are also associated with invasive carcinoma • Histologic type of invasive carcinoma may be different than that of the preinvasive component
IHC features	• Cases with *gastropancreatobiliary differentiation* label with MUC1, MUC5AC, and MUC6 • Cases with *intestinal differentiation* label with MUC2 and CDX2 • However, a significant proportion of the cases reveal mixed immunophenotype
Natural history	• Noninvasive IAPNs have a very good prognosis; however, recurrences can be seen even many years after surgery • IAPNs with an invasive carcinoma are associated with better survival than conventional invasive ampullary carcinomas (3-y survival of 69% vs 44%)

Abbreviations: CBD, common bile duct.

the lesion in the inner segment of the ampulla (the walls of the intra-ampullary CBD or intra-ampullary Wirsung). In fact, in some cases, it is located more proximally toward the upper CBD or pancreas proper.[113,114] For these reasons, these lesions do not seem to be amenable to ampullectomy for curative intent.

Special studies
IAPNs with intestinal differentiation express MUC2 and CDX2, whereas the ones with gastropancreatobiliary differentiation express MUC1, MUC5AC, and MUC6. However, a significant proportion of the cases reveal a mixed immunophenotype. Furthermore, morphologic immunohistochemical discordance is high.[113,130,131]

Differential diagnosis
Knowing the location and distribution of the lesion is essential to distinguish IAPNs from adenomas of the ampullary duodenum or intraductal neoplasms of the pancreas and bile ducts. Proper grossing of the specimens and correlation with the clinical, endoscopic, and radiologic findings can be helpful. As mentioned above, IAPNs are predominantly located within the ampullary channel with only minimal extension to the ampullary duodenum or proximal aspects of the common bile duct and the main pancreatic duct.[20,113] Microscopically, the presence of non-intestinal phenotype is also helpful because adenomas of the ampullary duodenum virtually always reveal intestinal differentiation.

Biologic behavior and treatment

Noninvasive IAPNs have a very good prognosis. However, recurrences of noninvasive examples can be seen even after many years of observation. In some resections, what is interpreted as noninvasive IAPN shows lymph node metastasis, which prompts the additional sectioning of the primary lesion only to reveal small invasive carcinomas. This underscores the complete removal of IAPNs and the ampullectomy would in fact be an inadequate operation if there is curative intent. Also, important to keep in mind that even IAPNs with minimal invasion may reveal lymph node metastasis. Therefore, long-term follow-up is warranted for all IAPNs.[113]

IAPNs with an invasive carcinoma are associated with better survival than invasive ampullary carcinomas without an associated IAPN (3-year survival of 69% vs 44%).[113] This survival advantage is likely attributable to early detection and smaller size of invasion, but differences in tumor biology is also a possibility (**Table 3**).[19,113,132]

SUMMARY

Pancreatic and ampullary preinvasive neoplasms represent a spectrum of early-stage abnormalities that can give rise to malignancies in the pancreas and ampulla of Vater, respectively. These lesions include PanIN, IPMNs, IOPN, ITPN, MCN, and simple mucinous cyst in the pancreas, as well as adenoma and IAPN in the ampulla. These preinvasive stages are crucial to understand as they precede the development of invasive cancers, offering a window of opportunity for early detection and intervention. Studying the histopathological and molecular characteristics of these preinvasive neoplasms is essential for advancing our knowledge of pancreatic and ampullary cancer progression and improving diagnostic and therapeutic strategies for these challenging malignancies.

CLINICS CARE POINTS

- The main-duct-type intraductal papillary mucinous neoplasms (IPMNs) have a greater risk of having high-grade dysplasia or invasive carcinoma. In contracts, branch-duct-type IPMNs may not require surgical resection if they are small (<3 cm) and lack worrisome features such as mural nodules and growth during follow-up. Therefore, classifying IPMNs as main-duct versus branch-duct type has value in preoperative algorithms.

- When reporting intraductal neoplasms or a mucinous cystic neoplasm, the presence of invasive carcinoma should always be mentioned in the diagnosis (such as "IPMN or MCN with an associated invasive carcinoma"), and the type and extent of invasive carcinoma should also be specified.

- High-grade dysplasia or associated invasive carcinoma may be focal and grossly invisible in intraductal neoplasms or a mucinous cystic neoplasm. Therefore, careful evaluation and thorough sampling are essential for accurate diagnosis.

- *DNAJB1-PRKACA* fusions, which had been thought specific for fibrolamellar hepatocellular carcinoma, may also be seen in intraductal papillary oncocytic neoplasms.

- Patients with an IPMN of any grade and any margin status need to be followed carefully after surgery.

- Morphology of intraductal tubulopapillary neoplasm (ITPN) and acinar cell carcinoma may mimic each other. Therefore, the possibility of an acinar cell carcinoma must be excluded by immunohistochemical staining before a case is classified as ITPN.

- Knowing the location and distribution of the lesion is essential to distinguish intra-ampullary papillary-tubular neoplasms from adenomas of the ampullary duodenum or intraductal neoplasms of the pancreas and bile ducts.

ACKNOWLEDGMENTS

The authors would like to thank Dr Zeynep Tarcan for her contributions in the preparation of this manuscript.

DISCLOSURE

O. Basturk has been supported in part by the Cancer Center Support Grant of the National Institutes of Health, United States/National Cancer Institute, United States under award number P30CA008748.

REFERENCES

1. Adsay NV, Merati K, Andea A, et al. The dichotomy in the preinvasive neoplasia to invasive carcinoma sequence in the pancreas: differential expression of MUC1 and MUC2 supports the existence of two separate pathways of carcinogenesis. Mod Pathol 2002;15(10):1087–95.
2. Basturk O, Hong SM, Wood LD, et al. A Revised Classification System and Recommendations From the Baltimore Consensus Meeting for Neoplastic Precursor Lesions in the Pancreas. Am J Surg Pathol 2015;39(12):1730–41.
3. Adsay V, Mino-Kenudson M, Furukawa T, et al. Pathologic Evaluation and Reporting of Intraductal Papillary Mucinous Neoplasms of the Pancreas and Other Tumoral Intraepithelial Neoplasms of Pancreatobiliary Tract Recommendations of Verona Consensus Meeting. Ann Surg 2016;263(1):162–77.
4. Hruban RH, Adsay NV, Albores-Saavedra J, et al. Pancreatic intraepithelial neoplasia: a new nomenclature and classification system for pancreatic duct lesions. Am J Surg Pathol 2001;25(5):579–86.
5. Basturk O. Pancreatic Intraepithelial Neoplasia. In: Klimstra DS, Nagtegaal ID, Rugge M, et al, editors. WHO classification of tumours of the digestive system. Lyon, France: IARC; 2019. p. 307–9.
6. Andea A, Sarkar F, Adsay VN. Clinicopathological correlates of pancreatic intraepithelial neoplasia: a comparative analysis of 82 cases with and 152 cases without pancreatic ductal adenocarcinoma. Mod Pathol 2003;16(10):996–1006.
7. Brat DJ, Lillemoe KD, Yeo CJ, et al. Progression of pancreatic intraductal neoplasias to infiltrating adenocarcinoma of the pancreas. Am J Surg Pathol 1998;22(2):163–9.
8. Stelow EB, Adams RB, Moskaluk CA. The prevalence of pancreatic intraepithelial neoplasia in pancreata with uncommon types of primary neoplasms. Am J Surg Pathol 2006;30(1):36–41.
9. Shi C, Klein AP, Goggins M, et al. Increased Prevalence of Precursor Lesions in Familial Pancreatic Cancer Patients. Clin Cancer Res 2009;15(24):7737–43.
10. Klein WM, Hruban RH, Klein-Szanto AJ, et al. Direct correlation between proliferative activity and dysplasia in pancreatic intraepithelial neoplasia (PanIN): additional evidence for a recently proposed model of progression. Mod Pathol 2002;15(4):441–7.
11. Lemoine NR, Jain S, Hughes CM, et al. Ki-ras oncogene activation in preinvasive pancreatic cancer. Gastroenterology 1992;102(1):230–6.
12. Moskaluk CA, Hruban RH, Kern SE. p16 and K-ras gene mutations in the intraductal precursors of human pancreatic adenocarcinoma. Cancer Res 1997;57(11):2140–3.

13. Springer S, Wang Y, Dal Molin M, et al. A combination of molecular markers and clinical features improve the classification of pancreatic cysts. Gastroenterology 2015;149(6):1501–10.
14. Hruban RH, Takaori K, Klimstra DS, et al. An illustrated consensus on the classification of pancreatic intraepithelial neoplasia and intraductal papillary mucinous neoplasms. Am J Surg Pathol 2004;28(8):977–87.
15. Longnecker DS, Adsay NV, Fernandez-del Castillo C, et al. Histopathological diagnosis of pancreatic intraepithelial neoplasia and intraductal papillary-mucinous neoplasms: interobserver agreement. Pancreas 2005;31(4):344–9.
16. Yachida S, Jones S, Bozic I, et al. Distant metastasis occurs late during the genetic evolution of pancreatic cancer. Nature 2010;467(7319):1114–7.
17. Konstantinidis IT, Vinuela EF, Tang LH, et al. Incidentally discovered pancreatic intraepithelial neoplasia: what is its clinical significance? Ann Surg Oncol 2013; 20(11):3643–7.
18. Adsay NV, Conlon KC, Zee SY, et al. Intraductal papillary-mucinous neoplasms of the pancreas: an analysis of in situ and invasive carcinomas in 28 patients. Cancer 2002;94(1):62–77.
19. Adsay V, Jang KT, Roa JC, et al. Intracholecystic Papillary-Tubular Neoplasms (ICPN) of the Gallbladder (Neoplastic Polyps, Adenomas, and Papillary Neoplasms That Are >= 1.0 cm) Clinicopathologic and Immunohistochemical Analysis of 123 Cases. Am J Surg Pathol 2012;36(9):1279–301.
20. Kloppel G, Adsay V, Konukiewitz B, et al. Precancerous lesions of the biliary tree. Best Pract Res Clin Gastroenterol 2013;27(2):285–97.
21. Pehlivanoglu B, Adsay V. Intraductal tubulopapillary neoplasms of the bile ducts: identity, clinicopathologic characteristics, and differential diagnosis of a distinct entity among intraductal tumors. Hum Pathol 2023;132:12–9.
22. Roa JC, Basturk O, Adsay V. Dysplasia and carcinoma of the gallbladder: pathological evaluation, sampling, differential diagnosis and clinical implications. Histopathology 2021;79(1):2–19.
23. Schlitter AM, Jang KT, Klöppel G, et al. Intraductal tubulopapillary neoplasms of the bile ducts: clinicopathologic, immunohistochemical, and molecular analysis of 20 cases. Mod Pathol 2016;29(1):93.
24. Wang T, Askan G, Ozcan K, et al. Tumoral Intraductal Neoplasms of the Bile Ducts Comprise Morphologically and Genetically Distinct Entities, Arch Pathol Lab Med, 147(12), 2023, 1390-1401.
25. Zen Y, Adsay NV, Bardadin K, et al. Biliary intraepithelial neoplasia: an international interobserver agreement study and proposal for diagnostic criteria. Mod Pathol 2007;20(6):701–9.
26. Adsay, V, O. Basturk, Pre-cancerous lesions of the gallbladder and extrahepatic bile ducts: concepts, terminology, and significance. Gastroenterol Clin. in press.
27. Pehlivanoglu B, Balci S, Basturk O, et al. Intracholecystic tubular non-mucinous neoplasm (ICTN) of the gallbladder: a clinicopathologically distinct, invasion-resistant entity. Virchows Arch 2021;478(3):435–47.
28. Basturk O, Aishima S, Esposito I. Intracholecystic Papillary Neoplasm. In: Borad WCoTE, editor. WHO classifications of tumours, digestive system tumours. Lyon (France): International Agency for Research on Cancer; 2019. p. 276–7.
29. Azar C, Van de Stadt J, Rickaert F, et al. Intraductal papillary mucinous tumours of the pancreas. Clinical and therapeutic issues in 32 patients. Gut 1996;39(3): 457–64.
30. Loftus EV Jr, Olivares-Pakzad BA, Batts KP, et al. Intraductal papillary-mucinous tumors of the pancreas: clinicopathologic features, outcome, and nomenclature.

Members of the Pancreas Clinic, and Pancreatic Surgeons of Mayo Clinic. Gastroenterology 1996;110(6):1909–18.

31. Paal E, Thompson LD, Przygodzki RM, et al. A clinicopathologic and immuno-histochemical study of 22 intraductal papillary mucinous neoplasms of the pancreas, with a review of the literature. Mod Pathol 1999;12(5):518–28.

32. Klöppel G. Clinicopathologic view of intraductal papillary-mucinous tumor of the pancreas. Hepato-Gastroenterology 1998;45(24):1981–5.

33. Ozcan K, Klimstra DS. A Review of Mucinous Cystic and Intraductal Neoplasms of the Pancreatobiliary Tract. Arch Pathol Lab Med 2022;146(3):298–311.

34. Terris B, Ponsot P, Paye F, et al. Intraductal papillary mucinous tumors of the pancreas confined to secondary ducts show less aggressive pathologic fea-tures as compared with those involving the main pancreatic duct. Am J Surg Pathol 2000;24(10):1372–7.

35. Irie H, Yoshimitsu K, Aibe H, et al. Natural history of pancreatic intraductal papil-lary mucinous tumor of branch duct type: follow-up study by magnetic reso-nance cholangiopancreatography. J Comput Assist Tomogr 2004;28(1):117–22.

36. White R, D'Angelica M, Katabi N, et al. Fate of the remnant pancreas after resec-tion of noninvasive intraductal papillary mucinous neoplasm. J Am Coll Surg 2007;204(5):987–93, discussion 993-5.

37. Chari ST, Yadav D, Smyrk TC, et al. Study of recurrence after surgical resection of intraductal papillary mucinous neoplasm of the pancreas. Gastroenterology 2002;123(5):1500–7.

38. Adsay NV, Longnecker DS, Klimstra DS. Pancreatic tumors with cystic dilatation of the ducts: intraductal papillary mucinous neoplasms and intraductal onco-cytic papillary neoplasms. Semin Diagn Pathol 2000;17(1):16–30.

39. Furukawa T, Klöppel G, Volkan Adsay N, et al. Classification of types of intraduc-tal papillary-mucinous neoplasm of the pancreas: a consensus study. Virchows Arch 2005;447(5):794–9.

40. Askan G, Bagci P, Memis B, et al. Intraductal Neoplasms of the Pancreas: An Update. Turk Patoloji Derg 2017;33(2):87–102.

41. Furukawa T, Hatori T, Fujita I, et al. Prognostic relevance of morphological types of intraductal papillary mucinous neoplasms of the pancreas. Gut 2011;60(4): 509–16.

42. Waters JA, Schnelldorfer T, Aguilar-Saavedra JR, et al. Survival after resection for invasive intraductal papillary mucinous neoplasm and for pancreatic adeno-carcinoma: a multi-institutional comparison according to American Joint Com-mittee on Cancer Stage. J Am Coll Surg 2011;213(2):275–83.

43. Hirono S, Shimizu Y, Ohtsuka T, et al. Recurrence patterns after surgical resec-tion of intraductal papillary mucinous neoplasm (IPMN) of the pancreas; a multi-center, retrospective study of 1074 IPMN patients by the Japan Pancreas Society. J Gastroenterol 2020;55(1):86–99.

44. Adsay NV, Pierson C, Sarkar F, et al. Colloid (mucinous noncystic) carcinoma of the pancreas. Am J Surg Pathol 2001;25(1):26–42.

45. Seidel G, Zahurak M, Iacobuzio-Donahue C, et al. Almost all infiltrating colloid carcinomas of the pancreas and periampullary region arise from in situ papillary neoplasms: a study of 39 cases. Am J Surg Pathol 2002;26(1):56–63.

46. Adsay NV, Merati K, Nassar H, et al. Pathogenesis of colloid (pure mucinous) carcinoma of exocrine organs: Coupling of gel-forming mucin (MUC2) produc-tion with altered cell polarity and abnormal cell-stroma interaction may be the key factor in the morphogenesis and indolent behavior of colloid carcinoma in the breast and pancreas. Am J Surg Pathol 2003;27(5):571–8.

47. D'Angelica M, Brennan MF, Suriawinata AA, et al. Intraductal papillary mucinous neoplasms of the pancreas: an analysis of clinicopathologic features and outcome. Ann Surg 2004;239(3):400–8.

48. Terada T, Ohta T, Kitamura Y, et al. Cell proliferative activity in intraductal papillary-mucinous neoplasms and invasive ductal adenocarcinomas of the pancreas: an immunohistochemical study. Arch Pathol Lab Med 1998;122(1):42–6.

49. Nagai E, Ueki T, Chijiiwa K, et al. Intraductal papillary mucinous neoplasms of the pancreas associated with so-called "mucinous ductal ectasia". Histochemical and immunohistochemical analysis of 29 cases. Am J Surg Pathol 1995; 19(5):576–89.

50. Basturk O, Khayyata S, Klimstra DS, et al. Preferential expression of MUC6 in oncocytic and pancreatobiliary types of intraductal papillary neoplasms highlights a pyloropancreatic pathway, distinct from the intestinal pathway, in pancreatic carcinogenesis. Am J Surg Pathol 2010;34(3):364–70.

51. Biankin AV, Biankin SA, Kench JG, et al. Aberrant p16(INK4A) and DPC4/Smad4 expression in intraductal papillary mucinous tumours of the pancreas is associated with invasive ductal adenocarcinoma. Gut 2002;50(6):861–8.

52. Iacobuzio-Donahue CA, Klimstra DS, Adsay NV, et al. Dpc-4 protein is expressed in virtually all human intraductal papillary mucinous neoplasms of the pancreas: comparison with conventional ductal adenocarcinomas. Am J Pathol 2000;157(3):755–61.

53. Sato N, Rosty C, Jansen M, et al. STK11/LKB1 Peutz-Jeghers gene inactivation in intraductal papillary-mucinous neoplasms of the pancreas. Am J Pathol 2001; 159(6):2017–22.

54. Wu J, Jiao Y, Dal Molin M, et al. Whole-exome sequencing of neoplastic cysts of the pancreas reveals recurrent mutations in components of ubiquitin-dependent pathways. Proc Natl Acad Sci U S A 2011;108(52):21188–93.

55. Wu J, Matthaei H, Maitra A, et al. Recurrent GNAS mutations define an unexpected pathway for pancreatic cyst development. Sci Transl Med 2011;3(92): 92ra66.

56. Tan MC, Basturk O, Brannon AR, et al. GNAS and KRAS Mutations Define Separate Progression Pathways in Intraductal Papillary Mucinous Neoplasm-Associated Carcinoma. J Am Coll Surg 2015;220(5):845–54.e1.

57. Springer S, Masica DL, Dal Molin M, et al. A multimodality test to guide the management of patients with a pancreatic cyst. Sci Transl Med 2019;11(501): eaav4772.

58. Tanaka M, Fernández-del Castillo C, Adsay V, et al. International consensus guidelines 2012 for the management of IPMN and MCN of the pancreas. Pancreatology 2012;12(3):183–97.

59. Sohn TA, Yeo CJ, Cameron JL, et al. Intraductal papillary mucinous neoplasms of the pancreas: an updated experience. Ann Surg 2004;239(6):788–97, discussion 797-9.

60. Grutzmann R, Niedergethmann M, Pilarsky C, et al. Intraductal papillary mucinous tumors of the pancreas: biology, diagnosis, and treatment. Oncol 2010;15(12): 1294–309.

61. Kim HS, Han Y, Kang JS, et al. Fate of Patients With Intraductal Papillary Mucinous Neoplasms of Pancreas After Resection According to the Pathology and Margin Status: Continuously Increasing Risk of Recurrence Even After Curative Resection Suggesting Necessity of Lifetime Surveillance. Ann Surg 2022;276(4):e231–8.

62. Muraki T, Jang KT, Reid MD, et al. Pancreatic ductal adenocarcinomas associated with intraductal papillary mucinous neoplasms (IPMNs) versus pseudo-IPMNs: relative frequency, clinicopathologic characteristics and differential diagnosis. Mod Pathol 2021;35(1):96–105.

63. Tanaka M, Chari S, Adsay V, et al. International consensus guidelines for management of intraductal papillary mucinous neoplasms and mucinous cystic neoplasms of the pancreas. Pancreatology 2006;6(1–2):17–32.

64. European Study Group on Cystic Tumours of the, P. European evidence-based guidelines on pancreatic cystic neoplasms Gut 2018;67(5):789–804.

65. Tanaka M, Fernández-Del Castillo C, Kamisawa T, et al. Revisions of international consensus Fukuoka guidelines for the management of IPMN of the pancreas. Pancreatology 2017;17(5):738–53.

66. Vege SS, Ziring B, Jain R, et al. American gastroenterological association institute guideline on the diagnosis and management of asymptomatic neoplastic pancreatic cysts. Gastroenterology 2015;148(4):819–22, quize12-3.

67. Miyakawa S, Horiguchi A, Hayakawa M, et al. Intraductal papillary adenocarcinoma with mucin hypersecretion and coexistent invasive ductal carcinoma of the pancreas with apparent topographic separation. J Gastroenterol 1996; 31(6):889–93.

68. Basturk O, Esposito I, Fukushima N, et al. Pancreatic Intraductal Papillary Mucinous Neoplasm. In: Board WcoTE, editor. WHO classification of tumours, digestive system tumours. Lyon (France): International Agency for Research on Cancer; 2019. p. 310–4.

69. Lucocq J, Hawkyard J, Robertson FP, et al. Risk of Recurrence after Surgical Resection for Adenocarcinoma Arising from Intraductal Papillary Mucinous Neoplasia (IPMN) with Patterns of Distribution and Treatment: An International, Multicentre, Observational Study. Ann Surg 2023. https://doi.org/10.1097/SLA.0000000000006144.

70. Marchegiani G, Andrianello S, Dal Borgo C, et al. Adjuvant chemotherapy is associated with improved postoperative survival in specific subtypes of invasive intraductal papillary mucinous neoplasms (IPMN) of the pancreas: it is time for randomized controlled data. HPB (Oxford) 2019;21(5):596–603.

71. Yamada S, Fujii T, Hirakawa A, et al. Comparison of the Survival Outcomes of Pancreatic Cancer and Intraductal Papillary Mucinous Neoplasms. Pancreas 2018;47(8):974–9.

72. Al Efishat M, Attiyeh MA, Eaton AA, et al. Progression Patterns in the Remnant Pancreas after Resection of Non-Invasive or Micro-Invasive Intraductal Papillary Mucinous Neoplasms (IPMN). Ann Surg Oncol 2018;25(6):1752–9.

73. Pfluger MJ, Griffin JF, Hackeng WM, et al. The Impact of Clinical and Pathological Features on Intraductal Papillary Mucinous Neoplasm Recurrence After Surgical Resection: Long-Term Follow-Up Analysis. Ann Surg 2022;275(6):1165–74.

74. Nara S, Shimada K, Kosuge T, et al. Minimally invasive intraductal papillary-mucinous carcinoma of the pancreas: clinicopathologic study of 104 intraductal papillary-mucinous neoplasms. Am J Surg Pathol 2008;32(2):243–55.

75. Adsay NV, Adair CF, Heffess CS, et al. Intraductal oncocytic papillary neoplasms of the pancreas. Am J Surg Pathol 1996;20(8):980–94.

76. Bosman F, Carneiro F, Hruban RH, et al. In: WHO classification of tumours of the digestive system. 4th edition. Lyon, France: IARC; 2010.

77. Chung SM, Hruban RH, Iacobuzio-Donahue C, et al. An analysis of molecular alterations and differentiation pathways in intraductal oncocytic papillary neoplasm of the pancreas. Mod Pathol 2005;18:277A–8A.

78. Jyotheeswaran S, Zotalis G, Penmetsa P, et al. A newly recognized entity: intra-ductal "oncocytic" papillary neoplasm of the pancreas. Am J Gastroenterol 1998;93(12):2539–43.

79. Noji T, Kondo S, Hirano S, et al. Intraductal oncocytic papillary neoplasm of the pancreas shows strong positivity on FDG-PET. Int J Gastrointest Cancer 2002; 32(1):43–6.

80. Patel SA, Adams R, Goldstein M, et al. Genetic analysis of invasive carcinoma arising in intraductal oncocytic papillary neoplasm of the pancreas. Am J Surg Pathol 2002;26(8):1071–7.

81. Basturk O. Pancreatic Intraductal Oncocytic Papillary Neoplasm. In: WHO classi-fication of tumours of the digestive system. Lyon, France: IARC; 2019. p. 315–6.

82. Basturk O, Tan M, Bhanot U, et al. The oncocytic subtype is genetically distinct from other pancreatic intraductal papillary mucinous neoplasm subtypes. Mod Pathol 2016;29(9):1058–69.

83. Vyas M, Hechtman JF, Zhang Y, et al. DNAJB1-PRKACA fusions occur in onco-cytic pancreatic and biliary neoplasms and are not specific for fibrolamellar he-patocellular carcinoma. Mod Pathol 2020;33(4):648–56.

84. Wang T, Askan G, Adsay V, et al. Intraductal Oncocytic Papillary Neoplasms: Clinical-Pathologic Characterization of 24 Cases, With An Emphasis on Associ-ated Invasive Carcinomas. Am J Surg Pathol 2019;43(5):656–61.

85. Nakaya M, Nakai Y, Takahashi M, et al. Intraductal oncocytic papillary neoplasm of the pancreas: clinical and radiological features compared to those of intra-ductal papillary mucinous neoplasm. Abdom Radiol (NY) 2023;48(8):2483–93.

86. Basturk O, Chung SM, Hruban RH, et al. Distinct pathways of pathogenesis of intraductal oncocytic papillary neoplasms and intraductal papillary mucinous neoplasms of the pancreas. Virchows Arch 2016;469(5):523–32.

87. Xiao HD, Yamaguchi H, Dias-Santagata D, et al. Molecular characteristics and biological behaviours of the oncocytic and pancreatobiliary subtypes of intra-ductal papillary mucinous neoplasms. J Pathol 2011;224(4):508–16.

88. Marchegiani G, Mino-Kenudson M, Ferrone CR, et al. Oncocytic-type intraductal papillary mucinous neoplasms: a unique malignant pancreatic tumor with good long-term prognosis. J Am Coll Surg 2015;220(5):839–44.

89. Basturk O, Esposito I, Fukushima N, et al. Pancreatic Intraductal Tubulopapillary Neoplasm. In: Board WCoTE, editor. WHO classification of tumours of the diges-tive system. Lyon, France: IARC; 2019.

90. Basturk O, Adsay V, Askan G, et al. Intraductal Tubulopapillary Neoplasm of the Pancreas: A Clinicopathologic and Immunohistochemical Analysis of 33 Cases. Am J Surg Pathol 2017;41(3):313–25.

91. Yamaguchi H, Shimizu M, Ban S, et al. Intraductal tubulopapillary neoplasms of the pancreas distinct from pancreatic intraepithelial neoplasia and intraductal papillary mucinous neoplasms. Am J Surg Pathol 2009;33(8):1164–72.

92. Tajiri T, Tate G, Inagaki T, et al. Intraductal tubular neoplasms of the pancreas: histogenesis and differentiation. Pancreas 2005;30(2):115–21.

93. Tajiri T, Tate G, Kunimura T, et al. Histologic and immunohistochemical compar-ison of intraductal tubular carcinoma, intraductal papillary-mucinous carcinoma, and ductal adenocarcinoma of the pancreas. Pancreas 2004;29(2):116–22.

94. Yamaguchi H, Kuboki Y, Hatori T, et al. Somatic mutations in PIK3CA and acti-vation of AKT in intraductal tubulopapillary neoplasms of the pancreas. Am J Surg Pathol 2011;35(12):1812–7.

95. Basturk O, Berger MF, Yamaguchi H, et al. Pancreatic intraductal tubulopapillary neoplasm is genetically distinct from intraductal papillary mucinous neoplasm and ductal adenocarcinoma. Mod Pathol 2017;30(12):1760–72.
96. Klimstra DS, Adsay NV, Dhall D, et al. Intraductal tubular carcinoma of the pancreas: Clinicopathologic and immunohistochemical analysis of 18 cases. Mod Pathol 2007;20:285A.
97. Jang KT, Park SM, Basturk O, et al. Clinicopathologic characteristics of 29 invasive carcinomas arising in 178 pancreatic mucinous cystic neoplasms with ovarian-type stroma: implications for management and prognosis. Am J Surg Pathol 2015;39(2):179–87.
98. Zhelnin K, Xue Y, Quigley B, et al. Nonmucinous Biliary Epithelium Is a Frequent Finding and Is Often the Predominant Epithelial Type in Mucinous Cystic Neoplasms of the Pancreas and Liver. Am J Surg Pathol 2017;41(1):116–20.
99. Zamboni G, Scarpa A, Bogina G, et al. Mucinous cystic tumors of the pancreas: clinicopathological features, prognosis, and relationship to other mucinous cystic tumors. Am J Surg Pathol 1999;23(4):410–22.
100. Izumo A, Yamaguchi K, Eguchi T, et al. Mucinous cystic tumor of the pancreas: immunohistochemical assessment of "ovarian-type stroma". Oncol Rep 2003; 10(3):515–25.
101. Ridder GJ, Maschek H, Flemming P, et al. Ovarian-like stroma in an invasive mucinous cystadenocarcinoma of the pancreas positive for inhibin. A hint concerning its possible histogenesis. Virchows Arch 1998;432(5):451–4.
102. Goh BK, Tan YM, Chung YFA, et al. A review of mucinous cystic neoplasms of the pancreas defined by ovarian-type stroma: clinicopathological features of 344 patients. World J Surg 2006;30(12):2236–45.
103. Crippa S, Salvia R, Warshaw AL, et al. Mucinous cystic neoplasm of the pancreas is not an aggressive entity: lessons from 163 resected patients. Ann Surg 2008;247(4):571–9.
104. Muraki T, Reid MD, Basturk O, et al. Undifferentiated Carcinoma With Osteoclastic Giant Cells of the Pancreas: Clinicopathologic Analysis of 38 Cases Highlights a More Protracted Clinical Course Than Currently Appreciated. Am J Surg Pathol 2016;40(9):1203–16.
105. Warshaw AL, Rutledge PL. Cystic tumors mistaken for pancreatic pseudocysts. Ann Surg 1987;205(4):393–8.
106. Krasinskas AM, Oakley GJ, Bagci P, et al. Simple Mucinous Cyst" of the Pancreas: A Clinicopathologic Analysis of 39 Examples of a Diagnostically Challenging Entity Distinct From Intraductal Papillary Mucinous Neoplasms and Mucinous Cystic Neoplasms. Am J Surg Pathol 2017;41(1):121–7.
107. Tezcan N, Cengiz D, Muraki T, et al. Simple mucinous cysts are pre-cancerous neoplasms with distinct clinicopathologic and radiologic characteristics: further delineation of a rare entity. USCAP 2024 113rd Annual Meeting Laboratory Investigation, 2024: p. Accepted poster.
108. Thompson LD, Becker RC, Przygodzki RM, et al. Mucinous cystic neoplasm (mucinous cystadenocarcinoma of low-grade malignant potential) of the pancreas: a clinicopathologic study of 130 cases. Am J Surg Pathol 1999;23(1):1–16.
109. Ohta T, Nagakawa T, Fukushima W, et al. Immunohistochemical study of carcinoembryonic antigen in mucinous cystic neoplasm of the pancreas. Eur Surg Res 1992;24(1):37–44.
110. Lewis GH, Wang H, Bellizzi AM, et al. Prognosis of minimally invasive carcinoma arising in mucinous cystic neoplasms of the pancreas. Am J Surg Pathol 2013; 37(4):601–5.

111. Milanetto AC, Tonello AS, Valotto G, et al. Simple mucinous cyst: another potential cancer precursor in the pancreas? Case report with molecular characterization and systematic review of the literature. Virchows Arch 2021;479(1):179–89.
112. Attiyeh M, Zhang L, Iacobuzio-Donahue C, et al. Simple mucinous cysts of the pancreas have heterogeneous somatic mutations. Hum Pathol 2020;101:1–9.
113. Ohike N, Kim GE, Tajiri T, et al. Intra-ampullary papillary-tubular neoplasm (IAPN): characterization of tumoral intraepithelial neoplasia occurring within the ampulla: a clinicopathologic analysis of 82 cases. Am J Surg Pathol 2010; 34(12):1731–48.
114. Tarcan Z, Esmer R, Akar K, et al. Intra-Ampullary Papillary Tubular Neoplasm (IAPN): Clinicopathologic Analysis of 72 Cases Highlights the Distinctive Characteristics. Lab Invest 2023;103(3):S1530–1.
115. Albores-Saavedra J, Henson DE, Klimstra DS. Tumors of the gallbladder, extrahepatic bile ducts, and vaterian system, in Atlas of Tumor Pathology. Maryland: American Registyr of Pathology: Silver Spring; 2015.
116. Alexander JR, Andrews JM, Buchi KN, et al. High prevalence of adenomatous polyps of the duodenal papilla in familial adenomatous polyposis. Dig Dis Sci 1989;34(2):167–70.
117. Domizio P, Talbot IC, Spigelman AD, et al. Upper gastrointestinal pathology in familial adenomatous polyposis: results from a prospective study of 102 patients. J Clin Pathol 1990;43(9):738–43.
118. Noda Y, Watanabe H, Iida M, et al. Histologic follow-up of ampullary adenomas in patients with familial adenomatosis coli. Cancer 1992;70(7):1847–56.
119. Odze R, Gallinger S, So K, et al. Duodenal adenomas in familial adenomatous polyposis: relation of cell differentiation and mucin histochemical features to growth pattern. Mod Pathol 1994;7(3):376–84.
120. Yao T, Ida M, Ohsato K, et al. Duodenal lesions in familial polyposis of the colon. Gastroenterology 1977;73(5):1086–92.
121. Perzin KH, Bridge MF. Adenomas of the small intestine: a clinicopathologic review of 51 cases and a study of their relationship to carcinoma. Cancer 1981; 48(3):799–819.
122. Cattell RB, Pyrtek LJ. Premalignant lesions of the ampulla of Vater. Surg Gynecol Obstet 1950;90(1):21–30.
123. Oh C, Jemerin EE. Benign adenomatous polyps of the papilla of vater. Surgery 1965;57:495–503.
124. Rosenberg J, Welch JP, Pyrtek LJ, et al. Benign villous adenomas of the ampulla of Vater. Cancer 1986;58(7):1563–8.
125. Sobol S, Cooperman AM. Villous adenoma of the ampulla of Vater. An unusual cause of biliary colic and obstructive jaundice. Gastroenterology 1978;75(1):107–9.
126. Shemesh E, Bat L. A prospective evaluation of the upper gastrointestinal tract and periampullary region in patients with Gardner syndrome. Am J Gastroenterol 1985;80(11):825–7.
127. Blackman E, Nash SV. Diagnosis of duodenal and ampullary epithelial neoplasms by endoscopic biopsy: a clinicopathologic and immunohistochemical study. Hum Pathol 1985;16(9):901–10.
128. Yamaguchi K, Enjoji M. Adenoma of the ampulla of Vater: putative precancerous lesion. Gut 1991;32(12):1558–61.
129. Adsay NV, Basturk O, Saka B, et al. Whipple Made Simple For Surgical Pathologists: Orientation, Dissection, and Sampling of Pancreaticoduodenectomy Specimens For a More Practical and Accurate Evaluation of Pancreatic, Distal Common Bile Duct, and Ampullary Tumors. Am J Surg Pathol 2014;38(4):480–93.

130. Reid MD, Balci S, Ohike N, et al. Ampullary carcinoma is often of mixed or hybrid histologic type: an analysis of reproducibility and clinical relevance of classification as pancreatobiliary versus intestinal in 232 cases. Mod Pathol 2016;29(12):1575–85.
131. Xue Y, Reid MD, Balci S, et al. Immunohistochemical Classification of Ampullary Carcinomas: Critical Reappraisal Fails to Confirm Prognostic Relevance for Recently Proposed Panels, and Highlights MUC5AC as a Strong Prognosticator. Am J Surg Pathol 2017;41(7):865–76.
132. Cubilla LA, Fitzgerald PJ. Tumors of the exocrine pancreas, in atlas of tumor pathology, 2nd series, fascicle 19. Washington, DC: Armed Forces Institute of Pathology; 1984.

Dysplasia and Early Carcinoma of the Gallbladder and Bile Ducts
Terminology, Classification, and Significance

N. Volkan Adsay, MD[a],*, Olca Basturk, MD[b]

KEYWORDS

- Gallbladder • Bile duct • Dysplasia • Intracholecystic • Intraductal • ICPN • ICTN
- IPN

KEY POINTS

- Tumoral intraepithelial neoplasms (intracholecystic neoplasms of gallbladder and intraductal neoplasms of the bile ducts) present as clinically detectable (papillary/polypoid) masses and account for 5% to 10% of the invasive cancers in this region.
- Flat (non-tumoral) type dysplasia are clinically unapparent incidental lesions; high-grade examples are commonly associated with invasive carcinoma, whereas low-grade ones seem to be clinically insignificant.
- Inflammation/injury–precancer–cancer sequence is well established in the biliary tract (with gallstones, parasites, primary sclerosing cholangitis, and hyalinizing cholecystitis as known risk factors). However, anatomic/chemical carcinogenesis model is also being increasingly appreciated (manifested in choledochal cysts, pancreatobiliary maljunction, and low-union of common hepatic duct with the cystic duct).
- Early (ie, in-situ and minimally invasive pTis/T1) gallbladder cancers have a very good prognosis with the 10-year survival above 90%, provided that a pT2 carcinoma has been ruled out with complete sampling. However, some cases develop biliary cancers many years after the diagnosis, attributable to the field-effect phenomenon.
- Field-effect phenomenon appears to be a significant concern for multifocal carcinogenesis in the biliary tract especially in patients with risk conditions.

---

[a] Department of Pathology, Koc University School of Medicine, Koç Üniversitesi Hastanesi, Davutpaşa Cd. No:4, Zeytinburnu, İstanbul 34010, Turkey; [b] Department of Pathology and Laboratory Medicine, Memorial Sloan Kettering Cancer Center, 1275 York Avenue, New York, NY 10065, USA
* Corresponding author.
E-mail address: vadsay@kuh.ku.edu.tr

Gastroenterol Clin N Am 53 (2024) 85–108
https://doi.org/10.1016/j.gtc.2023.10.001
0889-8553/24/© 2023 Elsevier Inc. All rights reserved.

INTRODUCTION
Incidence and Significance

Premalignant and cancerous lesions of gallbladder (GB) and bile ducts are relatively rare but present a major clinical challenge as they are highly prone to be missed or misdiagnosed because they are commonly mimicked and hidden by the inflammatory/injurious conditions such as stones, parasites, and sclerosing cholangitis, which, paradoxically, are also their main instigators.

The majority of the pre-malignant lesions encountered in these organs is of the "flat" type; that is, do not form clinically, radiologically, and even grossly detectable masses.[1–4] Since these do not form tumoral lesions by themselves, they are typically discovered incidentally next to established cancers, or in procedures performed for other conditions such as gallstones, cholecystitis, or choledochal cysts. Because cholecystectomy is 1 of the most frequently performed operations, and since premalignant processes are incidentally found in about 1% to 5% of the GBs,[5] they are in fact encountered with respectable regularity in daily practice. In contrast, bile ducts are seldom removed unless there is compelling concern for cancer, and therefore these lesions are far less commonly detected in the bile ducts. Pathologic diagnosis of these non-tumoral lesions is highly challenging, especially because mucosal injury in this region is notorious for generating remarkable atypical changes that are very difficult (and at times impossible) to distinguish from true dysplastic/neoplastic alterations.[1,6–10] Moreover, as cancerous transformation often develops in regenerative processes in these sites, it becomes very difficult to determine, where simple regeneration ends and true carcinomatous changes begin. This also leads to variable impressions about the true frequency of dysplastic lesions, especially in the lesser end of the spectrum.[11,12]

The other category of pre-malignant lesions is the tumoral type, that is, mass-forming preinvasive intra-epithelial/intra-mucosal neoplasia ("adenoma-carcinoma sequence"). They can be viewed as counterparts of pancreatic intraductal papillary mucinal neoplasms (IPMNs). These are less common, and manifest as radiologically, clinically, and grossly recognizable lesions, even when they are not invasive. They reveal various cell types, architectures with different biologic connotations, and spectrum of cancerous transformation. It is important to recognize this group because they are often curable if removed completely. They also offer a fascinating model of cancerous transformation for cancer researchers to analyze, with potential implications in carcinogenesis of other organs as well.

CLINICAL FEATURES
Clinical Presentation

As is the case for invasive cancers of most mucosal/epithelial organs, preinvasive lesions of these sites are also seen predominantly in elderly patients. However, at the same time, in most studies, the patients are almost a decade younger than the patients with invasive cancers, supporting the progression phenomenon.[12,13] Not surprisingly, in patients with risk factors such as choledochal cyst,[14] primary sclerosing cholangitis, and pancreatobiliary maljunction,[15–17] both the cancers as well as precancerous lesions occur in significantly younger patients.[11,12] In the populations with gallstones as the main risk factor such as parts of South America and India, GB carcinoma (GBC) shows striking predilection for women. However, this does not seem to hold as true for Far East,[18] for reasons that are not clearly understood.

"Flat" (non-tumoral) forms of dysplasia are by definition microscopic forms of dysplasia and therefore they do not by themselves cause any signs or symptoms if unaccompanied by invasive cancer.[1,10,13] As such, they are detected incidentally in specimens removed for other causes.[13] In contrast, tumoral forms of dysplasia, that is, "intracholecystic neoplasms" (in the GB)[19-21] or "intraductal neoplasms" (in the biliary tract) form clinically/radiologically visible masses (**Fig. 1**). Naturally there are overlaps between the non-tumoral and tumoral forms of dysplasia, and for their distinction a rule of thumb arbitrary criterion of 1 cm size is used.[19] As such, the latter often present with obstruction-related signs and symptoms.[20,22-26] Typically, they appear as filling defects in the lumen of the respective site and at times, they can be mistaken as stones. They can be multifocal; the entity previously known as papillomatosis, which can extensively involve biliary system, is also included in this category.[19] In fact, multifocality and the field-effect phenomenon creates a major issue for the long term management of these patients, in particular, when there is no or minimal invasive carcinoma and long term survival is expected.[19,26-29]

Terminology

The terms "dysplasia" and "preinvasive" (which is synonymous with intraepithelial neoplasia) are probably the best and most accurate to describe these lesions. Premalignant is also a commonly employed name. The term pre-neoplastic is inaccurate since they are fundamentally neoplastic lesions; this term can perhaps be reserved for metaplastic/hyperplastic changes that precede the dysplastic ones.[16]

It is important to acknowledge that in the uppermost end of the spectrum of these lesions is in-situ carcinoma, which is composed of cells that have molecularly and genetically undergone full "malignant transformation" at the cytologic level. However, they technically do not have the ability to exhibit malignant behavior such as metastasis due to their location and confinement by the histologic boundaries such as basement membrane and are thus still included in the "pre"-malignant category. Nevertheless, these lesions are classified as "pTis" within the cancer spectrum.

The spectrum of intraepithelial *neoplastic* transformation ranges from minimal alterations that can be difficult to distinguish from metaplasia/hyperplasia to all the way to

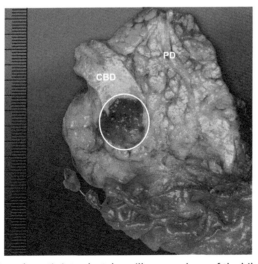

Fig. 1. Biliary IPN. Extra hepatic intraductal papillary neoplasm of the bile ducts, with friable papillary projections (circled), arising from the distal common bile duct (CBD). Main pancreatic duct (PD) is unremarkable.

those that can be qualified as intramucosal or "papillary" adenocarcinoma. Cases previously regarded as "papillomatosis" are also regarded in this spectrum in the tumoral intraepithelial neoplasm category (see later).[7,19,30]

In the World Health Organization (WHO) classification, these lesions are discussed under the heading of biliary intraepithelial neoplasm (BilIN)[31] although the term "dysplasia" is still the one used more widely, especially in the GB.[1] It is important to note here that the term "carcinoma in-situ (CIS)" is mostly abandoned in the WHO classification for the gastrointestinal (GI) tract and replaced by "high-grade dysplasia (HGD)" due to the fear of unwarranted over-interpretation and over-treatment caused by the term "carcinoma".[32] However, in many parts of the world (in particular Far East and South America) the terms CIS and intramucosal adenocarcinoma are widely and liberally used for the uppermost end of the spectrum. This causes controversies in diagnosis and management of these lesions and challenges in analyzing the literature. The authors here also agree that the most aggressive end of the spectrum indeed represents an intramucosal cancerous transformation, and thus should be recognized as such. As a result, bridging the conceptual gap between the East and the West, we use the term "HGD/CIS" together or parenthetically with a commentary for such cases. In fact, for the complex adenocarcinomatous changes confined to the mucosa, experts from Chile where GB cancer incidence is 1 of the highest in the world, the term early GBC (EGBC) is employed for both pTis and pT1 lesions.[27] See later management issues section for further discussion on this issue.

Traditionally, in the guidelines and main texts,[33,34] the proliferations included in this spectrum have been graded, based on the degree of microscopic cytoarchitectural atypia, into 3 tiers as low-grade, intermediate-grade, high-grade, which was later named as BilIN 1, 2, and 3.[35] However, in real life practice a 2-tiered approach have been more widely employed.[1,23] More recently, extrapolating from the modifications in the pancreas as well as in other organs, the 2-tiered approach as low-grade and high-grade has become more official, with the refined criteria that "low-grade" group encompasses the wide spectrum ranging from changes that are metaplasia/hyperplasia-like to convincing low/intermediate-grade dysplasia (ie, corresponding to BilINs 1 and 2), and the "high-grade" terminology is reserved essentially for only frank CIS type lesions.[23] Defined as such, low-grade cases detected incidentally in a resection specimen appear to be clinically insignificant whereas those HGD/CIS cases warrant careful attention because they are often in accompaniment of invasive cancer, or have a high risk of progressing into frank cancer if not treated.

As happened in the pancreas, the mass-forming preinvasive neoplasms (adenoma-carcinoma sequence) are now collected under the conceptual category of tumoral intraepithelial neoplasm and designated as "intracholecystic neoplasms" in the GB, and as "intraductal neoplasms" in the bile ducts. Included in this broad group are a spectrum of lesions including innocuous-appearing polypoid nodules that used to be called "pyloric gland adenomas" to all the way to "papillary adenocarcinoma" or "papillomatosis". Unfortunately, the term papillary adenocarcinoma is still used in some publications as a subset of cholangiocarcinoma, leading to confusion in classification and prognosis. In this broad conceptual group of tumoral intraepithelial neoplasms, distinct entities with different clinicopathologic, behavioral characteristics are being recognized. These include intracholecystic tubular non-mucinous neoplasms and adenomyoma-associated intracholecystic neoplasms in the GB and intraductal papillary neoplasms, intraductal oncocytic papillary neoplasms, and intraductal tubulopapillary neoplasms in the bile ducts.

Risk Factors

Etio-pathogenetically, there are 2 distinct pathways of carcinogenesis in the biliary tract. One is the inflammation-injury associated, which is the predominant one.[36] The other is the anatomic/chemical carcinogenesis pathway.

Inflammation-injury pathway

There are several important conditions that signify risk to develop GB/extrahepatic bile duct (EHBD) cancers through causing inflammation-injury. The common denominator to all these is that more or less they cause local injury that initiates the neoplastic transformation, which starts with regeneration/metaplasia/hyperplasia, and proceeds with dysplasia of various grades, and finally to frank carcinoma.[1,10,35] Some of these (such as gallstone-associated) seem to be more mechanically driven and the transformation takes place in the immediate area of the instigation.

Gallstones are found in association with a significant proportion of the dysplasia of the GB. In high-incidence regions like Chile, about 3% of cholecystectomies removed for gallstones reveal HGD/CIS and significantly higher percentage with precursor metaplastic changes and low-grade dysplasia.[5] While this figure is lower in the Western population, it is still about 1%, which makes up a respectable proportion of millions of cholecystectomies performed every year.[5,37] Of note, about 15% of cholecystectomies reveal epithelial atypia that falls in the differential diagnosis of dysplasia.[5-9,37] These present a major challenge for pathologists.

Parasites, established as risk factor for cancer, are also risk for dysplastic lesions.[38-40] There are various parasites implicated in the process, *Clonorchis sinensis* being the most famous.[41,42] Another one that is worth special mention is *Opistorchis viverrine*, which has been shown to cause intraductal neoplasms in some parts of parts of Thailand.[40] The exact risk of cancerous changes in patients with biliary flukes; however, is difficult to determine.

Primary sclerosing cholangitis is a well-established risk factor for preinvasive and invasive lesions of the biliary tract with substantial field-effect phenomenon.[43,44] In fact, in resections from these patients, dysplastic lesions and sub-clinical early cancers are not uncommonly discovered, even away from the strictures. This is also true for GBs removed with explants. These patients tend to be relatively younger.[45]

Hyalinizing Cholecystitis, a distinctive variant of chronic cholecystitis characterized by diffuse effacement of the GB wall by a thin band of paucicellular, fibrous tissue with a peculiar clefting pattern and minimal or no calcifications (ie, incomplete porcelain GB, **Fig. 2**) has a strong association with carcinoma.[36] Carcinomas that arise in this setting often have a subtle appearance. Extensive sampling is crucial to reveal the presence and extent of carcinoma.[36]

Anatomic/chemical carcinogenesis pathway

Choledochal cysts have now been well established to have a risk for carcinomatous transformation.[14] In fact, more than 15% of resected choledochal cysts are found to harbor HGD/CIS and half of these also have associated invasive carcinoma.[14] A subset of choledochal cysts appear to be closely related to pancreatobiliary maljunction discussed later, and in fact, may be a result of the latter condition, to an extent that Japanese classifications recognize this group as "dilated pancreatobiliary maljunction.[46,47]

Pancreatobiliary maljunction (also known as anomalous union of pancreatobiliary ducts), is in essence supra-Oddi conjunction of Wirsung and common bile duct that is typically associated with "long common channel" in the ampulla.[15-17] This anomaly allows the reflux of pancreatic enzymes into the biliary tract as confirmed by chemical

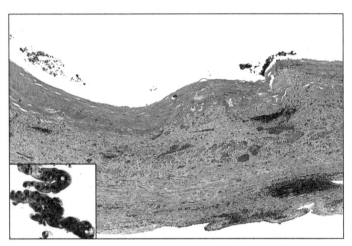

Fig. 2. Hyalinizing cholecystitis is characterized with at least partial hyaline sclerosis of the gallbladder wall. The surface epithelium is extensively, if not completely, denuded. Minimal and often mucosa-associated calcification may be present. Since hyalinizing cholecystitis is typically devoid of epithelium, any epithelial elements on the surface or within the wall should be regarded as a suspect for dysplasia or carcinoma. Hyalinizing cholecystitis with high-grade dysplasia (inset) is depicted here.

analysis of GB bile in these patients. This reflux is believed to be the cause of the very high incidence of GB and bile duct cancers seen in these patients, most proceeding through dysplastic lesions. Pancreatobiliary maljunction is a relatively rare condition in general population, but it accounts for about 8% of GBCs as well as a score of bile duct cancers.[15–17,48] Previously thought to be an Asian disorder, recent studies have shown that pancreatobiliary maljunction also accounts for about 8% of GBCs also in the United States.[16] Patients with pancreatobiliary maljunction exhibit substantial thickening of GB mucosa, which pathologically corresponds to a distinctive mucosal hyperplasia that has been termed reflux cholecystopathy (**Fig. 3**).[15] This

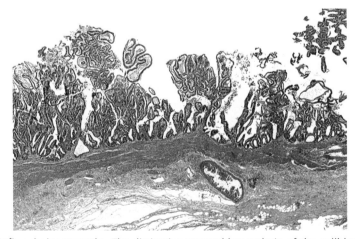

Fig. 3. Reflux cholecystopathy. The distinctive mucosal hyperplasia of the gallbladder seen in pancreatobiliary maljunction. The thick hyperplastic mucosa is continuously pushing into the tunica muscularis. Mucosal folds reveal characteristic bulbous dilatation of the tips.

hyperplasia can then undergo further dysplastic/carcinomatous transformation.[15] Guidelines published by the Japanese Study Group on pancreatobiliary maljunction, established 3 decades ago, recommend abdominal ultrasounds (mandated by the government as a part of general healthcare check-up) to include measurement of GB mucosal thickness. If thickened mucosa is discovered, then further studies are performed to investigate for pancreatobiliary maljunction. If pancreatobiliary maljunction is discovered, patients are taken to cholecystectomy and surveillance of biliary system. Numerous cancer patients have been discovered and many more presumably prevented by this approach.[46,47] Of note, about 25% of pancreatobiliary maljunction-associated cancers develop through intracholecystic neoplasms (and intraductal neoplasms of the bile ducts) whereas these tumoral intraepithelial neoplasms account for 5% to 10% of GBCs otherwise.[15–17] Also the frequency of unusual cancer types such as adenosquamous and neuroendocrine appears to be higher in this group.[49–51] As such, pancreatobiliary maljunction offers a fascinating model of carcinogenesis. It also establishes that reflux-associated chemical induction of carcinoma does occur in this region.[15]

   Low-union of common hepatic duct with the cystic duct (within or immediately adjacent to the pancreas) **(Fig. 4)** is an anatomic variation that is seen in less than 15% of the general population but was recently found to occur in more than 40% of periampullary cancers, and as high as 70% of upper EHBD cancers.[17] These figures seem to be beyond coincidence and bring the question of whether this anatomic variation (short common bile duct) leads to chemical milieu alteration in the biliary system

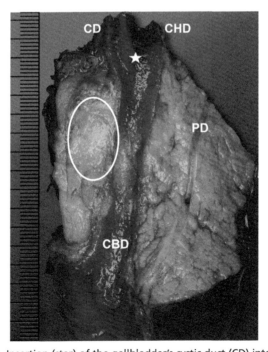

Fig. 4. Low-union. Insertion (star) of the gallbladder's cystic duct (CD) into the common hepatic duct (CHD) within or immediately above (within 5 mm of the pancreas border), known as low-union, is a rare anatomic variation that has been identified in a substantial subset of pancreatic, bile duct and ampullary cancers. A pancreatic ductal adenocarcinoma (circled) is depicted here.

and thus plays a role in carcinogenesis similar to reflux-associated gastroesophageal cancers or pancreatobiliary maljunction-associated cancers discussed earlier. In many cases diagnosed with "pancreatic cancer", the lesion is in the region of this low insertion. Pre-malignant lesions occurring in low-union patients require further scrutiny.

Field-Effect. As commonly observed in the patients with the risk factors discussed earlier, multifocality with synchronous and metachronous dysplastic lesions in different compartments of the biliary tract (including GB and any compartment of EHBD) is a substantial issue. Field-effect (field-defect), a concept well known for other mucosal organs such as the oral cavity and urothelium, seems to be as valid if not more so for the biliary tract.[52] In the literature, it is best documented for patients with primary sclerosing cholangitis,[43,45] although the phenomenon may be even more significant (though less well studied and appreciated) in pancreatobiliary maljunction cases and its associate choledochal cysts.[15–17] This field-effect phenomenon is also an important consideration when precancerous lesions are discovered incidentally. In particular, when an HGD/CIS is found in a cholecystectomy specimen, regardless of whether it is flat (non-tumoral) or tumoral type, there appears to be risk for the biliary tract, with some patients developing cancer in the bile ducts several years after the cholecystectomy.[2,3,19] If the same patient also has (or subsequently found to have) primary sclerosing cholangitis or pancreatobiliary maljunction, then this concern becomes much bigger.

Therefore, in a patient who is discovered to have a precancerous lesion in the GB or bile ducts, it is crucial to investigate the patient for these risk diseases and if found, then the patient should be placed under even-closer surveillance. Along those lines, if a patient with dysplasia or carcinoma in the biliary tract is undergoing a second operation of the region, we advocate to perform bile duct brushing of the remaining system to determine whether there are sub-clinical carcinomatous changes.

PATHOLOGY
Gallbladder

Flat (non-tumoral) dysplasia of gallbladder
These are typically detected incidentally in cholecystectomy specimens. (Pseudo)pyloric gland metaplasia occurs commonly in injured GBs and do not seem to have any recognizable association with dysplasia-carcinoma process, and does not even need to be reported.[1,35,53] Whereas, intestinal metaplasia is observed more commonly in the in background of carcinomatous changes and thus warrant more careful attention and additional examination.[53,54] A form of metaplasia-dysplasia sequence that is being increasingly recognized in the GI tract as "hypermucinous" and "foveolar", is also being characterized also in the GB.[35,37,55] This appears to occur more frequently in the high-incidence regions.[5,55] Transitioning with these metaplastic changes render low-grade dysplasia (LGD) difficult to define (**Fig. 5**). Moreover, LGD has substantial overlaps with atypical regenerative changes. As a result, the diagnosis of LGD is highly subjective and it is difficult to define widely-applicable criteria for it.[1,10,35] However, since LGD does not seem to have any clinical significance by itself, its recognition and accurate diagnosis seems to be of no clinical consequence.[1]

HGD/CIS of GB is detected in 1% to 3% of cholecystectomies depending on the population.[5,37] Importantly, HGD/CIS is seldom caught as a focal finding in otherwise normal mucosa. But rather, when it is diagnosed, it typically involves most of the preserved mucosa. This indicates when carcinomatous transformation takes place in the epithelium, it rapidly spreads to the remainder of the mucosa like a wildfire. HGD/CIS

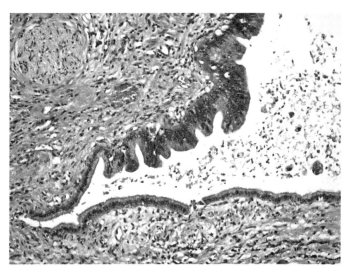

Fig. 5. Low-grade dysplasia (LGD) is difficult to distinguish from reactive atypia. However, pseudostratification of relatively uniform elongated nuclei involving the surface epithelium in the absence of any congestion, active inflammation, or stromal fibrosis is regarded as LGD by most authors.

is defined by diffuse and substantial cytologic atypia showing virtually all the attributes of cancers but by definition are still confined to the epithelium/mucosa (**Fig. 6**).[1,7,10] HGD/CIS display various architectural patterns as well as different cell types.[2–4,55] The significance of these patterns and cell types is still under investigation. Of note, foveolar/hypermucinous cell type, akin to their GI counterparts, is only beginning to be recognized as a form of dysplasia. While foveolar type dysplasia, like its GI kindreds, appears innocuous and is difficult to distinguish from metaplasia; it may be more sinister in biology than the other types.[5,37,55]

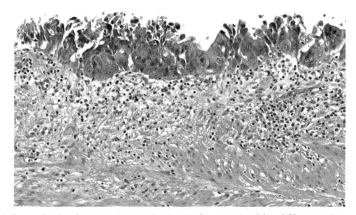

Fig. 6. High-grade dysplasia/carcinoma-in-situ is characterized by diffuse and severe architectural and/or cytologic atypia.

As discussed in the biologic behavior section, perhaps the most important problem regarding the literature on nature of HGD/CIS-only cases (and as an extension of that, of minimally invasive carcinoma cases), is that this diagnosis should not be rendered unless the entire specimen is examined to rule out more deeply invasive carcinomas.[2–4,27] Invasive carcinomas in the GB/EHBD can be extremely subtle as also evidenced by the fact that even close to half of advanced GBCs are diagnosed as "clinically/grossly unapparent".[13] Therefore, evolving guidelines emphasize the importance of total sampling of GB before the diagnosis of HGD/CIS-only is rendered.[1,19]

Tumoral intraepithelial (intracholecystic) neoplasms
These are characterized by papillary/polypoid (grossly and radiologically visible, typically >1 cm) mucosal masses that are distinct from the remaining mucosa and are fundamentally composed of dysplastic cells.[19,22] Essentially, they represent adenoma-carcinoma sequence.

Intracholecystic papillary tubular neoplasms (ICPNs, previously also called intracystic papillary neoplasm) are the prototype and the most common examples of intracholecystic neoplasms.[19] In the earlier literature regarded under 9 different names, they were later collected under 1 heading of ICPNs with the understanding that there are some subsets but there are also striking overlaps.[19,56] There is a spectrum of architectural patterns and spectrum of cell types, often in a mixture (**Fig. 7**). There is also spectrum in the degree of dysplastic transformation. In the lower-most end is the polypoid collection of normal-appearing pyloric type glands that had been dignified as pyloric gland adenoma, with the mean size in largest series being 0.6 and 0.8 cm, most of which are now regarded as polypoid metaplasia unless they form distinct visible polyps (preferably >1 cm).[19,57] The other end are those exuberant papillary tumors with HGD/CIS, which used to be called "papillary adenocarcinomas". Of note, "flat" (non-tumoral) dysplasia can have prominent papillary configuration that forms feathery change in the mucosa but are distinguished from the ICPNs by the lack of a visible tumor/polyp formation. Invasive carcinomas are detected in about 60% of resected ICPNs, and about 5% to 10% of GBCs arise in ICPNs.[19] Invasion can be microscopic and difficult to detect. Therefore, the sampling issues, and

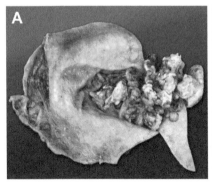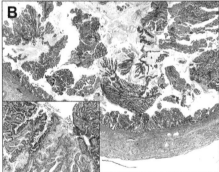

Fig. 7. (*A*) Intracholecystic papillary tubular neoplasms are characterized by a distinct polypoid or papillary mass(es) protruding into the lumen. (*B*) Intracholecystic papillary tubular neoplasms reveal an intraluminal growth of back-to-back papillary and/or tubular units with minimal intervening stroma. Due to their intramucosal nature, the base of the lesions is usually sharply demarcated. However, extension into the Aschoff-Rokitansky sinuses may be seen and mimic invasion. Transition from low-grade to high-grade dysplasia (inset) is evident in most cases. (Courtesy of Dr. Ryan Des Jean)

biologic behavior concepts discussed earlier including the potential concerns for field-effect and margin positivity are even more applicable to ICPNs.

Intracholecystic tubular non-mucinous neoplasm (ICTN) is a highly distinct and invasion-resistant type of intracholecystic neoplasms with specific molecular characteristics. It was previously regarded under the heading of ICPN as its "complex pyloric variant"[19] and also viewed by some in the spectrum of "pyloric gland adenoma".[48,58,59] However, recently the distinctive characteristics of this group became more clearly elucidated.[20,60] These tumors appear to be arising in cholesterol polyps, showing the exact same pedunculated cauliflower-like configuration with very thin stalks. Microscopic examination reveals a complex proliferation with minimal/no mucin (which was recognized as "non-mucinous" in the main paper on this[45]) that readily warrants the diagnosis of "HGD/CIS". In addition to MUC6-positive pyloric differentiation, they also commonly exhibit scattered beta-catenin expressing morules and display Wnt signaling pathway alterations.[61] However, thus-far none of the well-characterized cases reported to have invasive carcinoma. As importantly, just like the cholesterol polyps, they typically occur in GBs without any injury in the GB, and without any dysplastic changes elsewhere. Emerging evidence leads to the conclusion that these most likely arise in cholesterol polyps. Accordingly, the field-effect phenomenon discussed earlier does not at all seem to be applicable to ICTNs.[45]

Intracholecystic neoplasms arising in adenomyomas (or "mural" ICNs) also appear to form a distinct group. By default, they form mural and submucosal-appearing nodules in the fundic region that can be missed. These show several analogies to branch-duct type IPMNs of the pancreas by their localized nature, often multicystic appearance, papillary elements lined by gastric-type epithelium, and carcinomatous changes in about 15%, as well as the lack of dysplastic lesions in the remainder of the luminal GB mucosa.[21] Similar to ICTNs, these intracholecystic neoplasms arising in adenomyomas do not appear to bear the detrimental field-effect that conventional ICPNs present.[19,21]

Extrahepatic Bile Ducts

Flat (non-tumoral) dysplasia
Flat dysplasia in EHBD is typically discovered as a side in resections performed for cancer or 1 of the risk lesions such as choledochal cyst, primary sclerosing cholangitis or pancreatobiliary maljunction.[13] For LGD, the association with metaplasia and regenerative atypia discussed earlier for the GB is also valid for the EHBD. Similarly, LGD of EHBD is by itself of no known clinical significance but should alert the search for higher grade lesions. HGD/CIS, on the other hand, is rarely discovered in isolation. Most of the cases show invasive carcinoma somewhere in the system, bringing up the question of whether they are true preinvasive lesions or post-invasive retrograde "colonization" (cancerization, a.k.a ductal spread of invasive carcinoma cells). Regardless, they warrant careful analysis and complete removal if possible. If HGD/CIS is discovered at a margin, further resection should be attempted, if clinically feasible.[31]

Tumoral intraepithelial (intraductal) neoplasms
Intraductal papillary neoplasms of the bile ducts (IPNBs) are, for all practical purposes, biliary counterparts of pancreatic IPMNs. The entities previously designated as pyloric gland adenoma, intestinal-type adenoma, papillomatosis, or papillary cholangiocarcinoma (papillary adenocarcinoma) of the bile ducts are now all collected under the heading of IPNB.[60,62] Many of the clinicopathologic and biologic characteristics described earlier for ICPNs of GB are also applicable to IPNBs. This includes spectrum

of patterns, cell types, and dysplasia; high frequency of association with invasive carcinoma; multifocality; and field-effect concerns.[19,60,62] Recently, sub-classification of IPNBs as Type A (less complex) versus Type B (more complex and variegated) has been proposed and appears to correlate with frequency of invasion and progression rates.[63–65] Type B lesion appear to have higher rates of progression and aggression.

Intraductal oncocytic papillary neoplasm (IOPN) was for a while regarded as a "variant" of IPNB but is now regarded as a separate category.[60,66] Unlike ordinary IPNBs, IOPNs typically present as complex multilocular cystic and solid masses that is radiologically classified as "cystadenocarcinoma". The papillae are florid and arborizing. However, there is a certain degree of organization and monotony, which, combined with the oncocytic cytology, imparts the distinctive appearance to these tumors (**Fig. 8**). Although they are highly complex and may even appear infiltrative and un-resectable due to their expansile nature, in fact many of the cases have a long protracted clinical course even if there is invasive carcinoma, with 10-year survival over 90% if completely resected.[60,67–70] In addition to their distinctive morphology and more benevolent behavior, these tumors were also found to carry a fusion of PRKACA and PRKACB genes, not seen in other intraductal neoplasms or cholangiocarcinomas.[71,72] They also lack the classical molecular make up of IPNBs and invasive carcinomas of the biliary system.

Intraductal tubulopapillary neoplasms (ITPNs) are another type of mass-forming intraductal neoplasm of the bile ducts.[24,26,60] Unlike the IPNBs, these have tubular architecture and with minimal or no mucin production by the cells (**Fig. 9**).[26,60,73,74] They are often invasive but even then, they appear to have a more indolent behavior. Due to their tubular configuration, they often receive the diagnosis of an ordinary "adenocarcinoma" (cholangiocarcinoma) in limited specimens. However, they lack the molecular genetic alterations typically present in cholangiocarcinomas, and they are also different from IOPNs and IPNBs at the molecular level.[60,73,74]

Mucinous cystic neoplasms (MCNs), similar to those in the pancreas and liver, characterized by the presence of ovarian-type stroma can also occur in the bile ducts and peri-GB region, and almost exclusively in women of perimenopausal age group.[75–77] They typically form multilocular cystic tumors but some may have an intraductal growth. These tumors also represent "adenoma-carcinoma" sequence with neoplastic transformation

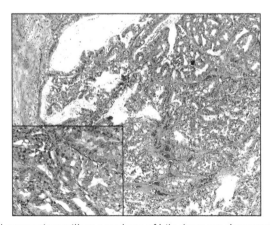

Fig. 8. Intraductal oncocytic papillary neoplasm of bile ducts are characterized with complex papillary projections lined by stratified cells. The cells have abundant eosinophilic granular cytoplasm and nuclei with single, prominent nucleoli (Inset).

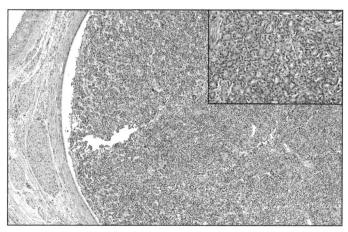

Fig. 9. Intraductal tubulopapillary neoplasm of bile ducts composed of back-to-back tubular glandular structures or punctuated solid areas. The tumor cells have modest amounts of cytoplasm and small and atypical nuclei. There is no obvious intracellular mucin (Inset).

from LGD to HGD to frank carcinoma. However, it appears that carcinomatous transformation is much less common (<5% of the cases) and is often limited in extent and not much clinical consequence as opposed to their pancreatic kindreds where about 15% of the cases show invasive carcinoma and is often mortal.[78]

PATHOLOGIC DIFFERENTIAL DIAGNOSES
Dysplasia Versus Reactive Changes

The differential diagnosis of dysplasia and reactive changes is a well-known problem in GB and EHBD pathology.[79] As discussed previously, pre-malignant lesions often develop in the context of injury and regeneration, and it can be impossible to know where one ends and the other one begins. Molecular studies to document abnormalities in cancer-associated genes (findings that could help to establish the neoplastic nature of lesions) have been limited. Therefore, dysplasia is defined and distinguished from other epithelial lesions based primarily on morphologic principles, drawing in part from experience with early neoplastic changes in the pancreatobiliary tract.

The architectural pattern of growth is helpful in diagnosing dysplasia. Nuclear enlargement and prominent, cherry-red nucleoli are also characteristic features of dysplasia, not seen in reactive lesions.[80] Mitotic figures, including atypical forms, can be prominent in areas of regeneration and are not helpful.

Of note, HGD shows a wildfire phenomenon in the GB, which means it is typically extensive at the time it is detected.[5,80,81] Therefore, focal epithelial atypia in a background of well-preserved non-dysplastic epithelium is more likely to represent reactive changes.

High-Grade Dysplasia Versus Early Invasive Carcinoma

The GB epithelium normally shows undulations and there is no muscularis mucosa to separate the mucosa from submucosa. More importantly, the tunica muscularis is highly irregular and porous.[82] Therefore, dysplastic glands can often be seen lying within or deep to the tunica muscularis. Also, there are no basal or myoepithelial cells that can help distinguish native epithelium from invasive carcinoma. Nevertheless, features that favor true invasive carcinoma include invasion of nerves or blood vessels, haphazard distribution pattern, lack of luminal bile and lack of a connection to benign epithelium at the surface. In the EHBD, pagetoid extension of HGD/CIS into the peri-biliary accessory glands can create a pseudo-invasive appearance. The lobular architecture and even size of units favor the process being non-invasive.

Tumoral Intraepithelial Neoplasms Versus Smaller/Lesser Lesions

Polypoid papillary proliferations, smaller than 1 cm, may occasionally be encountered. If these show clear-cut cytoarchitectural atypia of conventional dysplasia, then they should be acknowledged as pre-malignant. However, especially in the GB, small polypoid collections entirely composed of innocuous pyloric type glands should not be dignified as either "adenoma" or ICPN.[22]

ICPNs also ought to be distinguished from ordinary flat dysplasia, which may reveal epithelial proliferations forming small collections. But these cases should not be regarded as ICPN unless they form a distinct clinically evident and grossly visible mass.

ANCILLARY DIAGNOSTIC TESTS
Immunohistochemical and Molecular Features of Flat (Non-tumoral) Dysplasia

Immunohistochemically, mCEA and MUC1 typically shows staining at the apical border of dysplastic cells. However, intracytoplasmic labeling with mCEA and MUC1 is uncommon. Therefore, dense intracytoplasmic staining favors cancerization over dysplasia. TP53 nuclear staining occurs in more than 30% of cases of dysplasia and tends to be more common in HGD.[83] But it should be kept in mind that it can also be seen in areas of regenerative changes.[84] Similarly, although the Ki67 labeling index is high in cases of dysplasia and increases by grade, it can also be high in areas of regenerative changes.

Oncogenic *KRAS* mutations are uncommon in GB and proximal bile duct dysplasia.[85,86] However, they are identified in about 40% of distal bile duct lesions. *KRAS* mutation represents an early molecular event during the progression of bile duct dysplasia, whereas *TP53* mutation represents a late molecular event.[87,88] *Claudin 18 (CLDN18)* abnormalities are also common.[89] Alterations in cell cycle proteins, including *CDKN1A, cyclin D1* and *SMAD4 (DPC4)* may be detected in some bile duct dysplasia cases.[88]

Immunohistochemical and Molecular Features of Tumoral Intracholecystic Neoplasms

The immunophenotype of ordinary ICPNs[19,90] and IPNBs[60,91] corresponds to their line of differentiation. Most express mucin-related glycoproteins and oncoproteins, including mCEA. The MUC1 is typically confined to HGD. Microsatellite instability can be identified in 10% of IPNBs.[92,93]

Current evidence indicates that molecular alterations of ICPNs are different than those observed in the conventional dysplasia-carcinoma sequence in the GB. They are more similar to those described in intraductal neoplasms of the intrahepatic and extrahepatic bile ducts.[94] Although *KRAS* mutations are common in ICPNs,[83,95] they are uncommon in IPNBs, except for the gastric-type.[60,94] *GNAS* mutation, which is seen in about two-thirds of pancreatic IPMNs[96] is rarely seen in ICPNs[59,62,87] and IPNBs.[62] This disparity is presumably related to the rarity of the intestinal variant in western populations.

Recently, it has been reported that ICTN are associated with the Notch and Wnt/CTNNB1 signaling pathways alterations, harbor mutations in *APC2 and MLL2* (two known regulators of ß-catenin signaling) and reveal aberrant nuclear CTNNB1 protein expression.[61,97]

Immunohistochemical and Molecular Features of Mucinous Cystic Neoplasm

Immunohistochemically, actin, desmin and nuclear progesterone receptor expression is typical. Calretinin, inhibin and CD99 may also be positive. *KRAS* mutations are identified in 20% of MCNs, especially in cases with HGD. However, *GNAS, RNF43* and *PIK3CA* are wild-type in all cases.[75,98]

BIOLOGIC BEHAVIOR AND TREATMENT

Low-grade dysplasia (LGD) does not seem to have any clinical significance in any compartment of the biliary tract. For example, LGD discovered in a cholecystectomy specimen or in a choledochal cyst does not require any further attention provided that there is no other risk factor and the presence of in-situ or invasive carcinoma has been definitively excluded.[11,12,99] It should be acknowledged here that there are substantial subjectivity and reproducibility regarding the diagnosis of LGD and its distinction from regenerative changes. This also emphasizes the importance of second opinions if there is any possibility of a more clinically significant (higher grade) lesion (ie, HGD/CIS) in the differential diagnosis, because HGD/CIS has a very different connotation as discussed later. This also underscores the importance of thorough examination to rule out HGD/CIS in each case.[1,10,99]

Convincing examples of HGD/CIS has been proven to bear a major risk, not only for the same area (as a precursor) but also to the rest of the tract (as a marker, see earlier for field-effect discussion).[2–4,52] This concern of field-risk is higher if the process is extensive. One important aspect in the evaluation of the risk of HGD/CIS is the difficulty of distinguishing them from the "colonization" ("cancerization") phenomenon. Colonization/cancerization refers to the situation in which invasive carcinoma cells invade back into the mucosa retrogradely and mimicking CIS. This process can be impossible to distinguish from a true preinvasive process. They are fundamentally the same cells in different stages, and as of yet, there are no reliable markers to distinguish them.[1,35] These aspects signify the necessity to treat HGD/CIS as a full-blown, albeit curable, form of cancer if an accompanying invasive cancer can be definitively excluded. The presence of underlying risk disease multiplies the concern for progression. Along the same lines, if HGD/CIS is recorded at a margin of resection, the rest of the biliary tract should be regarded as under great risk for cancer development.

For uppermost end of the spectrum where carcinomatous transformation in the mucosa acquires more complex architecture, both the terminology and management become more problematic. he distinction of whether this is to be qualified as merely HGD, or pTis or even pT1a (intramucosal adenocarcinoma) or pT1b (minimally invasive) can often be quite subjective.[1,29,100] This has been most problematic in the GB where a combination of multiple factors have led to different views. First, lack of a complete and well-defined muscularis mucosa layer, as well as the common occurrence of mucosal invaginations (that are permitted by the porous tunica muscularis) allow CIS type changes to form complex invaginations without being truly invasive. Second, there are significant geographic variations in the way such lesions are evaluated by pathologists and treated by clinicians from different continents. To illustrate the magnitude of the issue, in an international consensus study, GBs that had been classified as HGD-only in the United States by multiple experts were actually classified by Asian and South American pathologists not only as CIS, but often as pT1 and even pT2 in close to half of the cases.[100] This is very similar to the issue in the early cancers of the stomach,[32] and it appears that practice-related cultural differences play a role in this. For example, in the Far East the term "carcinoma" does not carry the same concern because of the way pathologic diagnoses are shared with or explained to the patients, and moreover, in some countries patients prefer to receive the "carcinoma" designation because then the government takes on the treatment expenses. In contrast, in the West, the term carcinoma generates unnecessary social connotations including the possible loss of insurance, which oppositely drives the preference to avoidance of this term. As a result, WHO classification essentially eliminated the term "carcinoma in-situ (CIS)" in exchange with "high-grade dysplasia (HGD)" going along with the Western approach, although the concept obviously does exist and has various practical uses and is widely employed in Far East. Irrespective of the reasons for these variations, a case that is confidently classified as HGD in the United States may receive the diagnosis of pT1 uniformly in the East or South America, and unfortunately there are widely different views regarding the management of these 2 diagnoses.

For the GB, circumventing all these criterial variations, in Chile where the GBC incidence is 1 of the highest and GBCs are most well studied, the term early GB cancer (EGBC) has been employed for the spectrum of neoplastic transformation from simple HGD to more atypical forms qualifiable as CIS (pTis) to the frank intramucosal adenocarcinoma (pT1a) with demonstrable invasive carcinoma cells within the mucosa but not beyond. Studies on cohorts in which pT2 (perimuscular invasive) carcinoma has been ruled out with total sampling of GB have shown that in fact not only pTis (HGD/CIS) but also even more complex ones (pT1a) have very good prognosis.[27–29,101] Unfortunately, the literature from the Surveillance Epidemiology End Results (SEER) database, which is still commonly used in reference, draws a much more bleak picture for HGD/CIS indicating that 30% or more of cases succumb to cancer.[1,29,56] This is attributed to the fact that most of the cases in the SEER are based on "random sampling" and thus many are believed to represent under-staged pT2.[27–29,101] In fact, recent studies based on well sampled and well characterized cases have disclosed that not only pT1b cancers[29] but even very superficial pT2 carcinomas have a very good prognosis.[102,103] If a true pT2 GBC (with perimuscular invasion) has been ruled out with careful examination, the 10-year survival of HGD/CIS (and even early invasive cases[5,37]) is above 90%.[28] All of these recent observations serve as further assurance that lesser lesions (pTis cases, ie, HGD/CIS) are indeed much more benevolent than implied in the Western literature, which is mostly based on SEER.

In summary, it is becoming increasingly clear that in the GB, HGD/CIS and even its more complex forms have a very good prognosis, incomparably better than what has been indicated in the earlier literature. However, at the same time, about 5% of the cases show progression and dissemination. The early recurrences are believed to be mostly missed invasive carcinomas and emphasize the importance of sampling and exclusion of deeper lesions.[28,101] At the same time, there are late progressors, some 8 to 10 years after the cholecystectomy, and for these the field-effect and metachronous cancers in the remainder of the biliary tract are suspected to be the source. Extensiveness of HGD/CIS, cell type (for example, biliary), degree of papilla formation, margin positivity, suspect foci of invasion, involvement of Rokitansky-Aschoff sinuses, and especially history of a risk disease like pancreatobiliary maljunction are believed to bring higher risk for progression.

CLINICS CARE POINTS

- Low-grade dysplasia discovered in a cholecystectomy specimen or in a choledochal cyst does not require any further attention if there is no other risk factor, however, it is crucial that the presence of in-situ or invasive carcinoma has been definitively excluded by additional sampling.

- If high-grade dysplasia/carcinoma in-situ is recorded in any part of the biliary tract, the rest of the tract should be regarded as under risk for cancer development. Especially in patients with more extensive high-grade dysplasia/carcinoma in-situ, papillary configuration, biliary phenotype, margin positivity and the presence of an underlying risk factor like primary sclerosing cholangitis or pancreatobiliary maljunction, this risk is much greater, and long-term surveillance is warranted.

- Along those lines, if a patient with dysplasia or carcinoma in the biliary tract is undergoing a second operation of the region, we advocate to perform bile duct brushing of the remaining system to determine whether there are sub-clinical carcinomatous changes.

- *Hyalinizing Cholecystitis*, a distinctive variant of chronic cholecystitis, has a strong association with carcinoma. However, carcinomas arising in this setting often have a subtle appearance. Extensive, if not total, sampling is crucial to reveal the presence and extent of carcinoma.

- Patients with *pancreatobiliary maljunction* present an interesting model of carcinogenesis developing from a distinctive mucosal hyperplasia ("reflux cholecystopathy") to dysplasia (often tumoral type) and finally to invasive carcinoma, which occurs in a very significant proportion of the patients if untreated. It also connotes risk for entire biliary tract mucosa.

- SEER database draws a much more aggressive picture for in-situ and minimally invasive cancers, but this is attributable to the undersampled and underdiagnosed cases of more advanced cancers, because, the data are not supported in carefully crafted institutional studies. This underscores the importance of not rendering the diagnosis of high-grade dysplasia/carcinoma in-situ unless total sampling and careful exclusion of a more advanced carcinomatous process is conducted definitively.

ACKNOWLEDGMENTS

The authors are indebted to Drs. Juan Carlos Roa, Juan Carlos Araya, Hector Losada, and Enrique Bellolio from Chile; Drs. Juan Sarmiento and Jill Koshiol from the USA; Drs. Burcin Pehlivanoglu, Bahar Memis, Burcu Saka, Nevra Dursun, Pelin Bagci, Serdar Balci, Orhun Cig Taskin, and Zeynep Tarcan for their contributions to the studies that constitute the basis of most of the discussions provided in this text.

DISCLOSURE

O Basturk has been supported in part by the Cancer Center Support Grant of the National Institutes of Health, United States/National Cancer Institute, United States under award number P30CA008748.

REFERENCES

1. Roa JC, Basturk O, Adsay V. Dysplasia and carcinoma of the gallbladder: pathological evaluation, sampling, differential diagnosis and clinical implications. Histopathology 2021;79(1):2–19.
2. Bagci P, Dursun N, Saka B, et al. High grade dysplasia (intraepithelial neoplasia) of the gallbladder (GB): patterns, cell lineages and clinicopathologic associations in an analysis of 255 cases. Mod Pathol 2012;25:154a.
3. Bagci P, Saka B, Erbarut I, et al. Growth patterns of high-grade gallbladder dysplasia: clinicopathologic associations and diagnostic implications in an analysis of 318 cases. Mod Pathol 2013;26:422a.
4. Bagci P, Saka B, Erbarut I, et al. Cellular phenotypes in gallbladder dysplasia: diagnostic significance and clinical associations in an analysis of 318 cases. Lab Invest 2013;93:398a.

5. Koshiol J, Bellolio E, Vivallo C, et al. Distribution of dysplasia and cancer in the gallbladder: an analysis from a high cancer-risk population. Hum Pathol 2018; 82:87–94.

6. Hacihasanoglu E, Memis B, Pehlivanoglu B, et al. Factors impacting the performance characteristics of bile duct brushings a clinico-cytopathologic analysis of 253 patients. Arch Pathol Lab Med 2018;142(7):863–70.

7. Adsay V, Roa JC, Basturk O, et al. Epithelial atypia in the gallbladder: diagnosis and classification in an international consensus study. Mod Pathol 2016;29: 438a–9a.

8. Reid MD, Graham R, Memis B, et al. FISH'ing to verify the nature of different epithelial alterations in the gallbladder: molecular abnormalities are common in neoplastic but not in reactive lesions, thus validating the santiago criteria and potential usefulness of fish as an adjunct in diagnosis. Mod Pathol 2017; 30:450a.

9. Avadhani V, Hacihasanoglu E, Memis B, et al. Cytologic predictors of malignancy in bile duct brushings: a multi-reviewer analysis of 60 cases. Mod Pathol 2017;30(9):1273–86.

10. Adsay V, Saka B, Basturk O, et al. Criteria for pathologic sampling of gallbladder specimens. Am J Clin Pathol 2013;140(2):278–80.

11. Aloia TA, Jarufe N, Javle M, et al. Gallbladder cancer: expert consensus statement. Hpb 2015;17(8):681–90.

12. Balakrishnan A, Barmpounakis P, Demiris N, et al. Surgical outcomes of gallbladder cancer: the OMEGA retrospective, multicentre, international cohort study. Eclinicalmedicine 2023;59:101951.

13. Mazer LM, Losada HF, Chaudhry RM, et al. Tumor characteristics and survival analysis of incidental versus suspected gallbladder carcinoma. J Gastrointest Surg. Jul 2012;16(7):1311–7.

14. Mericoz CA, Hacihasanoglu E, Muraki T, et al. Evaluation and pathologic classification of choledochal cysts clinicopathologic analysis of 84 cases from the west. Am J Surg Pathol 2021;45(5):627–37.

15. Muraki T, Memis B, Reid MD, et al. Reflux-associated cholecystopathy analysis of 76 gallbladders from patients with supra-oddi union of the pancreatic duct and common bile duct (pancreatobiliary maljunction) elucidates a specific diagnostic pattern of mucosal hyperplasia as a prelude to carcinoma. Am J Surg Pathol 2017;41(9):1167–77.

16. Muraki T, Pehlivanoglu B, Memis B, et al. Pancreatobiliary maljunction-associated gallbladder cancer is as common in the west, shows distinct clinicopathologic characteristics and offers an invaluable model for anatomy-induced reflux-associated physio-chemical carcinogenesis. Ann Surg 2022;276(1): E32–9.

17. Muraki T, Reid MD, Pehlivanoglu B, et al. Variant anatomy of the biliary system as a cause of pancreatic and peri-ampullary cancers. HPB 2020;22(12): 1675–85.

18. Kwon W, Kim H, Han Y, et al. Role of tumour location and surgical extent on prognosis in T2 gallbladder cancer: an international multicentre study. Br J Surg 2020;107(10):1334–43.

19. Adsay V, Jang KT, Roa JC, et al. Intracholecystic papillary-tubular neoplasms (icpn) of the gallbladder (neoplastic polyps, adenomas, and papillary neoplasms that are >= 1.0 cm) clinicopathologic and immunohistochemical analysis of 123 cases. Am J Surg Pathol 2012;36(9):1279–301.

20. Pehlivanoglu B, Balci S, Basturk O, et al. Intracholecystic tubular non-mucinous neoplasm (ICTN) of the gallbladder: a clinicopathologically distinct, invasion-resistant entity. Virchows Arch 2021;478(3):435–47.
21. Rowan DJ, Pehlivanoglu B, Memis B, et al. Mural intracholecystic neoplasms arising in adenomyomatous nodules of the gallbladder an analysis of 19 examples of a clinicopathologically distinct entity. Am J Surg Pathol 2020;44(12): 1649–57.
22. Adsay V, Mino-Kenudson M, Furukawa T, et al. Pathologic evaluation and reporting of intraductal papillary mucinous neoplasms of the pancreas and other tumoral intraepithelial neoplasms of pancreatobiliary tract recommendations of verona consensus meeting. Ann Surg 2016;263(1):162–77.
23. Basturk O, Hong SM, Wood LD, et al. A revised classification system and recommendations from the baltimore consensus meeting for neoplastic precursor lesions in the pancreas. Am J Surg Pathol 2015;39(12):1730–41.
24. Katabi N, Torres J, Klimstra DS. Intraductal tubular neoplasms of the bile ducts. Am J Surg Pathol 2012;36(11):1647–55.
25. Kloppel G, Adsay V, Konukiewitz B, et al. Precancerous lesions of the biliary tree. Best Pract Res Cl Ga 2013;27(2):285–97.
26. Schlitter AM, Jang KT, Kloppel G, et al. Intraductal tubulopapillary neoplasms of the bile ducts: clinicopathologic, immunohistochemical, and molecular analysis of 20 cases. Mod Pathol 2016;29(1):93.
27. Roa JC, Tapia O, Manterola C, et al. Early gallbladder carcinoma has a favorable outcome but Rokitansky-Aschoff sinus involvement is an adverse prognostic factor (vol 463, pg 651, 2013). Virchows Arch 2013;463(6):851.
28. Patel K, Balci S, Saka B, et al. "Carcinoma In-Situ" of the gallbladder: the seer database perspective. Mod Pathol 2014;27:452a–3a.
29. Pehlivanoglu B, Akkas G, Memis B, et al. Reappraisal of T1b gallbladder cancer (GBC): clinicopathologic analysis of 473 in situ and invasive GBCs and critical review of the literature highlights its rarity, and that it has a very good prognosis. Virchows Arch 2023;482(2):311–23.
30. Adsay NV, Bagci P, Tajiri T, et al. Pathologic staging of pancreatic, ampullary, biliary, and gallbladder cancers: pitfalls and practical limitations of the current AJCC/UICC TNM staging system and opportunities for improvement. Semin Diagn Pathol 2012;29(3):127–41.
31. Basturk O, Aishima S, Esposito I. Biliary intraepithelial neoplasia. In: Klimstra DSLA, Paradis V, Schirmacher P, editors. WHO classification of tumours: digestive system tumours. 5th Edition. Lyon, France: International Agency for Research on Cancer; 2019. chap Tumours of the Gallbladder and Extrahepatic Bile Ducts.
32. Vieth M, Riddell RH, Montgomery EA. High-grade dysplasia versus carcinoma east is east and west is west, but does it need to be that way? Am J Surg Pathol 2014;38(11):1453–6.
33. Basturk O, Adsay NV. Benign and malignant tumors of the gallbladder and extrahepatic biliary tract. In: Odze R, Goldblum JR, editors. *Surgical pathology of the GI tract, liver, biliary tract, and pancreas*. 4th Edition. Philadelphia, PA: Elsevier; 2022.
34. Basturk O., Adsay N.V. Diseases of the gallbladder. In: L F, ed. MacSween's pathology of the liver. 8th Edition Elsevier; (In Press).
35. Zen Y, Adsay NV, Bardadin K, et al. Biliary intraepithelial neoplasia: an international interobserver agreement study and proposal for diagnostic criteria. Mod Pathol 2007;20(6):701–9.

36. Patel S, Roa JC, Tapia O, et al. Hyalinizing cholecystitis and associated carcinomas: clinicopathologic analysis of a distinctive variant of cholecystitis with porcelain-like features and accompanying diagnostically challenging carcinomas. Am J Surg Pathol 2011;35(8):1104–13.

37. Memis B, Reid MD, Bedolla G, et al. Pathologic findings in gallbladders: an analysis of the true frequency and distribution in 203 totally sampled and mapped gallbladders from a north american population. Mod Pathol 2017;30:447a.

38. Callea F, Sergi C, Fabbretti G, et al. Precancerous lesions of the biliary tree. J Surg Oncol Suppl 1993;3:131–3.

39. Parkin DM, Ohshima H, Srivatanakul P, et al. Cholangiocarcinoma: epidemiology, mechanisms of carcinogenesis and prevention. Cancer Epidemiol Biomarkers Prev 1993;2(6):537–44.

40. Nitta T, Nakanuma Y, Sato Y, et al. Pathological characteristics of intraductal polypoid neoplasms of bile ducts in Thailand. Int J Clin Exp Pathol 2015;8(7):8284–90.

41. Purtilo DT. Clonorchiasis and hepatic neoplasms. Trop Geogr Med 1976;28(1):21–7.

42. Kim YI, Yu ES, Kim ST. Intraductal variant of peripheral cholangiocarcinoma of the liver with Clonorchis sinensis infection. Cancer 1989;63(8):1562–6.

43. Bergquist A, Glaumann H, Persson B, et al. Risk factors and clinical presentation of hepatobiliary carcinoma in patients with primary sclerosing cholangitis: a case-control study. Hepatology 1998;27(2):311–6.

44. Lewis JT, Talwalkar JA, Rosen CB, et al. Precancerous bile duct pathology in end-stage primary sclerosing cholangitis, with and without cholangiocarcinoma. Am J Surg Pathol 2010;34(1):27–34.

45. Lewis JT, Talwalkar JA, Rosen CB, et al. Prevalence and risk factors for gallbladder neoplasia in patients with primary sclerosing cholangitis: evidence for a metaplasia-dysplasia-carcinoma sequence. Am J Surg Pathol 2007;31(6):907–13.

46. Kamisawa T, Ando H, Hamada Y, et al. Diagnostic criteria for pancreaticobiliary maljunction 2013. J Hepatobiliary Pancreat Sci 2014;21(3):159–61.

47. TJSGoPMJTCoJfD Criteria. Diagnostic criteria of pancreaticobiliary maljunction. J Hepatobiliary Pancreat Surg 1994;1:219–21.

48. Fukumura Y, Rong L, Maimaitiaili Y, et al. Precursor lesions of gallbladder carcinoma: disease concept, pathology, and genetics. Diagnostics 28 2022;12(2). https://doi.org/10.3390/diagnostics12020341.

49. Dursun N, Escalona OT, Roa JC, et al. Mucinous carcinomas of the gallbladder clinicopathologic analysis of 15 cases identified in 606 carcinomas. Arch Pathol Lab Med 2012;136(11):1347–58.

50. Roa JC, Tapia O, Cakir A, et al. Squamous cell and adenosquamous carcinomas of the gallbladder: clinicopathological analysis of 34 cases identified in 606 carcinomas. Mod Pathol 2011;24(8):1069–78.

51. Reid MD, Roa JC, Memis B, et al. Neuroendocrine neoplasms of the gallbladder. an immunohistochemical and clinicopathologic analysis of 29 cases. Mod Pathol 2017;30:196a.

52. Reid M, Losada H, Muraki T, et al. Field risk ("field-effect"/"field-defect") in the gallbladder and biliary tree: an under-recognized phenomenon with major implications for management and carcinogenesis. Lab Invest 2019;99.

53. Basturk O, Tapia O, Roa JC, et al. Metaplasia in the gallbladder: populational differences in the incidence of intestinal metaplasia supports its association with carcinoma. Modern Pathol. Jan 2009;22:307a–8a.

54. Dursun N, Roa JC, Tapia O, et al. Metaplasia in the gallbladder: an analysis of clinicopathologic associations in 1218 cholecystectomies. Lab Invest 2011;91: 147a.

55. Memis B, Roa JC, Araya J, et al. Frequency of dysplasia/carcinoma and foveolar atypia associated with gallbladder cancer risk: comparative analysis in mapped/totally sampled gallbladders from high-risk versus low-risk regions. Lab Invest 2019;99.

56. Albores-Saavedra J, Henson DE, Klimstra DS, et al. Tumors of the gallbladder, extrahepatic bile ducts, and vaterian system. AFIP atlas of tumor pathology fourth series, fasc 23. American Registry of Pathology 2015;xix:614, pages : illustrations (black and white, and colour).

57. Taskin OC, Basturk O, Reid MD, et al. Gallbladder polyps: Correlation of size and clinicopathologic characteristics based on updated definitions. PLoS One 2020;15(9):e0237979.

58. Nakanuma Y, Sugino T, Nomura K, et al. Pathological features of pyloric gland adenoma of the gallbladder in comparison with gastric subtype of intracholecystic papillary neoplasm. Ann Diagn Pathol 2022;56:151879.

59. He C, Fukumura Y, Toriyama A, et al. Pyloric gland adenoma (PGA) of the gallbladder: a unique and distinct tumor from pgas of the stomach, duodenum, and pancreas. Am J Surg Pathol 2018;42(9):1237–45.

60. Wang T, Askan G, Ozcan K, et al. Tumoral intraductal neoplasms of the bile ducts comprise morphologically and genetically distinct entities. Arch Pathol Lab Med 2023. https://doi.org/10.5858/arpa.2022-0343-OA.

61. Robinson B, Fisher K, Pehlivanoglu B, et al. CTNNB1-Mutations define a subset of preinvasive mass-forming lesions in the gallbladder with reduced malignant potential. Mod Pathol 2018;31:687.

62. Matthaei H, Wu J, Dal Molin M, et al. GNAS codon 201 mutations are uncommon in intraductal papillary neoplasms of the bile duct. HPB (Oxford) 2012;14(10): 677–83.

63. Kubota K, Jang JY, Nakanuma Y, et al. Clinicopathological characteristics of intraductal papillary neoplasm of the bile duct: a Japan-Korea collaborative study. J Hepatobiliary Pancreat Sci 2020;27(9):581–97.

64. Nakanuma Y, Jang KT, Fukushima N, et al. A statement by the Japan-Korea expert pathologists for future clinicopathological and molecular analyses toward consensus building of intraductal papillary neoplasm of the bile duct through several opinions at the present stage. J Hepato-Bil-Pan Sci 2018;25(3):181–7.

65. Zen Y, Akita M. Neoplastic Progression in Intraductal Papillary Neoplasm of the Bile Duct. Arch Pathol Lab Med 2023. https://doi.org/10.5858/arpa.2022-0407-RA.

66. Rouzbahman M, Serra S, Adsay NV, et al. Oncocytic papillary neoplasms of the biliary tract: a clinicopathological, mucin core and Wnt pathway protein analysis of four cases. Pathology 2007;39(4):413–8.

67. Basturk O, Tan M, Bhanot U, et al. The oncocytic subtype is genetically distinct from other pancreatic intraductal papillary mucinous neoplasm subtypes. Mod Pathol 2016;29(9):1058–69.

68. Marchegiani G, Mino-Kenudson M, Ferrone CR, et al. Oncocytic-type intraductal papillary mucinous neoplasms: a unique malignant pancreatic tumor with good long-term prognosis. J Am Coll Surg 2015;220(5):839–44.

69. Adsay NV, Adair CF, Heffess CS, et al. Intraductal oncocytic papillary neoplasms of the pancreas. Am J Surg Pathol 1996;20(8):980–94.

70. Basturk O, Chung SM, Hruban RH, et al. Distinct pathways of pathogenesis of intraductal oncocytic papillary neoplasms and intraductal papillary mucinous neoplasms of the pancreas. Virchows Arch 2016;469(5):523–32.

71. Vyas M, Hechtman JF, Zhang Y, et al. DNAJB1-PRKACA fusions occur in oncocytic pancreatic and biliary neoplasms and are not specific for fibrolamellar hepatocellular carcinoma. Mod Pathol 2020;33(4):648–56.

72. Singhi AD, Wood LD, Parks E, et al. Recurrent rearrangements in PRKACA and PRKACB in intraductal oncocytic papillary neoplasms of the pancreas and bile duct. Gastroenterology 2020;158(3):573–582 e2.

73. Basturk O, Berger MF, Yamaguchi H, et al. Pancreatic intraductal tubulopapillary neoplasm is genetically distinct from intraductal papillary mucinous neoplasm and ductal adenocarcinoma. Mod Pathol 2017;30(12):1760–72.

74. Pehlivanoglu B, Adsay V. Intraductal tubulopapillary neoplasms of the bile ducts: identity, clinicopathologic characteristics, and differential diagnosis of a distinct entity among intraductal tumors. Hum Pathol 2023;132:12–9.

75. Quigley B, Reid MD, Pehlivanoglu B, et al. Hepatobiliary mucinous cystic neoplasms with ovarian type stroma (so-called "hepatobiliary cystadenoma/cystadenocarcinoma") clinicopathologic analysis of 36 cases illustrates rarity of carcinomatous change. Am J Surg Pathol 2018;42(1):95–102.

76. Armutlu A, Quigley B, Choi H, et al. Hepatic cysts reappraisal of the classification, terminology, differential diagnosis, and clinicopathologic characteristics in 258 cases. Am J Surg Pathol 2022;46(9):1219–33.

77. Zhelnin K, Xue Y, Quigley B, et al. Nonmucinous biliary epithelium is a frequent finding and is often the predominant epithelial type in mucinous cystic neoplasms of the pancreas and liver. Am J Surg Pathol 2017;41(1):116–20.

78. Jang KT, Park SM, Basturk O, et al. Clinicopathologic characteristics of 29 invasive carcinomas arising in 178 pancreatic mucinous cystic neoplasms with ovarian-type stroma: implications for management and prognosis. Am J Surg Pathol 2015;39(2):179–87.

79. Katabi N. Neoplasia of gallbladder and biliary epithelium. Arch Pathol Lab Med 2010;134(11):1621–7.

80. Bagci P, Saka B, Erbarut I, et al. Cellular phenotypes in gallbladder Dysplasia: Diagnostic significance and clinical associations in an analysis of 318 cases (Abstract). Mod Pathol 2013;26:398A.

81. Bagci P, Saka B, Erbarut I, et al. Growth patterns of high-grade gallbladder dysplasia: Clinicopathologic associations and diagnostic implications in an analysis of 318 cases (Abstract). Mod Pathol 2013;26:422A.

82. Raparia K, Zhai QJ, Schwartz MR, et al. Muscularis mucosae versus muscularis propria in gallbladder, cystic duct, and common bile duct: smoothelin and desmin immunohistochemical study. Ann Diagn Pathol 2010;14(6):408–12.

83. Wistuba II, Miquel JF, Gazdar AF, et al. Gallbladder adenomas have molecular abnormalities different from those present in gallbladder carcinomas. Hum Pathol 1999;30(1):21–5.

84. Priya TP, Kapoor VK, Krishnani N, et al. Fragile histidine triad (FHIT) gene and its association with p53 protein expression in the progression of gall bladder cancer. Cancer Invest 2009;27(7):764–73.

85. Rijken AM, van Gulik TM, Polak MM, et al. Diagnostic and prognostic value of incidence of K-ras codon 12 mutations in resected distal bile duct carcinoma. J Surg Oncol 1998;68(3):187–92.

86. Suto T, Habano W, Sugai T, et al. Aberrations of the K-ras, p53, and APC genes in extrahepatic bile duct cancer. J Surg Oncol 2000;73(3):158–63.

87. Hsu M, Sasaki M, Igarashi S, et al. KRAS and GNAS mutations and p53 overexpression in biliary intraepithelial neoplasia and intrahepatic cholangiocarcinomas. Cancer 2013;119(9):1669–74.

88. Nakanishi Y, Zen Y, Kondo S, et al. Expression of cell cycle-related molecules in biliary premalignant lesions: biliary intraepithelial neoplasia and biliary intraductal papillary neoplasm. Hum Pathol 2008;39(8):1153–61.

89. Shinozaki A, Shibahara J, Noda N, et al. Claudin-18 in biliary neoplasms. Its significance in the classification of intrahepatic cholangiocarcinoma. Virchows Arch 2011;459(1):73–80.

90. WCoTE Board. Digestive System Tumours. WHO classification of tumours series. 5th edition1. Lyon (France): International Agency for Research on Cancer; 2019. WHO classification of tumours series.

91. Zen Y, Sasaki M, Fujii T, et al. Different expression patterns of mucin core proteins and cytokeratins during intrahepatic cholangiocarcinogenesis from biliary intraepithelial neoplasia and intraductal papillary neoplasm of the bile duct–an immunohistochemical study of 110 cases of hepatolithiasis. J Hepatol 2006; 44(2):350–8.

92. Abraham SC, Lee JH, Hruban RH, et al. Molecular and immunohistochemical analysis of intraductal papillary neoplasms of the biliary tract. Hum Pathol 2003;34(9):902–10.

93. Abraham SC, Lee JH, Boitnott JK, et al. Microsatellite instability in intraductal papillary neoplasms of the biliary tract. Mod Pathol 2002;15(12):1309–17.

94. Schlitter AM, Born D, Bettstetter M, et al. Intraductal papillary neoplasms of the bile duct: stepwise progression to carcinoma involves common molecular pathways. Mod Pathol 2014;27(1):73–86.

95. Pai RK, Mojtahed K, Pai RK. Mutations in the RAS/RAF/MAP kinase pathway commonly occur in gallbladder adenomas but are uncommon in gallbladder adenocarcinomas. Appl Immunohistochem Mol Morphol 2011;19(2):133–40.

96. Wu J, Matthaei H, Maitra A, et al. Recurrent GNAS mutations define an unexpected pathway for pancreatic cyst development. Sci Transl Med 2011;3(92): 92ra66.

97. Robinson B, Fisher K, Xu J, et al. Comparative Genetic analysis of invasion-resistant (complex non-mucinous pyloric) and invasion-prone types of intracholecytstic papillary-tubular neoplasms of the gallbladder (abstract). Mod Pathol 2015;28:187A.

98. Fujikura K, Akita M, Abe-Suzuki S, et al. Mucinous cystic neoplasms of the liver and pancreas: relationship between KRAS driver mutations and disease progression. Histopathology 2017;71(4):591–600.

99. Adsay NV, Basturk O, Roa JC, et al. Standardization of pathologic sampling and evaluation of gallbladder specimens: recommendations of the international study group on gallbladder cancer (ISG-GBC) of international hepato-pancreato-biliary association (IHPBA). Lab Invest 2022;102(Suppl 1):1206.

100. Roa JC, Basturk O, Torres J, et al. Marked geographic differences in the pathologic diagnosis of non-invasive (Tis) vs minimally invasive (T1) gallbladder cancer: santiago consensus conference highlights the need for the unifying category "early gallbladder cancer" (EGBC). Mod Pathol 2016;29:447a.

101. Kim HS, Park JW, Kim H, et al. Optimal surgical treatment in patients with T1b gallbladder cancer: An international multicenter study. J Hepato-Bil-Pan Sci 2018;25(12):533–43.

102. Chu J, Jang KT, Roa JC, et al. Prognostic validation of T2-Substaging of gall-bladder carcinomas: survival analysis of 127 korean cases with T2 substaging and survival correlation. Mod Pathol 2017;30:443a.
103. Memis B, Roa JC, Muraki T, et al. Not all T2 gallbladder carcinomas (GBC) are equal: proposal for sub-staging of T2 GBC with significant prognostic value. Mod Pathol 2016;29:445a.

Hepatic Precancerous Lesions and Early Hepatocellular Carcinoma

Kwun Wah Wen, MD, PhD*, Sanjay Kakar, MD

KEYWORDS

- Dysplastic nodule • Hepatocellular adenoma • Atypical hepatocellular neoplasm

KEY POINTS

- High-grade dysplastic nodule is the main precursor lesion for hepatocellular carcinoma (HCC) in cirrhotic liver and is distinguished from early HCC by stromal invasion, diffuse glutamine synthetase, and glypican-3 expression.
- Genomic features that favor HCC over high-grade dysplastic nodule include mutations in telomerase reverse transcriptase (TERT) promoter, CTNNB1, and TP53, as well as copy number alterations (1q, 8q gains).
- Risk factors for HCC in hepatocellular adenoma (HCA) include size >5 cm, male gender, and β-catenin activation; the risk varies by subtype being the lowest in hepatocyte nuclear factor 1α (HNF1A)-inactivated HCA and slightly higher (5%–10%) in inflammatory HCA (I-HCA), whereas the risk in sonic hedgehog and unclassified types is not fully known.
- β-catenin-activated adenomas (especially those with CTNNB1 exon 3 mutation) have a high risk of concurrent or subsequent HCC leading to the suggestion that this diagnosis should be avoided in biopsy and the designation of "atypical hepatocellular neoplasm" should be used.
- Diffuse staining with glutamine synthetase (GS) is an excellent marker for β-catenin activation for cases with CTNNB1 exon 3 mutation, whereas GS shows peripheral accentuation and is usually not diffuse in cases with CTNNB1 exon 7/8 mutation due to weak activation of wingless/integrated (Wnt) signaling.

INTRODUCTION

Hepatocellular carcinogenesis in the setting of cirrhosis is a multistep process that begins with large regenerative nodules (LRNs) (**Fig. 1**), which then may progress to high-grade dysplastic (HGD) nodule and finally to hepatocellular carcinoma (HCC). In non-cirrhotic livers, hepatocellular adenomas (HCAs) may lead to complications, such as bleeding, but some may also transform to HCC, with the risk determined by the clinical setting and the adenoma subtype. There has been progress in understanding of the

505 Parnassus Avenue, M545, Box #0102, San Francisco, CA 94143, USA
* Corresponding author.
E-mail address: Kwun.Wen@ucsf.edu

Gastroenterol Clin N Am 53 (2024) 109–132
https://doi.org/10.1016/j.gtc.2023.11.005
0889-8553/24/© 2023 Elsevier Inc. All rights reserved.

gastro.theclinics.com

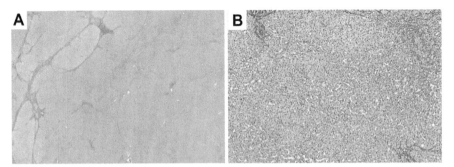

Fig. 1. Large regenerative nodule (LRN). (*A*) The LRN (*right*) stands out compared with the smaller cirrhotic nodules (*left*) (10x). There is no cytoarchitectural atypia. (*B*) Reticulin stain (100x) shows largely intact reticulin framework.

molecular basis of HCAs that has led to recognition of several subtypes, some of which can be aided with the use of immunohistochemistry. Accurate diagnosis of HCC and its precursor lesions is imperative for effective treatment and patient outcomes. This review focuses specifically on HCC precursor lesions and focuses morphology, immunohisto-chemical, and molecular tools that may help pathologists diagnose these lesions.

HEPATOCELLULAR CARCINOMA PRECURSOR LESIONS IN CIRRHOSIS
Terminology and Clinical Features

There are a variety of neoplastic precursor lesions that may develop in patients with cirrhosis that pose a risk for malignant progression. These are both at the cellular (microscopic) level and also visible, often as nodules at the gross (macroscopic) level. At the microscopic level, lesions such as large and small cell change and dysplastic foci are often used. In contrast, *LRNs*, also known as macroregenerative nodules, are defined as nodular lesions with a diameter of $\geq$ 1 cm.[1] They may be detected radiologically or in explants, but these are not considered neoplastic.

The term *large cell change* (**Fig. 2**A) refers to cells with nuclear atypia characterized by large cell size, hyperchromasia, pleomorphism, and multinucleation. The cytoplasmic size increases proportionally with the nuclear size, which results in maintenance of the nuclear-to-cytoplasmic (N:C) ratio. The term "large cell dysplasia" may

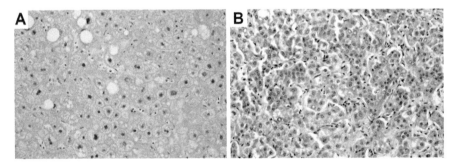

Fig. 2. Large cell and small cell changes. (*A*) Large cell change is characterized by nuclear enlargement, hyperchromasia, and preserved N:C ratio (200x). (*B*) Small cell change is characterized by cells smaller than normal hepatocytes with crowding, mild cytologic atypia, and high N:C ratio (200x).

be used for this lesion as well, but it is not preferred. The term *small cell change* (**Fig.** 2B) refers to hepatocytes with decreased cell volume, increased N:C ratio, mild nuclear atypia, and cytoplasmic basophilia, which gives the impression of nuclear crowding at a low power microscopic magnification. This is a definite neoplastic precursor lesion and may form visible nodules (see further as follows). *Dysplastic focus* refers to a lesion with dysplastic changes that measures less than 1 cm and, thus, is difficult to identify on gross examination. A dysplastic focus may show large cell or small cell change. *Dysplastic nodule* refers to a lesion with dysplastic hepatocytes that is ≥ 1 cm in size.

Dysplastic nodules are exclusively present in cirrhosis and exhibit cytoarchitectural atypia that is insufficient for a definitive diagnosis of HCC. They are classified into low and high grade based on the degree of cellular atypia. *Low-grade dysplastic (LGD) nodules* are thought to be composed of clonal proliferation of hepatocytes that lack high-grade features. *HGD nodules* (**Figs. 3** and **4**), by definition, show cytoarchitectural atypia that is insufficient for a definite diagnosis of HCC. They may be detected

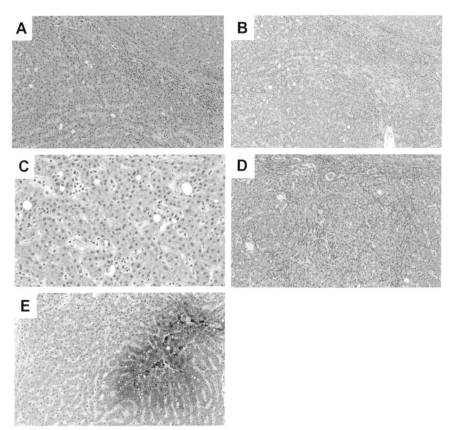

Fig. 3. High-grade dysplastic nodule. (*A*) Small cell change, mild cytologic atypia, and focally thick cell plates; mild ductular reaction can be seen at the interface with the adjacent liver (*top right*) (200x). (*B*) Ductular reaction is present at the interface of the HGD nodule and the background liver (*top right*) (100x). (*C*) Focal pseudoacinar architecture in HGD nodule (400x). (*D*) Reticulin stain highlights small cell change and focally thick cell plates with no significant loss of reticulin framework (200x). (*E*) Glutamine synthetase stain shows perivenular staining without diffuse staining typical of β-catenin activation (200x).

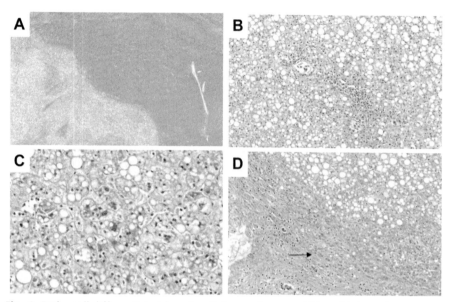

Fig. 4. Early well-differentiated hepatocellular carcinoma within a high-grade dysplastic nodule. (*A*) Nodule of steatotic HCC (*left*) arising in the background of HGD nodule (*right*) imparting a "nodule-in-nodule" appearance (40x). (*B*) Early HCC is often diffusely steatotic and may show minimal cytologic atypia similar to HGD nodule (200x). (*C*) Focal area with less fat and more prominent cytologic atypia in early HCC (400x). (*D*) Stromal invasion (*arrow*) characterized by extension of neoplastic hepatocytes into the adjacent fibrous stroma with no ductular reaction (200x).

radiologically or in explants. The distinction of HGD nodule from HCC can be challenging on imaging. Early HCC (see **Fig. 4**; **Fig. 5**) may be difficult to distinguish from HGD nodule on biopsy as some of the diagnostic features, such as stromal invasion may not be sampled. The distinction of HGD nodule from progressed HCC can be established by biopsy in most cases. Even when the radiologic features are typical of HCC and lesions are classified as LR-5 (in the LIRADS scheme), the reported error rate is 5% to 15%.[2,3] Both EASL and AASLD guidelines state the importance of biopsy when a higher level of certainty is required.[2,4] A more accurate diagnosis is essential for trials as well as for many systemic therapies. Eligibility of transplantation and consideration of resection are also reserved for cases with confirmed diagnosis of HCC and not applicable to HGD nodules.

Once lesions are considered malignant they are classified as either small or large. *Small HCCs* are HCCs with diameter of less than 2 cm and are associated with better survival.[5] Small HCC can be further subclassified into early HCC (see **Figs. 4** and **5**) and progressed HCC.[6] Other terms that have been used to describe early HCC include early well-differentiated HCC, vaguely nodular HCC, and HCC with indistinct margins/borders. On MRI, progressed HCCs are typically hypointense on T1-weighted and variably hyperintense on T2-weighted images, and a capsule is often present. On contrast-enhanced imaging, typical features of HCC are arterial hyperenhancement and wash out in the venous phase. In contrast, HGD nodule and early HCC show similar features including lack of a capsule, lack of typical arterial enhancement with isointense or hypointense appearance in arterial phase, and lack of typical washout in the venous phase.[7] The use of hepatobiliary-specific contrast agents can be helpful as regenerative

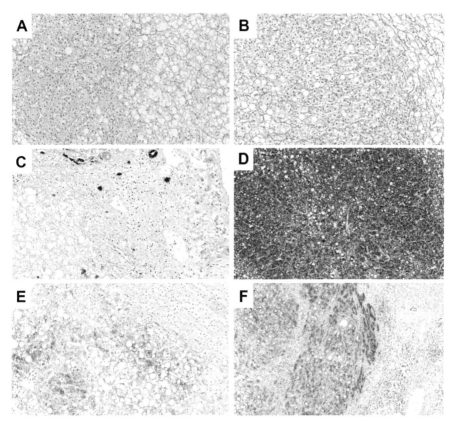

Fig. 5. Early well-differentiated hepatocellular carcinoma. (*A*) Reticulin stain in early HCC highlights focal loss of reticulin framework and focally thick cell plates in the non-steatotic area (*left*) (200x). Reticulin framework is often fragmented in steatotic areas even in non-neoplastic liver and hence reticulin pattern in these areas is not helpful. (*B*) Reticulin stain in early HCC demonstrates crowding and focally thick cell plates (200x). (*C*) CK7 stain demonstrates the lack of ductular reaction at interface of steatotic early HCC (*left*) and the adjacent portal tract (*right*) (200x). (*D*) Glutamine synthetase stain shows diffuse homogeneous staining in early HCC (100x). (*E*) Glypican-3 stain is positive in the early HCC but negative in the adjacent HGD nodule (200x). (*F*) Glypican-3 is positive in the early HCC but negative in the adjacent background liver (200x).

nodules are usually iso- or hyperintense in the hepatocyte phase, whereas HGD nodule and HCC can by hypointense.[8] Overall, the radiologic features that favor HCC are hypo-intensity on T1-weighted images, hyperintensity on T2- and diffusion-weighted images, hyperenhancement on the arterial phase, and hypointensity on the portal venous and hepatocyte phases.[8] However, there can be overlap in imaging features of regenerative nodules, HGD nodule, and early HCC.

Risk Factors and Pathogenesis

The pathogenesis of HCC in patients with cirrhosis is a progressive and multistep process, which starts from LRNs and progresses through LGD and HGD nodules and finally to HCC. It has been argued that large cell change is a predictive marker for HCC in chronic HBV patients, but is itself not preneoplastic.[9] Other studies have demonstrated abnormal DNA content[10] and increased labeling index in large cell change suggesting that it may be a preneoplastic phenomenon.[9]

Small cell change is typical of HGD nodules and well-differentiated HCC. DNA content abnormalities, increased proliferative index, and p53 overexpression have been identified in small cell change.[10–12] Small cell change is detected more frequently in cirrhosis with HCC than in cirrhosis without HCC.[13] The term "small cell dysplasia" is not preferred because this can also be observed in regenerative foci or areas with cellular senescence.[14,15] Small cell change may be a clonal process (with inactivation of cell cycle checkpoints) secondary to DNA damage and telomere shortening.[11,16]

Both LRNs and LGD nodules most often arise in cirrhosis,[10,11] but they can also be seen in other settings such as portal vein thrombosis or Budd–Chiari syndrome in non-cirrhotic livers. HGD nodules are associated with chronic liver disease with cirrhosis. For example, the etiologies and risks factors include hepatitis B or C infection, alcohol, nonalcoholic steatohepatitis, and metabolic syndrome.

HGD nodules have some molecular abnormalities that overlap with HCC: Mutations in *TERT* promoter are thought to be one of the earliest somatic genetic alterations in the transformation to HCC[17] and have been reported in approximately 5% LGD nodules, 20% of HGD nodules, 60% of early HCC, 40% of small HCC, and 65% in progressed HCC.[18–20] Mutations in *CTNNB1*, most commonly involving exon 3, are observed in 20% to 30% of all HCC with higher numbers (40%) in those with hepatitis C (HCV) infection.[21,22] *CTNNB1* mutations are rare or absent in HGD nodule.[23–25] Mutations on other components of the Wnt signaling pathway such as *AXIN1* and *APC* have been reported in 25% to 55% and 2% of HCC, respectively, but not in dysplastic nodules.[26–28] *TP53 mutations* occur in 25% to 45% of HCCs and are associated with worse prognosis.[20,26,29] *TP53* mutations are not observed in HGD nodules.[29] Copy number alterations, such as gains of 1q, 8p, and 8q and loss of 8p, 8q, and 22q, are common even in early HCC and occur in 5% to 8% of HGD nodules.[25,30] Gene expression profiling using reverse transcription-polymerase chain reaction (RT-PCR) has showed that 12 genes were differentially expressed in early HCCs compared with dysplastic nodule.[31] A three-gene set composed of GPC-3, LYVE1 (a lymphatic vessel endothelial receptor), and survivin demonstrated a discriminative accuracy of 94%.[31] However, these results need to be further validated before they can be recommended for clinical practice.

In summary, *TERT* promoter mutations and some of the copy number alterations occur early in hepatocarcinogenesis and are present in a small subset of HGD nodules, whereas *TP53* mutations and Wnt signaling alterations are later steps in progression and are usually not observed in HGD nodules.[25] Other genomic alterations observed in HCC such as *CDKN2A* loss, *MYC* amplification, *PTEN* mutation, and *ARID1A* mutation also occur later in HCC progression and are not seen in HGD nodules.[25]

Pathologic Features of Preneoplastic Lesions in Cirrhosis

LRNs may have a softer texture and may show outward bulging compared with other cirrhotic nodules. Microscopically, LRNs are similar to other cirrhotic nodules except for their size and comprise 1 to 2 cell thick hepatic plates with intact reticulin framework, interspersed portal tracts, and no cytoarchitectural atypia.

The gross features of LGD nodules are similar to those of LRNs. The hepatocytes of LGD nodules may be slightly smaller in size and may show distinctive findings compared with the background cirrhotic nodules such as fat, Mallory hyaline, bile stasis, clear cytoplasmic, iron, or copper deposits.

HGD nodules may grossly and microscopically show a "nodule-in-nodule" phenomenon in which a nodule of higher grade lesion (such as HCC) is present within a larger outer nodule of lower grade lesion (such as HGD nodules). Cytologic abnormalities manifest as small cell change, higher cell density, and mild nuclear atypia, whereas architectural changes include thick cell plates (usually 2–3 cells thick), focal pseudoacini, few unpaired arterioles, and focal fragmentation or loss of reticulin framework.[6]

Early HCC is characterized by indistinct margins, lack of capsule, and often shows morphologic features similar to HGD nodule.

ANCILLARY DIAGNOSTIC TESTS AND DIFFERENTIAL DIAGNOSIS
Ancillary Diagnostic Tests

There are a variety of immunohistochemical and molecular tests that may be used by pathologists to help diagnose and differentiate neoplastic precursor lesions.

CD34
Patchy sinusoidal staining with cluster of differentiation (CD)34 often at the periphery is typical of HGD nodules, whereas diffuse sinusoidal staining favors HCC.[32] CD34 staining can be more diffuse in some HGD nodules, whereas a prominent increase in sinusoidal staining with CD34 is not seen in a subset of HCC. Increased CD34 is also seen in other lesions, such as HCAs and focal nodular hyperplasia (FNH), although it is usually patchy in those entities. CD34 stain is more useful to identify lesional tissue than to distinguish HGD nodules from HCC.[33]

Glypican-3
Glypican-3 (GPC-3) is a cell surface heparin sulfate proteoglycan that is an oncofetal antigen expressed in embryonal/fetal tissue. Staining is negative in normal adult liver[34] and benign conditions such as FNH, HCA, and cirrhotic nodules. Staining patterns include cytoplasmic and/or membranous pattern.[35]

GPC-3 is positive in 60% to 80% of HCCs with a high sensitivity in poorly differentiated HCC, whereas positive staining is observed in less than 10% of HGD nodules and tends to be focal.[34–37] The sensitivity is low (<50%) for well-differentiated HCC. Occasional positive result can occur in regenerative nodules and active hepatitis C.[35,38]

Glutamine synthetase
As a downstream target of β-catenin signaling, GS is more sensitive than nuclear β-catenin for immunohistochemical detection of Wnt/β-catenin pathway activation. Diffuse staining is seen in the setting of β-catenin activation in 30% to 40% of HCC[22] and up to 70% of early HCC.[37] Diffuse GS staining (moderate to strong staining in more than half of the tumor cells) is rare in HGD nodules.[37] However, the absence of diffuse GS staining does not exclude HCC.

Heat shock protein 70
Heat shock protein 70 (HSP70) is a chaperone protein involved in cell cycle regulation and apoptotic activity. Positive staining has been reported in 90% of early HCC, whereas positive results in HGD nodules are rare.[37] HSP70 staining tends to be focal in HCC, and diffuse staining is seen in less than one-third of early HCC.[37] Variable degree of HSP70 expression can occur in non-neoplastic hepatocytes, often at the edge of mass lesions.[39] In our experience, HSP70 is not useful for diagnosis in most cases. HSP70 is also not specific for HCC and can be seen in a wide variety of non-hepatocellular tumors, including intrahepatic cholangiocarcinoma and metastatic carcinoma.[34,37,40,41]

CK7/CK19
Ductular reaction (CK7/CK19 positive) is usually present at the parenchymal–stromal interface in regenerative nodules. The absence of ductular reaction at the periphery is

a feature of stromal invasion that is characteristic of HCC. Cytokeratin (CK)7 and CK19 stains can help in demonstrating the lack of ductular reaction at the interface in HCC nodules.[42] Ductular reaction is usually present at the interface in HGD nodules: Stromal invasion can be focal and may not be sampled in a biopsy. Ductular reaction can be focally absent in HGD nodules.

Other markers
Several other markers such as *clathrin heavy chain* and *enhancer of zeste homologue* have been reported to be helpful.[43] Sensitivity of 93% for the diagnosis of early HCC has been reported with the use of these markers in conjunction with GPC-3, HSP70, and GS.[43] However, these are not widely used or available and need further validation before being adopted for routine diagnosis.

Genetic changes
CTNNB1 and *TP53* mutations are not observed in HGD nodules, whereas p*TERT* mutations are seen in 20% of HGD nodules (vs 60% of early HCC). Hence, the presence of these genomic changes favors HCC. Chromosomal gains/losses (eg, chromosomes 1q, 8q gains) are uncommon in HGD nodules and favor HCC.[44,45]

Differential Diagnosis of Key Lesions

Low-grade dysplastic nodule versus large regenerative nodule
In most instances, LGD nodules are indistinguishable from LRNs without clonality testing. The distinction of LRNs and LGD nodules can be arbitrary based on morphology and is not clinically relevant. We do not make the diagnosis of LGD nodule in our practice.

High-grade dysplastic nodule versus large regenerative nodule
The presence of small cell change, focally thick cell plates, focal pseudoacini, patchy increase in CD34 sinusoidal staining, and focal loss of reticulin favor HGD nodule.

High-grade dysplastic nodule versus early hepatocellular carcinoma
Stromal invasion is the earliest feature of HCC and is one of the most important distinguishing features from HGD nodules (**Table 1**). In contrast to early HCC, progressed HCC has a capsule, well-delineated margins/borders and morphologic features similar to conventional HCC that are greater than 2 cm.

Morphologic features
The histologic changes are a continuum from HGD nodule to early HCC. The most important distinguishing feature is the presence of stromal invasion in early HCC. This is characterized by invasion of neoplastic hepatocytes beyond the confines of the nodule into the stroma of portal tracts, fibrous septa, or adjacent parenchyma. However, this feature can be challenging to discern in a needle biopsy. Early HCC shows more cytoarchitectural atypia (increased cellularity, high N:C ratios, increased mitotic activity/proliferative index, pseudoglands, loss of portal tracts) than HGD nodule.

Histochemistry and immunohistochemistry
Reticulin framework abnormalities tend to be higher in early HCC. Diffuse CD34 sinusoidal staining, diffuse staining with glutamine synthetase (GS), and aberrant expression of glypican-3, HSP70, and nuclear β-catenin are more often seen in HCC.[34,37,40] The lack of ductular reaction at the leading edge of stromal invasion can be highlighted by CK7 and CK19. Because none of these results are specific for HCC, a combination of stains can be more helpful. HGD nodules can occasionally show some expression in any one of the markers.[37] The combination of GPC-3, CD34, and HSP70 has been

Table 1
Key distinctive features between high-grade dysplastic nodule and well-differentiated hepatocellular carcinoma

	High-Grade Dysplastic Nodule	Well-Differentiated Hepatocellular Carcinoma
Size	Usually <2 cm	Most >2 cm, early HCC is <2 cm.
Degree of atypia	Minimal	Mild; atypia is more evident in progressed HCC but can be minimal in early HCC
Extent of atypia	May be focal or diffuse	Usually diffuse
Reticulin framework	Intact or focal loss/fragmentation	Multifocal loss/fragmentation in progressed HCC; may be focal in early HCC
Stromal invasion	Absent	Present, but may be difficult to assess on biopsy
Ductular reaction at interface of nodule with adjacent liver (CK7/CK19)	Usually present circumferentially	Often absent in some areas of the interface
CD34 sinusoidal staining	Focal and often confined to the periphery	Diffuse in most cases of progressed HCC; may be focal in early HCC
Diffuse GS staining (β-catenin activation)	Absent	Can be present
Glypican-3 (GPC-3)	Absent or focal positive	Can be positive
HSP70	Usually negative	Can be positive
TERT promoter mutation	Present in <20%	Present in 50%–60%
TP53 mutation CTNNB1 mutation	Not present	Can be present
Chromosomal gains (1q, 8q, 7q)	Present in <10%	One or more changes present in most cases

Abbreviations: GS, glutamine synthetase; HSP, heat shock protein; *TERT*, telomerase reverse transcriptase.

advocated for distinguishing HGD nodules and early HCC with a specificity of 100% for HCC if two of these three markers are positive[37,40] (including early and well-differentiated HCC). The sensitivity was 72% in resections and 50% in biopsies.[37,40] In our experience, GS is the most helpful stain and diffuse staining strongly points toward HCC. GPC-3 is helpful if positive but has low sensitivity in this setting. In our experience, HSP70 stain is rarely helpful in these situations.

Prognosis

The risk of progression of LRNs and LGD nodules to HCC is similar or slightly higher compared with cases with smaller cirrhotic nodules.[46,47] HGD nodules are associated with a fourfold higher risk of HCC progression, with the reported malignant transformation rates of 12.5% to 80%.

Treatment and Outcome

There are no guidelines for treatment or follow-up for LRN and LGD nodules.[18] Ablation or resection is not required for LRNs and LGD nodules. HGD nodules are often treated with radiofrequency ablation but increased surveillance or resection is not recommended based on current guidelines. Because biopsy result of an HGD nodule does not exclude unsampled HCC, further management such as ablation versus repeat biopsy is based on correlation with radiologic features. This is contrast to HCC, for which resection is preferred unless the HCC tumor is unresectable.

PRECURSOR LESIONS IN PATIENTS WITHOUT CIRRHOSIS
Hepatocellular Adenoma

Clinical features
HCA, or hepatic adenoma, is a clonal hepatocellular neoplasm that most often arises in the non-cirrhotic setting. Five major subtypes have been described based on morphologic, immunohistochemical, and molecular features.[48] They include hepatocyte nuclear factor-1α (HNF1α)-inactivated HCA (H-HCA), inflammatory HCA (I-HCA), β-catenin-activated HCA (B-HCA), sonic hedgehog HCA (shHCA), and unclassified HCA (U-HCA)[49] (**Table 2**). There are many good reviews and studies on the various different subtypes of HCA.[30,50–53]

All HCA subtypes except the B-HCA with *CTNNB1* exon 3 deletion are uncommon in men. Most are associated with oral contraceptive pill usage. I-HCA is the most common subtype, representing 40% to 50% of sporadic HCAs followed by H-HCA which comprises 30% to 40% of cases. B-HCAs comprise approximately 5% to 10% of all HCAs. The relatively new subtype shHCA accounts for approximately 4% of all HCAs. About 5% to 10% of HCAs do not fit into the morphologic, immunohistochemical, or molecular features of the defined subtypes and have been designated as unclassified (U-HCAs).

The term "atypical hepatocellular neoplasm" (AHN) (see **Figs. 8** and **10**) has been proposed for well-differentiated hepatocellular neoplasms in non-cirrhotic livers that have atypical morphologic, immunohistochemical, and/or molecular features that are insufficient for a definite diagnosis of HCC.[30,52–54] Other terms such as "hepatocellular neoplasm of uncertain malignant potential" and "borderline lesion" have also been used.[52,55] We do not advocate the use of the term "atypical adenoma" and prefer to designate tumors with minor degree of atypia that is within the spectrum of adenoma as HCA without using the term "atypical." We use the term "AHN" if the atypia is sufficiently concerning but not severe enough for HCC. We also categorize all β-catenin-activated tumors either with or without atypia as AHN (at least on biopsy) due to the high risk of concurrent or subsequent HCC (**Table 3**).

Risk factors and pathogenesis
H-HCA shows an association with oral contraceptive usage/estrogen exposure as well as maturity-onset diabetes of the young type 3 (MODY3).[56,57] Familial hepatic adenomatosis and microadenomas have been associated with this HCA variant. I-HCA is strongly associated with oral contraceptive pill and estrogen exposure, and this is more common in females. Other clinical factors include risk factors for metabolic syndrome (eg, obesity, fatty liver disease, glycogenosis, increased alcohol consumption) and older age. The *CTNNB1* exon 3 deletion mutational subtype is associated with male gender (~40%), androgen usage, and hepatic vascular disease. The shHCA variant is less studied but has been reported to be associated with obesity.

Pathologic features
Hepatocyte nuclear factor 1α-inactivated hepatocellular adenoma. H-HCA is defined by biallelic inactivation of the gene *TCF1/HNF1A* that encodes HNF1α[56] (**Figs. 6** and **7**). HNF1α is a transcription factor regulating gluconeogenesis and lipogenesis

Table 2
Clinical and pathologic features of hepatocellular adenomas

Hepatocellular Precursors	Sex	Clinical Features and Risk Factors	Pathogenesis	Pathologic Features	GS	β-Catenin	CRP	SAA	LFABP	HCC Risk
I-HCA	F	OCP, DM, steatotic liver disease	JAK/STAT activation; 10% with β-catenin activation	Sinusoidal dilatation, inflammation, dystrophic vessels, ductular reaction	Perivenular	Membranous	Diffuse	Diffuse	Retained	Low
H-HCA	F	OCP, MODY3, adenomatosis	HNF1A inactivation	Steatosis, occasional pseudoglands	Perivenular	Membranous	Not increased	Not increased	Retained	Very low
B-HCA (CTNNB1 exon 3 deletion)	F/M	Young, androgen use	β-catenin activation (strong to intermediate)	Cytologic and architectural atypia, cholestasis	Diffuse homogeneous or heterogeneous	Nuclear, may be focal	Not increased	Not increased	Retained	High
B-HCA (CTNNB1 exon 7/8)	F	OCP	β-catenin activation (weak)	Not unique	Peripheral enhancement	Membranous	Not increased	Not increased	Retained	Low
shHCA	F	OCP, obesity	Sonic hedgehog activation	Hemorrhage	Perivenular	Membranous	Not increased	Not increased	Retained	Rare
U-HCA	F	Not known	Others	Not unique	Perivenular	Membranous	Not increased	Not increased	Retained	Low

Abbreviations: B, β-catenin; CRP, C-reactive protein; DM, diabetes mellitus; GS, glutamine synthetase; H, HNF1A inactivated; HCA, hepatocellular adenoma; HNF, hepatocyte nuclear factor; I, inflammatory; JAK/STAT, Janus kinase/signal transducers and activators of transcription; LFABP, liver fatty acid binding protein; MODY3, maturity-onset diabetes of the young type 3; OCP, oral contraceptive pill; SAA, serum amyloid A; sh, sonic hedgehog; U, unclassified.

Table 3
High-risk features in hepatocellular adenomas

Feature	Description	Significance
Clinical setting	Male gender, size >5 cm	Resection recommended
Focal atypical morphologic features	Cytoarchitectural atypia and/or reticulin abnormalities present but not sufficient for HCC	Consider resection or molecular testing if clinically necessary
Atypical morphologic features in H-HCA	Myxoid change, prominent pseudoacini, marked lipofuscin pigment	Consider resection or molecular testing if clinically necessary
β-catenin activation	Diffuse GS staining, nuclear beta-catenin, and/or CTNNB1 exon 3 mutation	Resection is recommended

in hepatocytes.[58] In H-HCA, mutation in *TCF1* results in downregulation of liver fatty acid-binding protein (LFABP) expression, leading to large and small droplet steatosis in the lesion. There is usually no significant inflammation. Immunohistochemistry for LFABP shows a lack of expression in the tumor cells, whereas the background liver and other HCA variants show retained LFABP expression.[59] Reticulin stain often shows a packeting pattern with the reticulin fibers wrapping around small groups of hepatocytes but the overall reticulin framework is largely intact (see **Fig. 6**).

In H-HCA, the presence of myxoid change, abundant lipofuscin pigment, prominent pseudoglandular architecture, and absence of steatosis have been identified as high-risk features[60,61] (see **Fig. 7**). Fat is a typical feature of H-HCA but may be sparse or absent in 10% to 15% of cases.[61] These cases show a characteristic morphology with an admixture of cells with lightly eosinophilic cytoplasm and cells with cytoplasmic clearing (see **Fig. 7**A). Focal pseudoglandular architecture is common but can be prominent in a minority of cases (see **Fig. 7**D). Rare H-HCA cases exhibit a highly characteristic morphology with prominent loose eosinophilic matrix between plates of neoplastic cells. This morphologic pattern has been referred to as "myxoid" change. Reticulin fibers encircling small groups of hepatocytes ("packeting") is a common feature in H-HCA (see **Fig. 6**C), but overt loss of reticulin framework should raise the possibility of HCC (see **Fig. 7**C). LFABP-negative HCC can be very well-differentiated and can closely resemble H-HCA. If the diagnosis is not clear based on morphology and reticulin

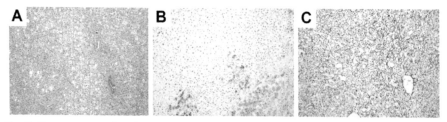

Fig. 6. Hepatocyte nuclear factor-1α-inactivated hepatocellular adenoma (H-HCA). (*A*) Well-differentiated hepatocellular proliferation with an admixture of eosinophilic and clear cells and patchy cytoplasmic fat (100x). (*B*) Loss of liver fatty acid binding protein (LFABP) in the tumor cells by immunohistochemistry (100x). (*C*) Reticulin stain shows encircling of small groups of tumor cells by reticulin fibers ("packeting") without overt loss of reticulin framework (100x).

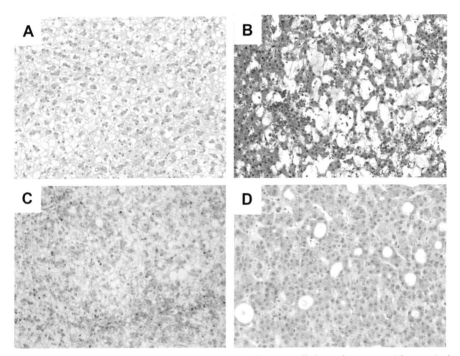

Fig. 7. Hepatocyte nuclear factor-1α-inactivated hepatocellular adenoma with atypical features. (*A*) Prominent lipofuscin pigment (200x) in lesional hepatocytes is considered a high-risk feature in H-HCA. (*B*) Neoplastic cells in H-HCA separated by abundant loose eosinophilic matrix ("myxoid change") are also considered a high-risk feature (200x). (*C*) Reticulin stain in an LFABP-negative HCC highlights loss of reticulin framework; these tumors can be extremely well differentiated and difficult to distinguish from H-HCA (200x). (*D*) H-HCA with prominent pseudoacinar pattern (10x). This was a focal finding, and the remaining areas did not show this pattern.

stain, demonstration of genomic abnormalities in addition to *HNF1A* mutations can help to distinguish H-HCA from LFABP-negative HCC.[61]

Diffuse GS staining has been reported in a small minority of cases but genetic alterations in Wnt signaling or nuclear β-catenin has not been detected. The significance of diffuse GS in H-HCA is unclear and may not be a high-risk feature.[61]

Inflammatory hepatocellular adenoma. The key signature of I-HCA is the constitutive activation of the Janus kinase/signal transducers and activators of transcription (JAK/STAT) signaling pathway with mutations in *IL6ST*, *JAK1*, *STAT3*, *FRK*, and *GNAS* (**Figs. 8** and **9**). The lesional tissue typically shows sinusoidal dilatation/telangiectasia, ductular reaction, inflammation, dystrophic arterioles, and hemorrhage. Although the background liver may show steatosis and hepatocellular ballooning, the lesional tissue shows no or minor amount of fat in most cases.

Immunohistochemistry for the acute phase reactants serum amyloid-associated (SAA) protein and C-reactive protein (CRP) (more sensitive but less specific than SAA) is diffusely positive. The main differential diagnosis is FNH, which shows ductular reaction and fibrous septa with thick vessels and can be positive for SAA (rare) and CRP (usually patchy). The classic map-like staining for GS in FNH helps in distinguishing it from I-HCA. Although SSA and CRP are useful to confirm I-HCA subtype, it is not helpful to distinguish it from HCC, as HCC can be positive for either or both markers.[50]

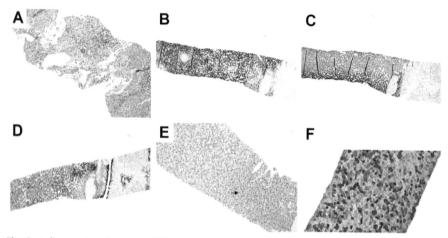

Fig. 8. Inflammatory hepatocellular adenoma (I-HCA) with β-catenin activation (atypical hepatocellular neoplasm) due to *CTNNB1* exon 3 deletion. (*A*) Well-differentiated hepatocellular proliferation with minima cytoarchitectural atypia, sinusoidal dilatation, inflammation, and dystrophic arterioles (100x). (*B*) Serum amyloid A (SAA) stain demonstrates diffuse staining in the tumor (40x). (*C*) C-reactive protein (CRP) stain demonstrates diffuse staining in the adenoma (40x). (*D*) Glutamine synthetase stain shows diffuse strong staining in the tumor (*left*) indicating β-catenin activation, whereas perivenular staining is seen in the adjacent normal liver (*right*) (40x). (*E*) Reticulin stain highlights focal loss of reticulin framework (*arrow*) (40x). Owing to focal reticulin loss and β-catenin activation, this was designated as AHN on biopsy and resection was recommended. (*F*) GS stain on a different I-HCA case with S45 mutation demonstrates diffuse heterogeneous staining ("starry sky") pattern (200x).

β-catenin activation due to *CTNNB1* mutations has been noted in 10% of IHCA ("mixed inflammatory/β-catenin" tumors) and approximately 50% of *CTTNB1* exon 3 mutated HCA exhibits activation of the inflammatory pathway[51,59] (see **Fig. 8**). Hence, GS stain should be obtained in all cases of I-HCA (see **Figs. 8** and **9**). If GS staining result is indeterminate, molecular assays for detecting activation of the Wnt/β-catenin pathway can be obtained.[62]

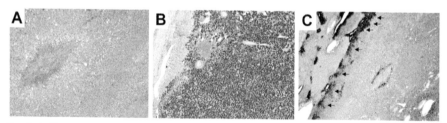

Fig. 9. Inflammatory hepatocellular adenoma (I-HCA) with *CTNNB1* exon 8 mutation. (*A*) I-HCA with focal sinusoidal dilatation, inflammation, dystrophic arterioles and no significant cytoarchitectural atypia (40x). (*B*) C-reactive protein (CRP) stain demonstrates diffuse staining in the tumor cells (40x). (*C*) Glutamine synthetase stain shows patchy weak staining in the tumor (*right*) with enhancement of staining at the rim (*arrows*) and normal perivenular staining in adjacent liver (*left*) (20x). *CTNNB1* exon 8 mutation leads to weak β-catenin activation and does not lead to diffuse GS staining but is associated with strong staining at the periphery of the tumor.

In rare instances, nodules with morphologic and immunohistochemical features similar to I-HCA can occur in alcoholic cirrhosis or cirrhosis due to other etiologies.[54,63] These nodules usually show mutations typical of I-HCA such as those involving *IL6ST*, *STAT3*, and *GNAS*.[54] The rate of progression of I-HCA-like lesions in cirrhosis is not clear. From a practical standpoint, we recommend considering them equivalent to HGD nodules for management until more detailed outcome data becomes available.

β-catenin-activated hepatocellular adenomas fall in two categories. *CTNNB1* exon 3 mutated subtype (**Fig. 10**): These tumors harbor large in-frame deletions or mutations involving exon 3 and show moderate (T41A mutation) or high (most others) levels of β-catenin activation. This leads to diffuse homogeneous GS staining (moderate to strong staining in ≥90% of the tumor cells) in most of these tumors (**Table 4**). On the other hand, S45 mutations are associated with a low level of β-catenin activation and tend to show diffuse heterogeneous staining (moderate to strong staining in 50%–90% of the tumor cells) that has been referred to as the "starry sky" pattern[51,55,62,64,65] (see **Fig. 8F**) (see **Table 4**). Nuclear β-catenin is more common in cases with strong beta-catenin activation and absent or focal with S45 mutation.[55]

This subtype of B-HCA can occur in males and in the setting of androgen usage[66] and hepatic vascular diseases.[67] Cytologic atypia, small cell change, pseudoglands,

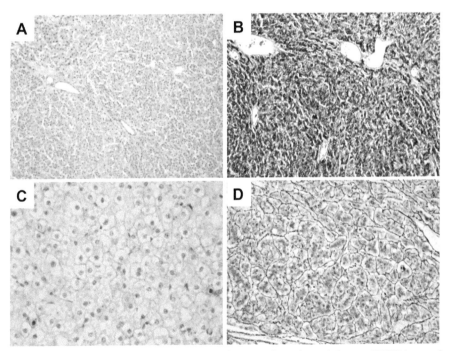

Fig. 10. Atypical hepatocellular neoplasm with β-catenin activated due to *CTNNB1* exon 3 deletion. (*A*) Well-differentiated hepatocellular neoplasm with small cell change, focally thick cell plates, and mild cytologic atypia (40x). (*B*) Glutamine synthetase stain demonstrates diffuse homogeneous staining indicating β-catenin activation (100x). (*C*) β-catenin stain highlights focal nuclear staining in lesional hepatocytes, supporting β-catenin activation (200x). (*D*) Reticulin stain (200x) shows irregular hepatic plate architecture with focal plate thickening (200x). Based on the morphologic features, reticulin abnormalities and β-catenin activation, this was designated as AHN.

Table 4
Patterns of staining with glutamine synthetase

Pattern	Description	Significance	CTNNB1 Mutation
Diffuse homogeneous	Moderate to strong cytoplasmic staining in >90% of tumor cells	High level of β-catenin activation	Exon 3 deletions and exon 3 non-S45 mutations
Diffuse heterogeneous	Moderate to strong cytoplasmic staining in 50%–90% of tumor cells	Intermediate level of β-catenin activation	Exon 3 mutations (T41, S45), rare cases with mutations in exon 7 and 8
Peripheral enhancement	Strong rim of staining at the periphery with patchy staining in the center	Weak level of β-catenin activation	Exon 7 and 8 mutations, some cases with exon 3 S45 mutation
Perivascular and/or patchy	Moderate to strong staining in perivascular regions and/or patchy staining in the lesion	No β-catenin activation (in most cases)	Exon 7 and 8 mutations or no mutations
Indeterminate	Difficult to determine diffuse vs patchy pattern	Not clear	Obtain molecular testing if clinically necessary

cholestasis, and variable loss of reticulin can occur in this subtype.[59] By definition, these features are insufficient for a diagnosis of HCC. The association with concurrent or subsequent HCC has been reported in 40% of cases.[59] In view of the atypical features and frequent association with HCC, it has been argued that these cases are better classified as AHNs rather than HCA, at least on biopsies.[52,53,62]

CTNNB1 exon 7/exon 8-mutated subtype: These tumors show mutations in *CTNNB1* exon 7 (codon 335, K335I and K335T) or exon 8 (codon 387, N387K) leading to weak activation of Wnt/β-catenin signaling pathway.[55,68] There are no distinctive morphologic features but most of these tumors do not show nuclear β-catenin or diffuse GS staining (see **Table 4**), although a minority of cases can show diffuse heterogeneous GS pattern.[55,65] Hence, these tumors are likely to be categorized as "unclassified" based on immunohistochemistry. These tumors often show peripheral accentuation of GS staining[55,65] (see **Fig. 9**C). In addition, diffuse CD34 sinusoidal staining is present in the central portion of these lesions but not close to the rim.[65] The combination of peripheral accentuation of GS and lack of sinusoidal CD34 at the periphery can help to identify this subtype (this can also occur with S45 mutation) but may be difficult to demonstrate on a biopsy. It has been proposed that these tumors have low malignant potential,[68] but these mutations have been identified in rare cases of HCC.[55,62]

Sonic hedgehog hepatocellular adenoma. This is a recently described subtype characterized by *INHBE:GLI1* fusion, leading to activation of the sonic hedgehog pathway and overexpression of prostaglandin D2 synthetase (PTGDS) and arginosuccinate synthase 1 (ASS1).[69] PTGDS and ASS1 immunohistochemical stains are not widely available for shHCA, and their sensitivity and specificity for this subtype are not fully established.[69,70]

Unclassified hepatocellular adenoma. This designation is used for 5% to 10% of HCAs that lack morphologic, immunohistochemical, and/or molecular features of recognized subtypes. When diagnosed based on immunohistochemistry, this category likely includes most shHCAs and *CTNNB1* exon 7/8-mutated B-HCAs.

Differential Diagnosis and Ancillary Diagnostic Features

Although immunohistochemistry is useful to determine the subtype of HCA (summarized in **Table 2** and will not be further elaborated in the text), it does not help distinguish HCA from HCC, because HCC can show LFABP loss,[60,61,71] positivity for SAA/CRP,[50] and diffuse GS staining/nuclear β-catenin.[30,51,55,59,64,68] In addition, there are various patterns of staining with GS that correlate with the different *CTNNB1* mutations and levels of β-catenin activation (see **Table 4**). However, there are three main clinicopathologic considerations aside from subtyping HCAs.

1. *Atypical hepatocellular neoplasm:* As mentioned earlier, the term can be used for a hepatocellular tumor with borderline or high-risk features but are insufficient for a definite diagnosis of HCC.[30,52,72] If a definite diagnosis is needed on biopsy, molecular analysis can be helpful. The presence of *TERT* promoter mutations, other molecular events (*TP53* mutation and *CDKN2A* loss), and/or chromosomal gains in 1q, 8q, and 7q strongly support HCC over HCA.[19,73,74]
2. *Hepatic adenomatosis:* This is a rare entity defined arbitrarily as 10 or more HCAs. Risk factors include advanced metabolic dysfunction-associated steatotic liver disease, metabolic syndrome, and obesity, especially for I-HCA. Other associations include oral contraceptive use, MODY3, McCune-Albright syndrome, Prader-Willi syndrome, congenital porto-systemic shunts/Abernethy malformation, and Fontan procedure.[75-77] In the setting of MODY3, biallelic inactivating mutations in *TCF1/*

HNF1A gene have been identified.[78] Transformation to HCC occurs in 2% to 3% of cases.[79,80] Similar to HCAs, nodules with size greater than 5 cm and/or *CTNNB1* mutations are associated with a higher propensity for malignant transformation[50] and hence should be considered for resection. Embolization and liver transplantation can be offered for unresectable high-risk nodules.

3. *Nodular lesions in patients with vascular disease:* A wide spectrum of nodular lesions can develop in the setting of vascular liver diseases, such as Budd-Chiari syndrome, Abernethy malformation, tetralogy of Fallot, hereditary hemorrhagic telangiectasia, and following Fontan procedure.[67,81,82] These lesions can be classified into nodular regenerative hyperplasia, LRN, FNH/FNH-like lesions, HCA/HCA-like lesions, HCC, and rarely hepatoblastoma.[81] These lesions can be multiple and even numerous and are thought to arise due to an imbalance between hepatic arterial and portal venous flow to the liver.[67,83] Histopathologic examination of these lesions is imperative for proper classification and management due to the risk of progression of HCC. The nodules with atypical features and/or β-catenin activation need complete resection.[64,67,84]

Prognosis

Risk factors of transformation of HCA to HCC include age greater than 50 years, male gender, anabolic steroid usage, metabolic syndrome, large tumor size (>5 cm), and activation of β-catenin pathway.[39,85,86] High proliferation index has also been suggested as a risk factor.[87] H-HCA has a very low risk for HCC transformation (<2%)[60,71] and may be higher in the setting of MODY3 and underlying hepatic vascular disease.[71] Inflammatory HCA, *CTNNB1* exon 7/8 variant of B-HCA, and U-HCA have low risk of malignant transformation to HCC. The *CTNNB1* exon 3 deletion variant of B-HCA carries a much higher HCC risk with concurrent or subsequent HCC in up to 40% of cases. shHCA has been reported to carry an increased risk of hemorrhage[70]; however, its hemorrhage risk did not seem higher compared with other HCA subtype in a recent study.[88] The risk of HCC in shHCA has not been well studied.

Treatment and Outcome

It has been recommended that HCAs associated with high-risk features such as size greater than 5 cm, male gender, and/or β-catenin activation (diffuse GS, nuclear β-catenin, or exon 3 *CTNNB1* mutation) should be resected[89] (see **Table 3**). Resection can also be considered for AHNs, which have atypical morphologic features that are suspicious but not diagnostic of HCC (see **Table 3**). The risk of recurrence or metastasis following resection is extremely low.

CLINICS CARE POINTS

- Small cell change, architectural changes such as focally thick plates and pseudoacini, occasional aberrant arterioles, and focal reticulin abnormalities distinguish high-grade dysplastic nodules from large regenerative nodules.

- Stromal invasion, absence of ductular reaction at periphery, slightly higher cytoarchitectural atypia, higher degree of abnormality on reticulin stain, more pronounced increase in sinusoidal CD34, diffuse glutamine synthetase (GS), and/or glypican-3 positivity can help to distinguish early hepatocellular carcinoma (HCC) from high-grade dysplastic nodule.

- Genomic changes (*TERT* promoter, *CTNNB1*, *TP53* mutations, and copy number alterations) can be obtained in challenging cases and favor HCC over high-grade dysplastic (HGD) nodules if present.

- Size greater than 5 cm, male gender, and β-catenin activation are risk factors of HCC in hepatocellular adenomas (HCAs).
- The risk of HCC is highest in β-catenin-activated HCA due to *CTNNB1* exon 3 mutations, which can be recognized by diffuse staining with glutamine synthetase.
- HCAs with *CTNNB1* exon 7/8 mutations have weak β-catenin-activation, have lower risk of HCC, lack diffuse GS staining and often show peripheral accentuation of GS staining.
- Atypical hepatocellular neoplasm (AHN) is used to describe hepatocellular neoplasms which resemble HCA but have atypical features that are not sufficient for an unequivocal diagnosis of HCC.
- Genomic features (*CTNNB1* mutation, *TERT* promoter mutation, other mutations, and copy number alterations) can help to distinguish HCA and AHN from HCC.

REFERENCES

1. Furuya K, Nakamura M, Yamamoto Y, et al. Macroregenerative nodule of the liver. A clinicopathologic study of 345 autopsy cases of chronic liver disease. Cancer 1988;61:99–105.
2. Singal AG, Llovet JM, Yarchoan M, et al. AASLD practice guidance on prevention, diagnosis, and treatment of hepatocellular carcinoma. Hepatology 2023; 78(6):1922–65.
3. Zou X, Luo Y, Morelli JN, et al. Differentiation of hepatocellular carcinoma from intrahepatic cholangiocarcinoma and combined hepatocellular-cholangiocarcinoma in high-risk patients matched to MR field strength: diagnostic performance of LI-RADS version 2018. Abdom Radiol (NY) 2021;46:3168–78.
4. European Association for the Study of the Liver, European Association for the Study of the Liver. Electronic address eee, European Association for the Study of the L. EASL Clinical Practice Guidelines: management of hepatocellular carcinoma. J Hepatol 2018;69:182–236.
5. Okuda K, Ohtsuki T, Obata H, et al. Natural history of hepatocellular carcinoma and prognosis in relation to treatment. Study of 850 patients. Cancer 1985;56: 918–28.
6. Roncalli M, Terracciano L, Di Tommaso L, et al, Gruppo Italiano Patologi Apparato Digerente GIPAD, Società Italiana di Anatomia Patologica e Citopatologia Diagnostica/International Academy of Pathology, Italian division SIAPEC/IAP. Gruppo italiano patologi apparato D, societa italiana di anatomia patologica e citopatologia diagnostica/international academy of pathology id. liver precancerous lesions and hepatocellular carcinoma: the histology report. Dig Liver Dis 2011;43(Suppl 4):S361–72.
7. Renzulli M, Braccischi L, D'Errico A, et al. State-of-the-art review on the correlations between pathological and magnetic resonance features of cirrhotic nodules. Histol Histopathol 2022;37:1151–65.
8. Scali EP, Walshe T, Tiwari HA, et al. A pictorial review of hepatobiliary magnetic resonance imaging with hepatocyte-specific contrast agents: uses, findings, and pitfalls of gadoxetate disodium and gadobenate dimeglumine. Can Assoc Radiol J 2017;68:293–307.
9. Niu ZS, Niu XJ, Wang WH, et al. Latest developments in precancerous lesions of hepatocellular carcinoma. World J Gastroenterol 2016;22:3305–14.
10. El-Sayed SS, El-Sadany M, Tabll AA, et al. DNA ploidy and liver cell dysplasia in liver biopsies from patients with liver cirrhosis. Can J Gastroenterol 2004;18:87–91.

11. Gong L, Li YH, Su Q, et al. Clonality of nodular lesions in liver cirrhosis and chromosomal abnormalities in monoclonal nodules of altered hepatocytes. Histopathology 2010;56:589–99.
12. Koskinas J, Petraki K, Kavantzas N, et al. Hepatic expression of the proliferative marker Ki-67 and p53 protein in HBV or HCV cirrhosis in relation to dysplastic liver cell changes and hepatocellular carcinoma. J Viral Hepat 2005;12:635–41.
13. Le Bail B, Bernard PH, Carles J, et al. Prevalence of liver cell dysplasia and association with HCC in a series of 100 cirrhotic liver explants. J Hepatol 1997;27:835–42.
14. Lee RG, Tsamandas AC, Demetris AJ. Large cell change (liver cell dysplasia) and hepatocellular carcinoma in cirrhosis: matched case-control study, pathological analysis, and pathogenetic hypothesis. Hepatology 1997;26:1415–22.
15. International Working P. Terminology of nodular hepatocellular lesions. Hepatology 1995;22:983–93.
16. Marchio A, Terris B, Meddeb M, et al. Chromosomal abnormalities in liver cell dysplasia detected by comparative genomic hybridisation. Mol Pathol 2001;54:270–4.
17. Nault JC, Ningarhari M, Rebouissou S, et al. The role of telomeres and telomerase in cirrhosis and liver cancer. Nat Rev Gastroenterol Hepatol 2019;16:544–58.
18. Nault JC, Calderaro J, Di Tommaso L, et al. Telomerase reverse transcriptase promoter mutation is an early somatic genetic alteration in the transformation of premalignant nodules in hepatocellular carcinoma on cirrhosis. Hepatology 2014;60:1983–92.
19. Pinyol R, Tovar V, Llovet JM. TERT promoter mutations: gatekeeper and driver of hepatocellular carcinoma. J Hepatol 2014;61:685–7.
20. Cancer Genome Atlas Research Network.. Comprehensive and integrative genomic characterization of hepatocellular carcinoma. Cell 2017;169:1327–41. e23.
21. Miyoshi Y, Iwao K, Nagasawa Y, et al. Activation of the beta-catenin gene in primary hepatocellular carcinomas by somatic alterations involving exon 3. Cancer Res 1998;58:2524–7.
22. Huang H, Fujii H, Sankila A, et al. Beta-catenin mutations are frequent in human hepatocellular carcinomas associated with hepatitis C virus infection. Am J Pathol 1999;155:1795–801.
23. Lee SE, Chang SH, Kim WY, et al. Frequent somatic TERT promoter mutations and CTNNB1 mutations in hepatocellular carcinoma. Oncotarget 2016;7:69267–75.
24. Park JY, Park WS, Nam SW, et al. Mutations of beta-catenin and AXIN I genes are a late event in human hepatocellular carcinogenesis. Liver Int 2005;25:70–6.
25. Craig AJ, von Felden J, Garcia-Lezana T, et al. Tumour evolution in hepatocellular carcinoma. Nat Rev Gastroenterol Hepatol 2020;17:139–52.
26. Kim YD, Park CH, Kim HS, et al. Genetic alterations of Wnt signaling pathway-associated genes in hepatocellular carcinoma. J Gastroenterol Hepatol 2008;23:110–8.
27. Ishizaki Y, Ikeda S, Fujimori M, et al. Immunohistochemical analysis and mutational analyses of beta-catenin, Axin family and APC genes in hepatocellular carcinomas. Int J Oncol 2004;24:1077–83.
28. Desjonqueres E, Campani C, Marra F, et al. Preneoplastic lesions in the liver: Molecular insights and relevance for clinical practice. Liver Int 2022;42:492–506.
29. Kang YK, Kim CJ, Kim WH, et al. p53 mutation and overexpression in hepatocellular carcinoma and dysplastic nodules in the liver. Virchows Arch 1998;432:27–32.

30. Evason KJ, Grenert JP, Ferrell LD, et al. Atypical hepatocellular adenoma-like neoplasms with beta-catenin activation show cytogenetic alterations similar to well-differentiated hepatocellular carcinomas. Hum Pathol 2013;44:750–8.
31. Llovet JM, Chen Y, Wurmbach E, et al. A molecular signature to discriminate dysplastic nodules from early hepatocellular carcinoma in HCV cirrhosis. Gastro-enterology 2006;131:1758–67.
32. Park YN, Yang CP, Fernandez GJ, et al. Neoangiogenesis and sinusoidal "capil-larization" in dysplastic nodules of the liver. Am J Surg Pathol 1998;22:656–62.
33. Dhillon AP, Colombari R, Savage K, et al. An immunohistochemical study of the blood vessels within primary hepatocellular tumours. Liver 1992;12:311–8.
34. Libbrecht L, Severi T, Cassiman D, et al. Glypican-3 expression distinguishes small hepatocellular carcinomas from cirrhosis, dysplastic nodules, and focal nodular hyperplasia-like nodules. Am J Surg Pathol 2006;30:1405–11.
35. Shafizadeh N, Ferrell LD, Kakar S. Utility and limitations of glypican-3 expression for the diagnosis of hepatocellular carcinoma at both ends of the differentiation spectrum. Mod Pathol 2008;21:1011–8.
36. Wang XY, Degos F, Dubois S, et al. Glypican-3 expression in hepatocellular tu-mors: diagnostic value for preneoplastic lesions and hepatocellular carcinomas. Hum Pathol 2006;37:1435–41.
37. Di Tommaso L, Destro A, Seok JY, et al. The application of markers (HSP70 GPC3 and GS) in liver biopsies is useful for detection of hepatocellular carcinoma. J Hepatol 2009;50:746–54.
38. Abdul-Al HM, Makhlouf HR, Wang G, et al. Glypican-3 expression in benign liver tissue with active hepatitis C: implications for the diagnosis of hepatocellular car-cinoma. Hum Pathol 2008;39:209–12.
39. Kakar S, Grenert JP, Paradis V, et al. Hepatocellular carcinoma arising in ade-noma: similar immunohistochemical and cytogenetic features in adenoma and hepatocellular carcinoma portions of the tumor. Mod Pathol 2014;27:1499–509.
40. Di Tommaso L, Franchi G, Park YN, et al. Diagnostic value of HSP70, glypican 3, and glutamine synthetase in hepatocellular nodules in cirrhosis. Hepatology 2007;45:725–34.
41. Shafizadeh N, Kakar S. Diagnosis of well-differentiated hepatocellular lesions: role of immunohistochemistry and other ancillary techniques. Adv Anat Pathol 2011;18:438–45.
42. Park YN, Kojiro M, Di Tommaso L, et al. Ductular reaction is helpful in defining early stromal invasion, small hepatocellular carcinomas, and dysplastic nodules. Cancer 2007;109:915–23.
43. Sciarra A, Di Tommaso L, Nakano M, et al. Morphophenotypic changes in human multistep hepatocarcinogenesis with translational implications. J Hepatol 2016; 64:87–93.
44. Maggioni M, Coggi G, Cassani B, et al. Molecular changes in hepatocellular dysplastic nodules on microdissected liver biopsies. Hepatology 2000;32:942–6.
45. Sun M, Eshleman JR, Ferrell LD, et al. An early lesion in hepatic carcinogenesis: loss of heterozygosity in human cirrhotic livers and dysplastic nodules at the 1p36-p34 region. Hepatology 2001;33:1415–24.
46. Sato T, Kondo F, Ebara M, et al. Natural history of large regenerative nodules and dysplastic nodules in liver cirrhosis: 28-year follow-up study. Hepatol Int 2015;9:330–6.
47. Cho YK, Wook Chung J, Kim Y, et al. Radiofrequency ablation of high-grade dysplastic nodules. Hepatology 2011;54:2005–11.

48. Bioulac-Sage P, Blanc JF, Rebouissou S, et al. Genotype phenotype classification of hepatocellular adenoma. World J Gastroenterol 2007;13:2649–54.

49. Liu L, Shah SS, Naini BV, et al. Immunostains Used to Subtype Hepatic Adenomas Do Not Distinguish Hepatic Adenomas From Hepatocellular Carcinomas. Am J Surg Pathol 2016;40:1062–9.

50. Zucman-Rossi J, Jeannot E, Nhieu JT, et al. Genotype-phenotype correlation in hepatocellular adenoma: new classification and relationship with HCC. Hepatology 2006;43:515–24.

51. Nault JC, Couchy G, Balabaud C, et al. Molecular Classification of Hepatocellular Adenoma Associates With Risk Factors, Bleeding, and Malignant Transformation. Gastroenterology 2017;152:880–894 e886.

52. Choi WT, Kakar S. Atypical Hepatocellular Neoplasms: Review of Clinical, Morphologic, Immunohistochemical, Molecular, and Cytogenetic Features. Adv Anat Pathol 2018;25:254–62.

53. Umetsu SE, Kakar S. Evaluating Liver Biopsies with Well-Differentiated Hepatocellular Lesions. Surg Pathol Clin 2023;16:581–98.

54. Calderaro J, Nault JC, Balabaud C, et al. Inflammatory hepatocellular adenomas developed in the setting of chronic liver disease and cirrhosis. Mod Pathol 2016; 29:43–50.

55. Rebouissou S, Franconi A, Calderaro J, et al. Genotype-phenotype correlation of CTNNB1 mutations reveals different ss-catenin activity associated with liver tumor progression. Hepatology 2016;64:2047–61.

56. Bluteau O, Jeannot E, Bioulac-Sage P, et al. Bi-allelic inactivation of TCF1 in hepatic adenomas. Nat Genet 2002;32:312–5.

57. Yamagata K, Oda N, Kaisaki PJ, et al. Mutations in the hepatocyte nuclear factor-1alpha gene in maturity-onset diabetes of the young (MODY3). Nature 1996;384: 455–8.

58. Rebouissou S, Imbeaud S, Balabaud C, et al. HNF1alpha inactivation promotes lipogenesis in human hepatocellular adenoma independently of SREBP-1 and carbohydrate-response element-binding protein (ChREBP) activation. J Biol Chem 2007;282:14437–46.

59. Bioulac-Sage P, Rebouissou S, Thomas C, et al. Hepatocellular adenoma subtype classification using molecular markers and immunohistochemistry. Hepatology 2007;46:740–8.

60. Putra J, Ferrell LD, Gouw ASH, et al. Malignant transformation of liver fatty acid binding protein-deficient hepatocellular adenomas: histopathologic spectrum of a rare phenomenon. Mod Pathol 2020;33:665–75.

61. Joseph NM, Blank A, Shain AH, et al. Hepatocellular neoplasms with loss of liver fatty acid binding protein: Clinicopathologic features and molecular profiling. Hum Pathol 2022;122:60–71.

62. Joseph NM, Umetsu SE, Shafizadeh N, et al. Genomic profiling of well-differentiated hepatocellular neoplasms with diffuse glutamine synthetase staining reveals similar genetics across the adenoma to carcinoma spectrum. Mod Pathol 2019;32:1627–36.

63. Sasaki M, Yoneda N, Kitamura S, et al. A serum amyloid A-positive hepatocellular neoplasm arising in alcoholic cirrhosis: a previously unrecognized type of inflammatory hepatocellular tumor. Mod Pathol 2012;25:1584–93.

64. Hale G, Liu X, Hu J, et al. Correlation of exon 3 beta-catenin mutations with glutamine synthetase staining patterns in hepatocellular adenoma and hepatocellular carcinoma. Mod Pathol 2016;29:1370–80.

65. Sempoux C, Gouw ASH, Dunet V, et al. Predictive Patterns of Glutamine Synthetase Immunohistochemical Staining in CTNNB1-mutated Hepatocellular Adenomas. Am J Surg Pathol 2021;45:477–87.
66. Gupta S, Naini BV, Munoz R, et al. Hepatocellular Neoplasms Arising in Association With Androgen Use. Am J Surg Pathol 2016;40:454–61.
67. Sempoux C, Paradis V, Komuta M, et al. Hepatocellular nodules expressing markers of hepatocellular adenomas in Budd-Chiari syndrome and other rare hepatic vascular disorders. J Hepatol 2015;63:1173–80.
68. Pilati C, Letouze E, Nault JC, et al. Genomic profiling of hepatocellular adenomas reveals recurrent FRK-activating mutations and the mechanisms of malignant transformation. Cancer Cell 2014;25:428–41.
69. Nault JC, Couchy G, Caruso S, et al. Argininosuccinate synthase 1 and periportal gene expression in sonic hedgehog hepatocellular adenomas. Hepatology 2018;68:964–76.
70. Henriet E, Abou Hammoud A, Dupuy JW, et al. Argininosuccinate synthase 1 (ASS1): A marker of unclassified hepatocellular adenoma and high bleeding risk. Hepatology 2017;66:2016–28.
71. Hechtman JF, Abou-Alfa GK, Stadler ZK, et al. Somatic HNF1A mutations in the malignant transformation of hepatocellular adenomas: a retrospective analysis of data from MSK-IMPACT and TCGA. Hum Pathol 2019;83:1–6.
72. Kakar S, Evason KJ, Ferrell LD. Well-differentiated hepatocellular neoplasm of uncertain malignant potential: proposal for a new diagnostic category–reply. Hum Pathol 2014;45:660–1.
73. Nault JC, Zucman-Rossi J. TERT promoter mutations in primary liver tumors. Clin Res Hepatol Gastroenterol 2016;40:9–14.
74. Kakar S, Chen X, Ho C, et al. Chromosomal abnormalities determined by comparative genomic hybridization are helpful in the diagnosis of atypical hepatocellular neoplasms. Histopathology 2009;55:197–205.
75. Gaujoux S, Salenave S, Ronot M, et al. Hepatobiliary and Pancreatic neoplasms in patients with McCune-Albright syndrome. J Clin Endocrinol Metab 2014;99:E97–101.
76. Grazioli L, Federle MP, Ichikawa T, et al. Liver adenomatosis: clinical, histopathologic, and imaging findings in 15 patients. Radiology 2000;216:395–402.
77. Dauleh H, Soliman A, Haris B, et al. Case Report: Hepatic Adenomatosis in a Patient With Prader-Willi Syndrome. Front Endocrinol 2022;13:826772.
78. Bacq Y, Jacquemin E, Balabaud C, et al. Familial liver adenomatosis associated with hepatocyte nuclear factor 1alpha inactivation. Gastroenterology 2003;125:1470–5.
79. Lammert C, Toal E, Mathur K, et al. Large Hepatic Adenomas and Hepatic Adenomatosis: A Multicenter Study of Risk Factors, Interventions, and Complications. Am J Gastroenterol 2022;117:1089–96.
80. Barbier L, Nault JC, Dujardin F, et al. Natural history of liver adenomatosis: a long-term observational study. J Hepatol 2019;71:1184–92.
81. Sempoux C, Balabaud C, Paradis V, et al. Hepatocellular nodules in vascular liver diseases. Virchows Arch 2018;473:33–44.
82. Brenard R, Chapaux X, Deltenre P, et al. Large spectrum of liver vascular lesions including high prevalence of focal nodular hyperplasia in patients with hereditary haemorrhagic telangiectasia: the Belgian Registry based on 30 patients. Eur J Gastroenterol Hepatol 2010;22:1253–9.
83. Lautz TB, Shah SA, Superina RA. Hepatoblastoma in Children With Congenital Portosystemic Shunts. J Pediatr Gastroenterol Nutr 2016;62:542–5.

84. Sorkin T, Strautnieks S, Foskett P, et al. Multiple beta-catenin mutations in hepatocellular lesions arising in Abernethy malformation. Hum Pathol 2016;53:153–8.
85. Dokmak S, Paradis V, Vilgrain V, et al. A single-center surgical experience of 122 patients with single and multiple hepatocellular adenomas. Gastroenterology 2009;137:1698–705.
86. Farges O, Ferreira N, Dokmak S, et al. Changing trends in malignant transformation of hepatocellular adenoma. Gut 2011;60:85–9.
87. Jones A, Kroneman TN, Blahnik AJ, et al. Ki-67 "hot spot" digital analysis is useful in the distinction of hepatic adenomas and well-differentiated hepatocellular carcinomas. Virchows Arch 2021;478:201–7.
88. Lehrke HD, Van Treeck BJ, Allende D, et al. Does Argininosuccinate Synthase 1 (ASS1) Immunohistochemistry Predict an Increased Risk of Hemorrhage for Hepatocellular Adenomas? Appl Immunohistochem Mol Morphol 2020;28:464–70.
89. European Association for the Study of the Liver.. EASL clinical practice guidelines on the management of benign liver tumours. J Hepatol 2016;65:386–98.

Pathology and Clinical Significance of Inflammatory Bowel Disease-Associated Colorectal Dysplastic Lesions

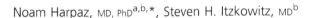

Noam Harpaz, MD, PhD[a,b,*], Steven H. Itzkowitz, MD[b]

KEYWORDS

- Inflammatory bowel disease • Crohn disease • Ulcerative colitis • Dysplasia
- Colorectal cancer

KEY POINTS

- The detection of dysplasia in endoscopic biopsies provides a means to identify patients with inflammatory bowel disease (IBD) who are at risk for developing colorectal cancer, evaluate their risk level, and manage their condition in a timely fashion before the development of incurable cancer.
- A large body of circumstantial evidence supports the efficacy of colonic surveillance as a cancer prevention strategy and its endorsement by major gastroenterology societies.
- Optimizing the management of patients with chronic IBD-associated colorectal dysplasia requires comprehensive evaluation of their clinical risk factors, endoscopic findings, and lesional pathologic condition.
- The histopathologic classification of dysplastic lesions based on their histologic grade (indefinite, low grade, and high grade) offers vital prognostic information concerning both current and future cancer risk.
- Dysplastic lesions that differ morphologically from conventional adenomatous lesions are increasingly recognized and appreciated for their contribution to neoplastic progression in IBD.

Continued

[a] Department of Pathology, Molecular and Cell-Based Medicine, Icahn School of Medicine at Mount Sinai; [b] Department of Medicine, Division of Gastroenterology, Icahn School of Medicine at Mount Sinai, Annenberg Building 5-12L, 1468 Madison Avenue, New York, NY 10029, USA
* Corresponding author. Department of Pathology, Molecular and Cell-Based Medicine, Icahn School of Medicine at Mount Sinai, Annenberg Building 15-38, 1468 Madison Avenue, New York, NY 10029.
E-mail address: noam.harpaz@mountsinai.org

Gastroenterol Clin N Am 53 (2024) 133–154
https://doi.org/10.1016/j.gtc.2023.09.005
0889-8553/24/© 2023 Elsevier Inc. All rights reserved.

gastro.theclinics.com

Continued

- Recent advances in imaging and endoscopic resection techniques make endoscopic detection and removal of dysplastic lesions more feasible, although surgery may still be unavoidable in some clinical situations.
- Optimal management of patients with dysplastic lesions is guided by their endoscopic classification as invisible versus invisible and endoscopically resectable versus nonresectable.

INTRODUCTION

Idiopathic inflammatory bowel disease (IBD), encompassing ulcerative colitis (UC) and Crohn disease (CD), currently affects up to 1.3% of North American and European populations and is increasing in prevalence worldwide.[1,2] Colitis associated with IBD is an established risk factor for the development of colorectal cancer (CRC), which is, in turn, a major contributor to IBD-associated mortality.[3,4] Compared with the general population, the peak age at which CRC is diagnosed in patients with IBD is 1 to 2 decades earlier, the age-adjusted incidence is 2-fold to 3-fold, and survival rates are lower,[5–12] making cancer prevention a clinical management priority in this population.

IBD-related CRC is the culmination of a colitis-dysplasia-cancer sequence, a complex series of progressive oncogenic molecular alterations of the intestinal epithelium that are initiated and sustained by the mutagenic effects of mucosal inflammation and are reflected by morphologic aberrations of the colorectal epithelium, termed dysplasia. As a predecessor of CRC, dysplasia detected in endoscopic biopsies can serve as a means to identify patients at high risk, evaluate their risk level, and manage their condition in a timely fashion before the emergence of incurable cancer. Endoscopic surveillance for detection of dysplasia, or early curable CRC, has been the cornerstone of cancer prevention in the IBD population for decades and is universally endorsed by major gastroenterological societies.[13–15] Although it is not feasible to confirm its efficacy in reducing cancer mortality by means of randomized controlled trials, the beneficial influence of endoscopic surveillance has been inferred from a substantial body of observational studies.[16]

Recent studies have suggested a trend toward decreasing incidence of CRC compared with earlier estimates, at least in certain populations, presumably reflecting improved therapeutic options to control inflammation, technological advances in endoscopic visualization, and broader implementation of surveillance.[5,17–19] Nonetheless, the risk exceeds 0.5% annually after 8 years of disease and about 20% during the course of a lifetime.[20] It is likely that further reductions in cancer mortality could be achieved by translating our growing understanding of the natural history of dysplasia and its pathologic and molecular underpinnings into improved treatment algorithms. This review aims to provide a contemporary overview of the pathologic and endoscopic classification of dysplasia in IBD, their roles in determining surveillance and management algorithms, and the emerging diagnostic and therapeutic approaches that might further enhance patient management.

RISK FACTORS FOR NEOPLASIA IN INFLAMMATORY BOWEL DISEASE

The risk of developing neoplasia in IBD arises from a combination of patient-related, disease-related, and pathology-related factors. The most consistent risk factors are those reflecting extensive colonic involvement (determined histologically), cumulative inflammatory burden (a metric that incorporates disease duration and inflammation severity), primary sclerosing cholangitis, prior dysplasia, and a history of CRC in a first-degree relative. Conversely, protective factors include the use of 5-aminosalicylic acid medications, statins, and surveillance colonoscopy.[21]

MACROSCOPIC CHARACTERISTICS AND ENDOSCOPIC CLASSIFICATION OF DYSPLASIA

Patients with extensive, or pan-colonic, disease are the major risk group, accounting for approximately 80% of UC-associated CRC cases, whereas those with left-sided UC face lower risks and those with ulcerative proctitis or proctosigmoiditis have little or no risk. The risk of cancer development among patients with colonic CD is similar to those with UC of equivalent disease duration and extent.

Dysplasia and CRC occur in parallel within chronically inflamed colorectal segments. In patients who undergo surgery for the management of CRC, dysplasia is present in the adjacent mucosa in approximately 90% of cases and in remote colonic locations in 30% to 75%, where its distribution may be unifocal, multifocal, or diffuse.[22,23] Although any segment of the colon can be affected, the highest prevalence of CRC and dysplasia has been reported in the distal colon and rectum.[22,24]

The macroscopic features of dysplasia in IBD are diverse. Most dysplastic lesions are described as nodules, plaques, patches, villiform growths, or broad-based exophytic masses but some are detectable only with enhanced visualization techniques such as chromoendoscopy, whereas others are detected only by chance in random endoscopic biopsies or histologic sections of resected colons.

The macroscopic classification and management of dysplasia have changed with the introduction of high-definition endoscopy. Terms such as "dysplasia-associated lesion or mass" and "adenoma-like" or "nonadenoma-like" polyps that were used in the past to classify dysplastic lesions based on their endoscopic appearances are no longer used because they lack precision, making it difficult to devise therapeutic protocols and to compare outcomes between studies.[25] The Surveillance for Colorectal Endoscopic Neoplasia Detection and Management in Inflammatory Bowel Disease (SCENIC) international consensus statement, published in 2015, represented an advance by providing definitions intended to standardize the classification and reporting of IBD-associated dysplasia (**Table 1**).[26] The SCENIC system classifies lesions as "visible" if they can be identified by means of targeted biopsies or "invisible" if they are identified in nontargeted biopsies, and as endoscopically resectable if they present

Table 1
SCENIC endoscopic classification of dysplasia[26]

Term	Definition
Visible	Identified in targeted biopsies from a visible lesion
Polypoid	Lesion protruding into lumen ≥2.5 mm
• Pedunculated	• Attached to the mucosa by a stalk
• Sessile	• No stalk; entire base is contiguous with mucosa
Nonpolypoid	Little (<2.5 mm) or no protrusion above the mucosa
• Superficial elevated	• Protrusion <2.5 mm
• Flat	• No protrusion
• Depressed	• At least a portion of lesion below mucosa
Invisible	No visible lesion, identified in random (nontargeted) biopsies

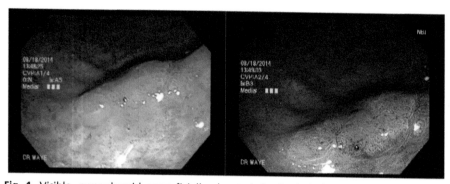

Fig. 1. Visible, nonpolypoid, superficially elevated dysplastic lesion in a patient with UC. Left; visualization under white light. Right; visualization under narrow band imaging reveals a sharply demarcated border, confirming that the lesion is endoscopically resectable. (*Courtesy of* Jerome D. Waye, M.D.)

clear borders and a manageable size (typically 2 cm or less), or nonresectable otherwise. Visible lesions can be further subdivided into polypoid and nonpolypoid categories, corresponding to sessile or pedunculated polyps, and to lesions that are superficially elevated, flat or depressed, respectively (**Fig. 1**). The SCENIC classification is well suited to contemporary enhanced endoscopic visualization techniques, including high-definition optics and chromoendoscopy, and supports a shift in the current therapeutic approach to dysplasia wherein local excision can provide a safe alternative to surgery.

DEFINITION AND CLASSIFICATION OF DYSPLASIA

Dysplasia is defined histologically as an unequivocal neoplastic alteration in the intestinal epithelium that remains confined within the original basement membrane.[27] Histologic abnormalities in IBD that are interpreted as, or suspected of being, reactive are thereby excluded.

The most widely used classification system for dysplasia is the grading system of Riddell and colleagues,[27] proposed in 1983, in which the epithelium is divided into 4 grades: negative for dysplasia (NEG), indefinite for dysplasia (IND), low-grade dysplasia (LGD), or high-grade dysplasia (HGD; **Table 2**; **Fig. 2**). The Vienna grading system, an alternative classification used by some pathologists in Europe and Asia, parallels the Riddell system in most respects.[28]

The NEG category encompasses normal mucosa, mucosa with postinflammatory features, such as crypt architectural distortion, and reactive epithelium in the setting of active or recent inflammation. Actively inflamed or ulcerated mucosa frequently exhibits cytologic atypia that resembles dysplasia, including enlarged, stratified, or variably sized nuclei, prominent nucleoli, increased mitotic activity, or reduced mucin. The distinction between reactive and dysplastic epithelium is usually not difficult because they each exhibit certain distinguishing characteristics. In reactive epithelium, the degree of cytologic atypia fluctuates across the epithelium in parallel with local variations in the intensity of inflammation. For example, maximal atypia usually occurs in the mucosa adjacent to erosions but diminishes gradually in less-inflamed surroundings. The epithelium that lines inflamed colonic crypts typically assumes a "maturation gradient" in which phenotypically immature, proliferative colonocytes located in the basal crypts gradually assume more mature characteristics, such as small, normochromatic nuclei, distinct absorptive and goblet phenotypes, and absent

Grade	Histologic Criteria
	Table 2 **Riddell grades and histologic criteria for dysplasia in inflammatory bowel disease[27]**
NEG	Normal Reactive to inflammatory surroundings: 　Reduced cytoplasmic mucin 　Nuclear atypia in basal crypt epithelium and adjacent to ulceration 　Decreasing nuclear size near surface (maturation) 　Normochromatic or mildly hyperchromatic nuclei 　Smooth, uniform nuclear membranes 　Nuclei may be stratified 　Nucleoli may be prominent 　Typical mitoses 　Cytoplasmic mucin vacuoles in regenerative goblet cells
IND	Cytologic atypia that eludes definitive classification as reactive or dysplastic 　Background of active inflammation or regeneration 　Atypia exceeding that of recognizably regenerative mucosa 　Inconspicuous surface maturation Technical obstacles to interpretation 　Tangential orientation 　Insufficient sample size 　Sectioning or staining artifacts
LGD	Preserved cellular polarity Nuclei confined to basal half of cells Uniform nuclear size and shape Relatively low nuclear to cytoplasmic ratios Few, typical mitotic figures Inconspicuous nucleoli
HGD	Loss of nuclear polarity Nuclear stratification involving luminal half of cells High nuclear to cytoplasmic ratios Marked nuclear hyperchromasia and pleomorphism Markedly enlarged nucleoli Atypical mitotic figures Intraluminal necrotic debris Complex architecture (fused or incomplete tubules, cribriform)

mitoses, as they approach the surface. A lack of goblet cells in regenerating epithelium may mimic some types of dysplastic epithelium but the presence of apical mucin droplets provides evidence of incipient goblet cell regeneration. In contrast, the presence of intensely stained, pleomorphic nuclei, macronucleoli, and especially sharply demarcated regions of atypia, or atypia of the surface epithelium equal to or even greater than in the crypt bases are features that suggest dysplasia.

The IND category refers to epithelium with cytologic atypia that eludes definitive classification for any one of several reasons. A common reason is an inability to differentiate inflamed reactive epithelium from true dysplasia. Another may be due to specimens that are difficult to interpret due to technical factors such as tangential orientation, small sample size, or tissue artifacts. When rendering a diagnosis of IND, it is advisable for the pathologist to append an interpretive statement indicating the specific points of doubt and conveying the pathologist's leanings if possible (eg, probably negative or probably positive for dysplasia) and to seek consultation with colleagues who have expertise in IBD pathologic conditions. Clinical guidelines suggest that therapeutic measures be used to mitigate the effects of active inflammation

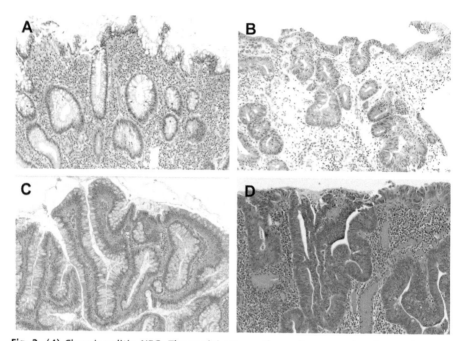

Fig. 2. (*A*) Chronic colitis, NEG. The nuclei are mostly small, nonoverlapping, and normochromatic. Mild nuclear enlargement and crowding in the basal crypt epithelium are typical regenerative changes. (*B*) Active chronic colitis, IND. Some of the crypt and surface epithelium shows mild nuclear atypia including crowding, enlargement, and hyperchromasia. In this setting, it is difficult to determine with certainty whether these changes are entirely regenerative. (*C*) Intestinal type low-grade dysplasia featuring tubular glands with enlarged, elongated nuclei that are confined to the basal half of the epithelial cells. Surface maturation is absent. (*D*) High-grade intestinal type dysplasia manifested by a complex epithelial growth pattern and moderately severe nuclear atypia, including enlargement, hyperchromasia, and stratification.

as much as possible to reduce their confounding effects on biopsy interpretation[29]; however, the mere presence of inflammation neither makes pathologic diagnoses unreliable nor does it justify dismissing a biopsy report of dysplasia when determining a patient's clinical management. In fact, dysplastic epithelium may be inflamed as well.

The category LGD is characterized by orderly growth patterns, mild cytologic atypia, and preserved epithelial cell polarity. Morphologically, the classic prototype resembles conventional adenomatous polyps. The epithelium maintains a uniform tubular, villous, or mixed growth pattern. The nuclei are enlarged, elliptical, and crowded; are oriented in parallel; and mostly occupy the basal cytoplasm. Their chromatin is mildly hyperchromatic or clumped, and they have smooth, delicate nuclear membranes, small nucleoli, and occasional mitotic figures. The cytoplasm is clear or eosinophilic, goblet cells are diminished or, in some cases, increased, and there are occasionally abundant Paneth-like or endocrine cells.

As dysplasia progresses from LGD to HGD, cytologic atypia increases, epithelial polarity is diminished or lost, and the growth pattern may become irregular. The nuclei are stratified or skewed, hyperchromatic, enlarged and pleomorphic. In some cases they are round and vesicular with irregularly thickened nuclear membranes, prominent nucleoli and an open chromatin pattern. The presence of atypical mitotic figures, dirty intraluminal necrosis, or complex growth patterns such as fused or cribriform crypts often accompanies the development of intramucosal adenocarcinoma, in which there is penetration of neoplastic cells or glands into the lamina propria or the muscularis mucosae, but not into the submucosa. Although this term does not fit the strict definition of dysplasia since the basement membrane has been breached, metastasis rarely if ever occurs and such lesions are grouped with HGD in the Riddell classification (and as a subcategory of HGD in the Vienna system). In contrast, lesions that feature desmoplastic stroma are considered to have invaded the submucosa and are classified as invasive carcinoma.

In addition to classification by grade, dysplasia can also be classified into distinct morphologic categories. Pathologists have long been aware of precancerous lesions in IBD that differ morphologically from the historical "adenomatous" prototype, some of which are uncommon or difficult to recognize. A newly developed comprehensive classification of dysplastic lesions in IBD based on uniform morphologic criteria and nomenclature has been advanced in provisional form[30] and, more recently, in final form,[31] by an international working group of pathologists with expertise in IBD. The classification encompasses 3 broad categories: intestinal, gastric, and mixed intestinal-gastric dysplasia and is further subclassified into 9 diagnostic categories based on serrated versus nonserrated growth patterns and other features (**Table 3**).

The utility of this classification has been confirmed in single and multi-institutional studies that have begun to apply it systematically to investigate pathologic correlations with IBD-associated cancer,[32,33] clinical outcome data,[34] endoscopic features[35,36] and genotype–phenotype correlations.[37,38] An expert interobserver agreement study confirmed its reproducibility, reporting that 67% of diagnoses rendered for a series of challenge cases were considered to be definitive and achieved substantial interrater agreement, and that 86% of the cases were graded as either LGD (75%) or HGD (11%) based on the Riddell system.[31]

The largest category is "intestinal" dysplasia, which encompasses 6 distinct diagnostic entities: tubular/villous (also termed "adenomatous"), goblet cell deficient, crypt cell, sessile-serrated lesion-like, traditional serrated adenoma-like, and serrated dysplasia not otherwise specified (NOS). Tubular/villous (adenomatous) dysplasia, the most commonly encountered category, resembles conventional sporadic adenomas morphologically (see above; see **Fig. 2**C). It encompasses several variants that are enriched in goblet cells (previously termed "hypermucinous" dysplasia), Paneth cells, or endocrine cells. The question whether or not these variants should be classified as separate entities remains to be determined in future studies.

Goblet cell-deficient dysplasia (GCDD), originally termed "dysplasia with incomplete goblet cell maturation,"[39] is characterized by noncrowded tubular crypts, low columnar epithelium with eosinophilic cytoplasm, and near-absent goblet cells (**Fig. 3**C). It was shown in an early study to predict progression to HGD or CRC at a similar actuarial rate as conventional dysplasia and to co-occur with conventional dysplasia in 50% of cases.[39] In a later multicenter cross-sectional study, it accounted for 6% of nonconventional dysplasia, showed HGD in 31% of cases, expressed aberrant p53 in 28% of cases and was associated longitudinally with the development of carcinoma in the same segment of colon.[32]

Crypt cell dysplasia (CCD) features noncrowded tubular crypts lined by epithelial cells that are phenotypically similar to those of normal large intestine but contain cytologically atypical nuclei (see **Fig. 3**A and B). GCDD and CCD are evidently uncommon and likely to be overlooked, especially in the setting of active inflammation. Nevertheless, the working group observed that CCD and GCDD were both diagnosed with high levels confidence and achieved substantial interobserver agreement. One study,

Table 3
Newly developed classification of dysplasia in inflammatory bowel disease[31]

Term	Histologic Features	Clinical Features
Intestinal type		
Tubular/villous adenoma-like	Tubular and/or villous architecture Enlarged, elongated, hyperchromatic, stratified nuclei Variable goblet cell density, may be predominant cell type (hypermucinous) May contain Paneth or endocrine cells Nuclear maturation in surface of villi	May be difficult to distinguish from sporadic adenoma in mucosa affected by colitis Potential precursor of mucinous adenocarcinoma (especially hypermucinous)[100]
Goblet cell–deficient	Noncrowded, uniform tubular growth pattern Flat surface Nonstratified, mildly hyperchromatic, round or oval nuclei Pale to intensely eosinophilic cytoplasm Absent or rare goblet cells	Frequently invisible[35,36] Potential precursor of tubuloglandular adenocarcinoma[100,101] High interobserver agreement[31]
Crypt cell	Noncrowded, uniform tubular growth pattern Flat surface Crypts lined by enterocytes interspersed with goblet cells; Paneth cells and endocrine cells often present but not required Round to oval, enlarged, hyperchromatic, or vesicular nuclei Atypical nuclei extend to surface epithelium	Frequently invisible[35,36] Frequent in patients with PSC[102] Frequent aneuploidy and p53 overexpression[102] Potential precursor of tubuloglandular adenocarcinoma[100,101] High interobserver agreement[31]
TSA-like	Resembles sporadic TSA Villiform Slit-like serrations, ectopic crypts Eosinophilic cytoplasm Pencillate nuclei, fine chromatin pattern	Slight male predominance (64%)[34] Polypoid, 80% located in distal colon Nonpolypoid variant distributed throughout colon[52] Frequent KRAS mutations[34,52] Progression rate to HGD and CRC similar to conventional LGD[34]

(continued on next page)

Table 3
(continued)

Term	Histologic Features	Clinical Features
SSL-like	Resembles sporadic SSL but flat crypt bases and lateral extension not required More irregular architecture and nuclear atypia Crypt serrations involving basal or superficial crypts Columnar epithelium with microvesicular cytoplasm and variable interspersed goblet cells Round-shaped to oval-shaped or slightly elongated, hyperchromatic, and may contain inconspicuous nucleoli	Male (83%) and left colon (78%) predominance, in contrast with female, right-sided predominance in nondysplastic SSL[34] Progression rate to HGD and CRC similar to conventional LGD[34]
Serrated NOS	Not classifiable as SSL or TSA-like Eosinophilic cytoplasm and round, vesicular nuclei	Insufficient data
Gastric type		
Tubular/villous	Apical foveolar-like neutral mucin Tubular and/or villous architecture Rare or no goblet cells Basally-oriented round, vesicular nuclei, reduced size near surface May have abundant mucin secretions (hypermucinous)	Insufficient data. Current data based on combined intestinal and gastric hypermucinous dysplasia
Serrated	Apical foveolar-like neutral mucin Serrated growth pattern Similar to tubular/villous but little or no reduction in nuclear size near the surface	Insufficient data. Current data based on combined intestinal and gastric hypermucinous dysplasia
Mixed intestinal-gastric type		
	Combination of columnar epithelia with foveolar and enteric or goblet cell features	Insufficient data

Abbreviations: IBD, inflammatory bowel disease; NOS, not otherwise specified; SSL, sessile serrated lesion; TSA, traditional serrated adenoma.

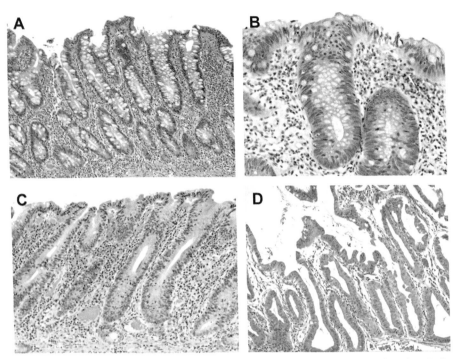

Fig. 3. (*A*) LGD, crypt cell type. (*B*) CCD at higher magnification. The mucosal surface is flat and the crypts are uniform and tubular. The pattern of goblet cells interspersed individually among enterocytes and rare endocrine cells is similar to that of normal crypts but the nuclei are enlarged and hyperchromatic, and there is little or no surface maturation. (*C*) LGD, goblet cell deficient type. Similarly to CCD, the surface is flat, the crypts are uniform and tubular, and there is nuclear atypia without surface maturation but the cytoplasm is uniformly eosinophilic and goblet cells are rare or absent. (*D*) serrated dysplasia NOS characterized by serrated eosinophilic epithelium with vesicular nuclei and prominent nucleoli.

published in abstract form, reported that GCCD and CCD accounted for most dysplastic biopsies associated with nontargeted endoscopic biopsies,[35] an observation that is not surprising in view of their flat growth patterns, and this association has been corroborated in recent multicenter[36] and single-center studies.[40]

Serrated epithelium is common in IBD and encompasses a diverse range of entities. Regenerative epithelial serration often occurs in mucosa adjacent to healing ulcers and in inflammatory polyps and has no recognized neoplastic potential. Patients with multiple inflammatory polyps have long been considered to be at increased risk for the development of CRC but a recent study demonstrated that inflammatory polyposis is merely a surrogate marker of chronic inflammation rather than an independent risk factor.[41] Serrated epithelial change without dysplasia in IBD has also been implicated as a risk factor for HGD and CRC[42–44] and may include a subset of potential high-risk lesions with aneuploidy[45] but its morphologic distinction from inflammatory polyposis and independent association with neoplasia require further exploration. Nondysplastic serrated polyps that resemble conventional hyperplastic polyps and sessile serrated lesions (SSLs) are frequently encountered in IBD. Studies have shown that they are morphologically and genetically similar to their counterparts in non-IBD patients and have negligible rates of progression to malignancy.[34,46,47]

Several types of dysplastic serrated polyps have been described in IBD.[34,48–51] The working group categorized them into 3 intestinal categories, SSL-like, traditional serrated adenoma (TSA)-like, and serrated NOS, and a separate category of gastric serrated dysplasia. SSL-like dysplasia in IBD resembles conventional sporadic SSLs morphologically but has a less regular growth pattern, may lack flat basal crypts with lateral L-shaped and T-shaped extensions, and contains cytologically atypical nuclei (**Fig. 4**A). TSA-like dysplasia is morphologically similar to sporadic TSA, featuring a villiform growth pattern with slit-like epithelial serrations, ectopic crypts, and tall columnar epithelial cells with eosinophilic cytoplasm and elongated (pencillate) nuclei (see **Fig. 4**B). Although TSA-like lesions are typically polypoid and occur in the distal large intestine,[34] a recent study described a subset of nonpolypoid TSA-like lesions in IBD that present as ill-defined, granular areas of mucosa that may occur anywhere in the colon and have higher rates synchronous and metachronous HGD and CRC.[52] The category serrated dysplasia NOS is reserved for serrated dysplastic lesions that do not fit into either the SSL-like or TSA-like categories, which most commonly feature eosinophilic cytoplasm and vesicular nuclei (see **Fig.** 2D).

Gastric dysplasia, another major morphologic category of dysplasia in IBD, is defined by epithelium with gastric foveolar-type mucinous differentiation defined by

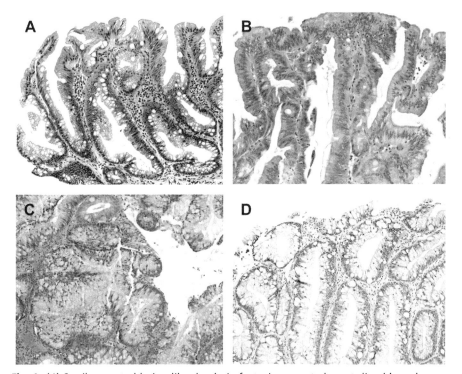

Fig. 4. (*A*) Sessile serrated lesion-like dysplasia featuring serrated crypts lined by columnar epithelium with microvesicular cytoplasm and atypical nuclei. The presence of flat crypt bases with lateral extensions is not a diagnostic requirement. (*B*) Traditional serrated adenoma-like dysplasia characterized by tall columnar epithelium with serrated configuration, slit-like spaces, occasional ectopic crypts, and pencillate nuclei. (*C*) Gastric serrated dysplasia featuring columnar epithelium with foveolar-like cytoplasm and neutral mucin content. (*D*) Mixed intestinal-gastric dysplasia characterized by gastric epithelium with pale eosinophilic cytoplasm admixed with goblet cells.

the presence of pale eosinophilic neutral mucin, either occupying the entire cytoplasm or forming an apical mucin cap. This category has been reported in the literature in several case series of IBD-associated carcinomas that described morphologically atypical mucosa, which expressed MUC5AC, a mucin apoprotein that is normally expressed in gastric foveolar epithelium, occurring in contiguity with cancer.[53–57] Nonetheless, only a few examples of this dysplasia category have been described as a distinct entity; rather, gastric dysplasia of this type has usually been combined in the literature with intestinal goblet cell-rich villous dysplasia under such designations as villous hypermucinous,[38,58] "mucinous"[37,59] and "hypermucinous"[32,36] to reflect the mucinous differentiation of the dysplastic cells. Further research will therefore be needed to compare the natural histories and biological characteristics of mucin-rich lesions with gastric versus intestinal differentiation.

Gastric dysplasia is subclassified into 2 subcategories, one characterized by a tubular, villous, or mixed architectural growth pattern and the other by a serrated growth pattern. The tubular/villous type features uncrowded crypts and villi that, when present, show surface tapering. The serrated type features serrations of both the basal and superficial crypts and surface epithelium, as well as occasional mucin-filled cystic glands but typically has no villi (see **Fig. 4**C). Both subcategories of gastric dysplasia feature enlarged, spindle to oval, vesicular nuclei that are oriented basally along the basement membrane without significant stratification. When villi are present, the nuclei often diminish in size near the villous tips.

The working group also recognized a category of mixed intestinal-gastric dysplasia that features an admixture of goblet cells, enterocytes, and gastric foveolar-like mucinous cells. This category may have a serrated, tubular, or villous architectural growth pattern (see **Fig. 4**D). Few examples of this category have been described morphologically in the literature; however, several studies of mucin expression in IBD-associated dysplastic lesions have described admixtures of epithelium with expression of MUC5AC and MUC2 (which is normally expressed by goblet cells), which imply mixed differentiation. Further studies will be needed to better delineate the morphologic and biological characteristics of this category.

PROGNOSTIC SIGNIFICANCE OF DYSPLASIA GRADE

Multiple surveillance and surgical studies have evaluated the risks of neoplastic progression associated with different grades of dysplasia but the effects of heterogeneity in study design, study populations, pathologist expertise, and surgical protocols make it difficult to compare findings across the literature. A recent single-institution study that adjusted for confounding factors such as PSC and inflammation, and which was based on diagnoses rendered by subspecialist gastrointestinal pathologists, reported incidence rates for the development of HGD or CRC of 0.4% per patient-year, 3.1% per patient-year, and 8.4% per patient-year following a diagnosis of no dysplasia, IND only, or LGD, respectively.[60] A more recent meta-analysis based on 38 studies reported the incidences of HGD or CRC in patients with IBD who received a biopsy diagnosis of LGD to be more than 1 in 10, with even higher rates among patients with multifocal LGD or invisible LGD.[61] Another finding was that patients diagnosed with IND progressed to HGD or CRC at a similar rate as those with LGD, confirming the findings of an earlier single-institution study.[62] The risk factors for progression identified in patients with IND were primary sclerosing cholangitis (PSC) and aneuploidy, and those identified in patients with LGD included, among others, PSC, previous IND, distal or multifocal lesions, and nonpolypoid/flat or invisible lesions.

MOLECULAR ALTERATIONS IN DYSPLASIA

The basic oncogenic pathways leading to dysplasia and CRC in IBD bear resemblance to those of sporadic CRC, including conservation of major pathways of chromosomal instability, microsatellite instability, and aberrant gene methylation, and, as expected, they involve similar driver genes. However, the vastly different inflammatory microenvironment in which tumorigenesis occurs in IBD is reflected by differences in the timing and prevalence of specific genetic alterations in the IBD setting. Studies have shown relatively low frequencies of mutations in Wnt-related genes and KRAS, and more frequent mutations in TP53, isocitrate dehydrogenase 1 (IDH1), and MYC compared with sporadic carcinogenesis.[63–68] Although loss of p53 tumor suppressor function in IBD is considered an early event in colitis-associated carcinogenesis, recent evidence suggests that it may be preceded by nongenomic events such as epigenetic changes, and that copy number changes reflecting chromosomal instability may play an important role in dysplasia progression.[67,69] Although molecular biomarkers hold promise for enabling personalized diagnosis and therapy in IBD-associated neoplasia, further research will be required to integrate them into the clinical management of high-risk patients.

INTEROBSERVER VARIATION AND ANCILLARY MARKERS

Interobserver variation among pathologists in interpreting and grading dysplasia in IBD has been a long-standing problem.[27,70–73] Typically, agreement levels among pathologists are fair to moderate even among experts, the highest levels of agreement being observed at the extremes of NEG and HGD and the lowest levels of agreement for LGD and IND. The potential implications were illustrated by a study in which central pathology experts performed a post hoc review and revision of diagnoses of indefinite and LGD dysplasia that had been rendered at 6 university-based pathology departments. Based on the revised classifications, the 5-year rates of progression from flat dysplasia to HGD or CRC increased from 12% to 37% and the progression rates from indefinite dysplasia to HGD or CRC decreased from 21% to 5%.[74]

Efforts to increase reproducibility by means of ancillary techniques have focused on histochemical and immunohistochemical markers,[52,75–78] ploidy measurements,[79] and molecular techniques, but immunohistochemistry is the most accessible method in pathology practice. Multiple studies have reported aberrant expression of TP53 in dysplastic lesions[52,76,77]; however, its diagnostic usefulness in distinguishing LGD from indefinite or reactive mucosa is limited by its lower sensitivity in lesions with LGD compared with HGD and by its occasional overexpression in the basal crypt epithelium of regenerative mucosa. Immunohistochemical expression of α-methylacyl-CoA racemase is relatively sensitive and specific for dysplasia in IBD, one study reporting expression in 90% of lesions with LGD, 80% with HGD and 71% of CRCs but not in nondysplastic regenerating epithelium.[78] More recently, loss of expression of special AT-rich sequence binding protein (SATB2), which is expressed in normal colorectal epithelium, was reported in 41% of IBD-associated dysplastic lesions, both visible and invisible types but not in sporadic adenomatous polyps. Despite this specificity, the low sensitivity (20%) of SATB2 loss in lesions with LGD limits its usefulness in diagnostically ambiguous situations.[80]

ENDOSCOPIC IDENTIFICATION OF DYSPLASIA

In the current era in which high-definition white light endoscopes (HD-WLE) have mostly replaced standard definition scopes, many, and perhaps most, dysplastic lesions in IBD are endoscopically visible. Nevertheless, chromoendoscopy, either using dye-spray techniques or image enhancing technology (virtual chromoendoscopy [VCE]) can further improve rates of dysplasia detection. Since the SCENIC statement, multiple studies and meta-analyses have been published comparing the effectiveness of dye chromoendoscopy (DCE), VCE, and HD-WLE without any firm agreement as to which technique is best.[81] Despite that DCE often detects more dysplastic lesions than HD-WLE, performing random biopsies is still justified. First, some studies report patients in whom dysplasia was detected only by random biopsies.[82] Second, lesions reported as IND are often invisible but important to detect because they predict heightened rates of progression to HGD or CRC compared with no dysplasia.[60] Third, as discussed earlier, some nonconventional forms of dysplasia are endoscopically invisible because the crypt architecture is normal, so they are often detected by random biopsies.

When performing DCE, some studies suggest that lesions with Kudo type III or IV pit patterns, and those greater than 7 mm, are likely to be dysplastic.[83] VCE is often found to be noninferior to DCE and might be more time-efficient. There are several techniques for performing VCE, adding to the confusion of how to choose which one to use for IBD surveillance.[81]

ROLE OF ENDOSCOPIC SURVEILLANCE AND MANAGEMENT

There are only minor differences among gastrointestinal societies with respect to the recommendations from medical societies for colonoscopic surveillance (**Fig. 5**).[13–15,26] Currently no reliable methods exist for detecting dysplasia in IBD other than colonoscopy with biopsy. Because the endoscopic appearance of IBD-associated dysplasia and CRC is often subtle, and classifying lesions to determine endoscopic resectability is so important for management, achieving adequate

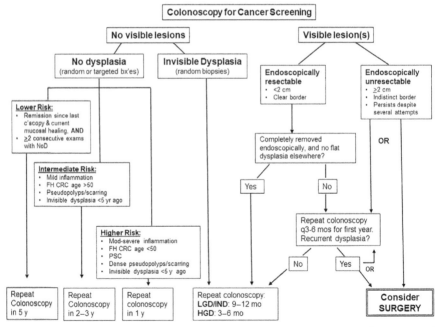

Fig. 5. Suggested algorithm for endoscopic surveillance and management of patients with chronic IBD.

colonoscopic quality metrics is critical. Therefore, screening and surveillance examinations should (1) ideally be performed with the patient in remission; (2) adhere to standard colonoscopic quality metrics; and (3) be performed by endoscopists with experience in IBD-associated neoplasia detection, especially for cases with a history of dysplasia. Standard of care is to use HD-WLE instead of standard-definition WLE. The use of dye-spray chromoendoscopy or VCE with imaging enhancing techniques should be left to the discretion of the endoscopist as to how experienced they are with such techniques. Our practice is to routinely perform HD-WLE with random biopsies while interrogating any visible lesions with natural band imaging and/or chromoendoscopy, reserving pan-colonic HD-CE for higher risk patients such as those with PSC, an earlier history of invisible or visible dysplasia, and mucosal scarring, atrophy, or pseudopolyps.

Dysplastic polyps that occur in nondiseased mucosa are considered to be sporadic adenomas and do not affect on the recommended frequency of endoscopic surveillance examinations after endoscopic polypectomy. Sporadic adenomas can presumably occur in mucosa affected by colitis as well. In the past, distinguishing them from "adenoma-like" dysplastic polyps associated with IBD was considered important because the latter often led to colectomy and was the subject of numerous histologic, immunohistochemical, and molecular studies.[84] However, this distinction is no longer relevant because short-term[85,86] and long-term[87,88] follow-up studies have shown that the probability of developing CRC after simple polypectomy is low provided there is no other background dysplasia.

More advanced endoscopic resection techniques can also be used to successfully treat most visible dysplastic lesions but should be entrusted to highly experienced endoscopists proficient in techniques such as endoscopic mucosal resection or endoscopic submucosal dissection (ESD) to ensure a complete resection with unambiguous resection margins and reduce the likelihood of local recurrence.[89,90] Both techniques have proven effective, with local recurrence rates of dysplasia of 3.5% to 4.4% and rates of metachronous CRC of less than 0.2% during an interval of 33 months.[89] ESD is increasingly being used to manage visible dysplastic lesions. A recent meta-analysis found the following rates associated with ESD: curative resection 81%, local recurrence 5%, bleeding 8%, perforation 6%, metachronous tumors 6%, and additional surgery 10%.[90] Thus, ESD can be considered an approach that manages dysplasia despite not necessarily always eliminating the need for future surgery. This can have a very important influence on patient management, as the patient (and their physician) adjusts to the possibility of colectomy to prevent CRC.

Patients whose dysplastic lesions have been completely removed via endoscopy, and where the adjacent flat mucosa is nondysplastic, are recommended to continue with regular endoscopic follow-ups because there is a high probability of metachronous dysplasia but a very low probability of CRC following endoscopic resection of dysplasia.[69,90] A diagnosis of HGD is of concern because the likelihood of synchronous CRC risk is approximately 15%.[91] Nonetheless, endoscopic excision of HGD lesions has proven effective, and the grade of dysplasia has been shown to have little influence on the rate of metachronous CRC.[90]

NEW DIAGNOSTIC AND THERAPEUTIC APPROACHES TO DYSPLASIA

The potential for innovative visualization methods and noninvasive surveillance methods to enhance the clinical management of IBD patients is beginning to be realized. Computer-aided polyp detection (CADe) systems are associated with higher adenoma and polyp detection rates in non-IBD settings.[92] Although studies using this technology have not yet been reported for IBD surveillance examination, it is tempting to speculate that CADe might enhance the detection of subtle endoscopic lesions in the chronically inflamed colon.

As for noninvasive approaches, a small feasibility study in patients with IBD reported that at a specificity of 89%, the combination of methylated BMP3 and NDRG4 genes in the stool detected 100% of 9 CRC and 80% of 10 dysplasias (4/4 HGD; 4/6 LGD).[93] A more recent study demonstrated the promise of using a multitarget stool DNA test without a hemoglobin component to detect IBD neoplasia. In that study, the sensitivity of mt-sDNAHgb-was 100% for detecting HGD, 84.6% for LGD greater than 1 cm, and 73.3% for colitis-associated CRC, with a specificity of 83.4%.[94]

SUMMARY

Optimization and comprehensive implementation of the management algorithms for the prevention of IBD-associated CRC remain unmet goals. Although reported declines in the incidence of IBD-associated CRC in Scandinavian countries and Canada are encouraging,[5,17–19] similar declines have not been observed in other Western countries with comparable health-care resources and surveillance programs,[95–97] and patients with IBD are still being diagnosed with CRC while under surveillance.[12,98,99] Addressing potential gaps in implementation and adherence to surveillance programs will require more personalized approaches to patient management and the development of noninvasive surveillance methods, likely based on genetic techniques. Greater insights into the pathology and molecular underpinnings of dysplasia may improve the effectiveness of our surveillance and promise better patient outcomes by increasing patient adherence and focusing our resources and attention on those patients who are at the highest risk.

CLINICS CARE POINTS

- Although inflammation can complicate the pathologic interpretation of dysplasia, a biopsy report of "IND" indicates a significant risk for the future development of HGD or carcinoma.
- Enhanced imaging techniques such as high-definition optics and chromoendoscopy can aid in targeting biopsies of inconspicuous dysplastic lesions during endoscopy but the recommendation for nontargeted biopsy sampling may still provide overall clinical benefit.
- Advanced endoscopic resection techniques can serve as a successful alternative to surgery for dysplastic lesions that meet certain criteria but they may not be applicable in some situations.
- Optimizing the surveillance intervals of high-risk patients with IBD requires a comprehensive assessment of their clinical risk factors and histologic and endoscopic findings at colonoscopy.

DISCLOSURE

The authors have no relevant disclosures to declare.

REFERENCES

1. Alatab S, Sepanlou SG, Ikuta K, et al. The global, regional, and national burden of inflammatory bowel disease in 195 countries and territories, 1990–2017: a systematic analysis for the Global Burden of Disease Study 2017. Lancet gastroenterology & hepatology 2020;5(1):17–30.

2. Zhao M, Gönczi L, Lakatos PL, et al. The burden of inflammatory bowel disease in Europe in 2020. Journal of Crohn's and Colitis 2021;15(9):1573–87.
3. Munkholm P. Review article: the incidence and prevalence of colorectal cancer in inflammatory bowel disease. Aliment Pharmacol Ther 2003;18:1–5.
4. Dyson JK, Rutter MD. Colorectal cancer in inflammatory bowel disease: What is the real magnitude of the risk? WJG 2012;18(29):3839.
5. Lutgens MW, van Oijen MG, van der Heijden GJ, et al. Declining risk of colorectal cancer in inflammatory bowel disease: an updated meta-analysis of population-based cohort studies. Inflamm Bowel Dis 2013;19(4):789–99.
6. Beaugerie L, Svrcek M, Seksik P, et al. Risk of colorectal high-grade dysplasia and cancer in a prospective observational cohort of patients with inflammatory bowel disease. Gastroenterology 2013;145(1):166–75.
7. Wetwittayakhlang P, Golovics PA, Gonczi L, et al. Stable incidence and risk factors of colorectal cancer in ulcerative colitis: A population-based cohort between 1977–2020. Clin Gastroenterol Hepatol 2023, in press.
8. Bogach J, Pond G, Eskicioglu C, et al. Age-related survival differences in patients with inflammatory bowel disease–associated colorectal cancer: A population-based cohort study. Inflamm Bowel Dis 2019;25(12):1957–65.
9. Lu C, Schardey J, Zhang T, et al. Survival outcomes and clinicopathological features in inflammatory bowel disease-associated colorectal cancer: A systematic review and meta-analysis. Ann Surg 2022;276(5):e319–30.
10. Arhi C, Askari A, Nachiappan S, et al. Stage at diagnosis and survival of colorectal cancer with or without underlying inflammatory bowel disease: Apopulation-based study. Journal of Crohn's and Colitis 2021;15(3):375–82.
11. Yaeger R, Paroder V, Bates DD, et al. Systemic chemotherapy for metastatic colitis-associated cancer has a worse outcome than sporadic colorectal cancer: matched case cohort analysis. Clin Colorectal Cancer 2020;19(4):e151–6.
12. Gordon C, Chee D, Hamilton B, et al. Root-cause analyses of missed opportunities for the diagnosis of colorectal cancer in patients with inflammatory bowel disease. Aliment Pharmacol Ther 2021;53(2):291–301.
13. Cairns SR, Scholefield JH, Steele RJ, et al. Guidelines for colorectal cancer screening and surveillance in moderate and high risk groups (update from 2002). Gut 2010;59(5):666–89.
14. Magro F, Gionchetti P, Eliakim R, et al. Third European evidence-based consensus on diagnosis and management of ulcerative colitis. Part 1: definitions, diagnosis, extra-intestinal manifestations, pregnancy, cancer surveillance, surgery, and ileo-anal pouch disorders. Journal of Crohn's and Colitis 2017;11(6):649–70.
15. Farraye FA, Odze RD, Eaden J, et al. AGA institute medical position panel on diagnosis and management of colorectal neoplasia in inflammatory bowel disease. Gastroenterology 2010;138(2):738–45.
16. Bye WA, Ma C, Nguyen TM, et al. Strategies for detecting colorectal cancer in patients with inflammatory bowel disease: a cochrane systematic review and meta-analysis. Am J Gastroenterol 2018;113(12):1801.
17. Loo SY, Vutcovici M, Bitton A, et al. Risk of malignant cancers in inflammatory bowel disease. Journal of Crohn's and Colitis 2019;13(10):1302–10.
18. Soderlund S, Brandt L, Lapidus A, et al. Decreasing time-trends of colorectal cancer in a large cohort of patients with inflammatory bowel disease. Gastroenterology 2009;136(5):1561–7.
19. Olen O, Erichsen R, Sachs MC, et al. Colorectal cancer in ulcerative colitis: a Scandinavian population-based cohort study. Lancet 2020;395(10218):123–31.

20. Beaugerie L, Itzkowitz SH. Cancers complicating inflammatory bowel disease. N Engl J Med 2015;372(15):1441–52.

21. Wijnands AM, de Jong ME, Lutgens MW, et al. Prognostic factors for advanced colorectal neoplasia in inflammatory bowel disease: systematic review and meta-analysis. Gastroenterology 2021;160(5):1584–98.

22. Connell WR, Talbot IC, Harpaz N, et al. Clinicopathological characteristics of colorectal carcinoma complicating ulcerative colitis. Gut 1994;35(10):1419–23.

23. Harpaz N, Talbot IC. Colorectal cancer in idiopathic inflammatory bowel disease. Semin Diagn Pathol 1996;13:339–57.

24. Goldstone R, Itzkowitz S, Harpaz N, et al. Dysplasia is more common in the distal than proximal colon in ulcerative colitis surveillance. Inflamm Bowel Dis 2012;18(5):832–7.

25. Chiu K, Riddell RH, Schaeffer DF. DALM, rest in peace: a pathologist's perspective on dysplasia in inflammatory bowel disease in the post-DALM era. Mod Pathol 2018;31(8):1180–90.

26. Laine L, Kaltenbach T, Barkun A, et al. SCENIC international consensus statement on surveillance and management of dysplasia in inflammatory bowel disease. Gastrointest Endosc 2015;81(3):489–501.

27. Riddell RH, Goldman H, Ransohoff DF, et al. Dysplasia in inflammatory bowel disease: Standardized classification with provisional clinical applications. Hum Pathol 1983;14(11):931–68.

28. Schlemper RJ, Riddell RH, Kato Y, et al. The Vienna classification of gastrointestinal epithelial neoplasia. Gut 2000;47(2):251–5.

29. Murthy SK, Feuerstein JD, Nguyen GC, et al. AGA clinical practice update on endoscopic surveillance and management of colorectal dysplasia in inflammatory bowel diseases: Expert review. Gastroenterology 2021;161(3):1043–51.e4.

30. Harpaz N, Goldblum JR, Shepherd N, et al. Novel classification of dysplasia in IBD. Mod Path 2017;30:174A.

31. Harpaz N, Goldblum JR, Shepherd NA, et al. Colorectal dysplasia in chronic inflammatory bowel disease: A contemporary consensus classification and interobserver study. Hum Pathol 2023;138:49–61.

32. Choi WT, Yozu M, Miller GC, et al. Nonconventional dysplasia in patients with inflammatory bowel disease and colorectal carcinoma: a multicenter clinicopathologic study. Mod Pathol 2020;33(5):933–43.

33. Iwaya M, Ota H, Tateishi Y, et al. Relationship between carcinoma subtype and overlying dysplasia in IBD-associated colorectal carcinoma. Lab Invest 2018; 98:271.

34. Ko HM, Harpaz N, McBride RB, et al. Serrated colorectal polyps in inflammatory bowel disease. Mod Pathol 2015;28(12):1584–93.

35. Ma YR, Sfreddo HJ, Ko HM, et al. Histological characteristics of Ibd-associated dysplasia in non-targeted colorectal biopsies. Gastroenterology 2017;152:S374.

36. Choi WT, Salomao M, Zhao L, et al. Hypermucinous, goblet cell-deficient and crypt cell dysplasias in inflammatory bowel disease are often associated with flat/invisible endoscopic appearance and advanced neoplasia on follow-up. J Crohn's Colitis 2022;16(1):98–108.

37. Gui X, Köbel M, Ferraz JG, et al. Histological and molecular diversity and heterogeneity of precancerous lesions associated with inflammatory bowel diseases. J Clin Pathol 2020;73(7):391–402.

38. Kamarádová K, Vošmiková H, Rozkošová K, et al. Non-conventional mucosal lesions (serrated epithelial change, villous hypermucinous change) are frequent

in patients with inflammatory bowel disease—results of molecular and immuno-histochemical single institutional study. Virchows Arch 2020;476(2):231–41.

39. Qin L, Zhu H, Raoufi M, et al. Incomplete goblet cell maturation: A distinctive form of flat dysplasia in IBD. Lab Invest 2011;91:164.

40. Bahceci D, Lauwers GY, Choi WT. Clinicopathologic features of undetected dysplasia found in total colectomy or proctocolectomy specimens of patients with inflammatory bowel disease. Histopathology 2022;81(2):183–91.

41. Mahmoud R, Shah SC, ten Hove JR, et al. No Association Between Pseudopolyps and Colorectal Neoplasia in Patients With Inflammatory Bowel Diseases. Gastroenterology 2019;156(5):1333–44.e3.

42. Parian A, Koh J, Limketkai BN, et al. Association between serrated epithelial changes and colorectal dysplasia in inflammatory bowel disease. Gastrointest Endosc 2016;84(1):87–95.

43. Parian AM, Limketkai BN, Chowdhury R, et al. Serrated epithelial change is associated with high rates of neoplasia in ulcerative colitis patients: a case-controlled study and systematic review with meta-analysis. Inflamm Bowel Dis 2021;27(9):1475–81.

44. Singhi AD, Waters KM, Makhoul EP, et al. Targeted next-generation sequencing supports serrated epithelial change as an early precursor to inflammatory bowel disease–associated colorectal neoplasia. Hum Pathol 2021;112:9–19.

45. Choi WT, Wen KW, Rabinovitch PS, et al. DNA content analysis of colorectal serrated lesions detects an aneuploid subset of inflammatory bowel disease-associated serrated epithelial change and traditional serrated adenomas. Histopathology 2018;73(3):464–72.

46. Odze RD, Brien T, Brown CA, et al. Molecular alterations in chronic ulcerative colitis-associated and sporadic hyperplastic polyps: a comparative analysis. Am J Gastroenterol 2002;97(5):1235–42.

47. Shen J, Gibson JA, Schulte S, et al. Clinical, pathologic, and outcome study of hyperplastic and sessile serrated polyps in inflammatory bowel disease. Hum Pathol 2015;46(10):1548–56.

48. Kilgore SP, Sigel JE, Goldblum JR. Hyperplastic-like mucosal change in Crohn's disease: an unusual form of dysplasia? Mod Pathol 2000;13(7):797–801.

49. Polydorides AD, Harpaz N. Serrated lesions in inflammatory bowel disease. Gastrointest Endosc 2017;85(2):461.

50. Bossard C, Denis MG, Bézieau S, et al. Involvement of the serrated neoplasia pathway in inflammatory bowel disease-related colorectal oncogenesis. Oncol Rep 2007;18(5):1093–7.

51. Rubio CA. Serrated neoplasias and de novo carcinomas in ulcerative colitis: a histological study in colectomy specimens. J Gastroenterol Hepatol 2007; 22(7):1024–31.

52. Miller GC, Liu C, Bettington ML, et al. Traditional serrated adenoma-like lesions in patients with inflammatory bowel disease. Hum Pathol 2020;97:19–28.

53. Sugimoto S, Shimoda M, Iwao Y, et al. Intramucosal poorly differentiated and signet-ring cell components in patients with ulcerative colitis-associated high-grade dysplasia. Dig Endosc 2019;31(6):706–11.

54. Ajioka Y, Iwanaga A, Watanabe J. Histogenesis of colorectal carcinoma in ulcerative colitis. Stomach Intestine 2008;43:1935–46.

55. Arpa G, Vanoli A, Grillo F, et al. Prognostic relevance and putative histogenetic role of cytokeratin 7 and MUC5AC expression in Crohn's disease-associated small bowel carcinoma. Virchows Arch 2021;479(4):667–78.

56. Borralho P, Vieira A, Freitas J, et al. Aberrant gastric apomucin expression in ulcerative colitis and associated neoplasia. J Crohn's Colitis 2007;1(1):35–40.
57. Tatsumi N, Kushima R, Vieth M, et al. Cytokeratin 7/20 and mucin core protein expression in ulcerative colitis-associated colorectal neoplasms. Virchows Arch 2006;448(6):756–62.
58. Andersen SN, Lovig T, Clausen OPF, et al. Villous, hypermucinous mucosa in long standing ulcerative colitis shows high frequency of K-ras mutations. Gut 1999;45(5):686–92.
59. Gui X, Köbel M, Ferraz JG, et al. Newly recognized non-adenomatous lesions associated with enteric carcinomas in inflammatory bowel disease–report of six rare and unique cases. Ann Diagn Pathol 2020;44:151455.
60. Mahmoud R, Shah SC, Torres J, et al. Association between indefinite dysplasia and advanced neoplasia in patients with inflammatory bowel diseases undergoing surveillance. Clin Gastroenterol Hepatol 2020;18(7):1518–27.
61. Wan J, Wang X, Zhang Y, et al. Systematic review with meta-analysis: incidence and factors for progression to advanced neoplasia in inflammatory bowel disease patients with indefinite and low-grade dysplasia. Aliment Pharmacol Ther 2022;55(6):632–44.
62. Choi C ho R, Ignjatovic-Wilson A, Askari A, et al. Low-grade dysplasia in ulcerative colitis: Risk factors for developing high-grade dysplasia or colorectal cancer. Am J Gastroenterol 2015;110(10):1461–71.
63. Yaeger R, Shah MA, Miller VA, et al. Genomic alterations observed in colitis-associated cancers are distinct from those found in sporadic colorectal cancers and vary by type of inflammatory bowel disease. Gastroenterology 2016;151(2):278–87.e6.
64. Rajamaki K, Taira A, Katainen R, et al. Genetic and epigenetic characteristics of inflammatory bowel disease–Associated colorectal cancer. Gastroenterology 2021;161(2):592–607.
65. Robles AI, Traverso G, Zhang M, et al. Whole-exome sequencing analyses of inflammatory bowel disease_associated colorectal cancers. Gastroenterology 2016;150(4):931–43.
66. Dienstmann R, Vermeulen L, Guinney J, et al. Consensus molecular subtypes and the evolution of precision medicine in colorectal cancer. Nat Rev Cancer 2017;17(2):79–92.
67. Chatila WK, Walch H, Hechtman JF, et al. Integrated clinical and genomic analysis identifies driver events and molecular evolution of colitis-associated cancers. Nat Commun 2023;14(1):110.
68. Dhir M, Montgomery EA, Glöckner SC, et al. Epigenetic regulation of WNT signaling pathway genes in inflammatory bowel disease (IBD) associated neoplasia. J Gastrointest Surg 2008;12(10):1745–53.
69. Wanders LK, Dekker E, Pullens B, et al. Cancer risk after resection of polypoid dysplasia in patients with longstanding ulcerative colitis: a meta-analysis. Clin Gastroenterol Hepatol 2014;12(5):756–64.
70. Melville DM, Jass JR, Morson BC, et al. Observer study of the grading of dysplasia in ulcerative colitis: comparison with clinical outcome. Hum Pathol 1989;20(10):1008–14.
71. Dixon MF, Brown LJ, Gilmour HM, et al. Observer variation in the assessment of dysplasia in ulcerative colitis. Histopathology 1988;13(4):385–97.
72. Odze RD, Goldblum J, Noffsinger A, et al. Interobserver variability in the diagnosis of ulcerative colitis-associated dysplasia by telepathology. Mod Pathol 2002;15(4):379–86.

73. Eaden J, Abrams K, McKay H, et al. Inter-observer variation between general and specialist gastrointestinal pathologists when grading dysplasia in ulcerative colitis. J Pathol 2001;194(2):152–7.
74. Van Schaik FDM, Ten Kate FJW, Offerhaus JGA, et al. Misclassification of dysplasia in patients with inflammatory bowel disease: Consequences for progression rates to advanced neoplasia. Inflamm Bowel Dis 2011;17(5):1108–16.
75. Xie H, Xiao SY, Pai R, et al. Diagnostic utility of TP53 and cytokeratin 7 immunohistochemistry in idiopathic inflammatory bowel disease-associated neoplasia. Mod Pathol 2014;27(2):303–13.
76. Sato A, MacHinami R. p53 immunohistochemistry of ulcerative colitis-associated with dysplasia and carcinoma. Pathol Int 1999;49(10):858–68.
77. Harpaz N, Peck AL, Yin J, et al. p53 protein expression in ulcerative colitis-associated colorectal dysplasia and carcinoma. Hum Pathol 1994;25(10):1069–74.
78. Dorer R, Odze RD. AMACR immunostaining is useful in detecting dysplastic epithelium in Barrett's esophagus, ulcerative colitis, and Crohn's disease. Am J Surg Pathol 2006;30(7):871–7.
79. Tsai JH, Rabinovitch PS, HuangD, et al. Association of aneuploidy and flat dysplasia with development of high-gradedysplasia or colorectal cancer in patients with inflammatory bowel disease. Gastroenterology 2017;153(6):1492–5.
80. Ma C, Henn P, Miller C, et al. Loss of SATB2 expression is a biomarker of inflammatory bowel disease–associated colorectal dysplasia and adenocarcinoma. Am J Surg Pathol 2019;43(10):1314.
81. Gabbiadini R, D'Amico F, De Marco A, et al. Colorectal cancer surveillance in patients with inflammatory bowel diseases: chromoendoscopy or non-chromoendoscopy, that is the question. J Clin Med 2022;11(3):509.
82. Moussata D, Allez M, Cazals-Hatem D, et al. Are random biopsies still useful for the detection of neoplasia in patients with IBD undergoing surveillance colonoscopy with chromoendoscopy? Gut 2018;67(4):616–24.
83. Lolli E, De Cristofaro E, Marafini I, et al. Endoscopic predictors of neoplastic lesions in inflammatory bowel diseases patients undergoing chromoendoscopy. Cancers 2022;14(18):4426.
84. Harpaz N, Polydorides AD. Colorectal dysplasia in chronic inflammatory bowel disease: pathology, clinical implications, and pathogenesis. Arch Pathol Lab Med 2010;134(6):876–95.
85. Rubin PH, Friedman S, Harpaz N, et al. Colonoscopic polypectomy in chronic colitis: conservative management after endoscopic resection of dysplastic polyps. Gastroenterology 1999;117(6):1295–300.
86. Engelsgjerd M, Farraye FA, Odze RD. Polypectomy may be adequate treatment for adenoma-like dysplastic lesions in chronic ulcerative colitis. Gastroenterology 1999;117(6):1288–94.
87. Odze RD, Farraye FA, Hecht JL, et al. Long-term follow-up after polypectomy treatment for adenoma-like dysplastic lesions in ulcerative colitis. Clin Gastroenterol Hepatol 2004;2(7):534–41.
88. Kisiel JB, Loftus EV Jr, Harmsen SW, et al. Outcome of sporadic adenomas and adenoma-like dysplasia in patients with ulcerative colitis undergoing polypectomy. Inflamm Bowel Dis 2012;18(2):226–35.
89. Mohapatra S, Sankaramangalam K, Lopimpisuth C, et al. Advanced endoscopic resection for colorectal dysplasia in inflammatory bowel disease: a meta-analysis. Endosc Int Open 2022;10(05):E593–601.

90. Mohan BP, Khan SR, Chandan S, et al. Endoscopic resection of colon dysplasia in patients with inflammatory bowel disease: a systematic review and meta-analysis. Gastrointest Endosc 2021;93(1):59–67.

91. Kabir M, Fofaria R, Arebi N, et al. Systematic review with meta-analysis: IBD-associated colonic dysplasia prognosis in the videoendoscopic era (1990 to present). Aliment Pharmacol Ther 2020;52(1):5–19.

92. Gimeno-García AZ, Hernández-Pérez A, Nicolás-Pérez D, et al. Artificial intelligence applied to colonoscopy: is it time to take a step forward? Cancers 2023;15(8):2193.

93. Kisiel JB, Yab TC, Nazer Hussain FT, et al. Stool DNA testing for the detection of colorectal neoplasia in patients with inflammatory bowel disease. Alimentary pharmacology & therapeutics 2013;37(5):546–54.

94. Itzkowitz S, Farraye FA, Limburg PJ, et al. Assessment of stool DNA markers to detect colorectal neoplasia in patients with inflammatory bowel disease: A multi-site case-control Study. J Crohn's Colitis 2023;17(9):1436–44.

95. Choi CHR, Rutter MD, Askari A, et al. Forty-year analysis of colonoscopic surveillance program for neoplasia in ulcerative colitis: an updated overview. Am J Gastroenterol 2015;110(7):1022.

96. Selinger CP, Andrews JM, Titman A, et al. Long-term follow-up reveals low incidence of colorectal cancer, but frequent need for resection, among australian patients with inflammatory bowel disease. Clin Gastroenterol Hepatol 2014; 12(4):644–50.

97. Hamilton B, Green H, Heerasing N, et al. Incidence and prevalence of inflammatory bowel disease in Devon, UK. Frontline Gastroenterol 2021;12(6):461–70.

98. Ballester MP, Mesonero F, Flórez-Diez P, et al. Adherence to endoscopic surveillance for advanced lesions and colorectal cancer in inflammatory bowel disease: an AEG and GETECCU collaborative cohort study. Aliment Pharmacol Ther 2022;55(11):1402–13.

99. Burke KE, Nayor J, Campbell EJ, et al. Interval colorectal cancer in inflammatory bowel disease: the role of guideline adherence. Dig Dis Sci 2020;65(1):111–8.

100. Akarca FG, Yozu M, Alpert L, et al. Non-conventional dysplasia is frequently associated with low-grade tubuloglandular and mucinous adenocarcinomas in inflammatory bowel disease. Histopathology, 2023, in press.

101. Levi GS, Harpaz N. Intestinal low-grade tubuloglandular adenocarcinoma in inflammatory bowel disease. Am J Surg Pathol 2006;30(8):1022–9.

102. Wen KW, Umetsu SE, Goldblum JR, et al. DNA flow cytometric and interobserver study of crypt cell atypia in inflammatory bowel disease. Histopathology 2019; 75(4):578–88.

Sporadic Polyps of the Colorectum

Ian Brown, MBBS, FRCPA[a,b,c,]*, Mark Bettington, MBBS, PhD, FRCPA[a,c,d]

KEYWORDS

- Polyp • Malignant polyp • Colorectal • Adenoma • Serrated neoplasia

KEY POINTS

- Large bowel polyps are a major part of gastrointestinal pathology practice.
- While much of large bowel polyp pathology can seem basic; polyp diagnoses are the cornerstone of surveillance guidelines and thus have meaningful clinical implications.
- Conventional adenomas are readily recognized but attention must be paid to the designation of high-grade dysplasia and villosity to improve reproducibility.
- Malignant polyps are uncommon but accurate diagnosis and risk stratification are critical to guiding clinical management decisions.
- Serrated polyps are common. Histologic emphasis should be directed to the distinction of hyperplastic polyp from sessile serrated adenoma.

INTRODUCTION

A colorectal polyp is defined as any lesion that is elevated above the surrounding mucosa or visible to the endoscopist. Polyps result from overgrowth of the native elements of the mucosa or underlying submucosa and are either epithelial or non-epithelial in nature. They can be classified based on the underlying nature of the overgrowth or infiltrate. Epithelial overgrowth accounts for most colorectal polyps, and essentially all cancer precursors in the large intestine. Two main pathways of colorectal carcinogenesis exist—the chromosomal instability pathway and the serrated pathway. Chromosomal instability accounts for approximately 70% of colorectal carcinogenesis and results from the progressive accumulation of mutations producing gains or losses of whole or significant portions of chromosomes.[1] These mutations result in activation of various oncogenes for example, *KRAS* and dysfunction of tumor

a Envoi Pathology, Brisbane; b Pathology Queensland, Royal Brisbane and Women's Hospital Cnr Herston and Bowen Bridge Roads, Herston Qld 4006, Australia; c University of Queensland, St Lucia, Qld 4072, Australia; d Queensland Institute of Medical Research, 300 Herston Road, Herston QLD 4006, Australia
* Corresponding author. Envoi Specialist Pathologists, 5, 38 Bishop Street, Kelvin Grove, QLD 4059, Australia.
E-mail address: ianbrown@envoi.com.au

Gastroenterol Clin N Am 53 (2024) 155–177
https://doi.org/10.1016/j.gtc.2023.10.002
0889-5553/24/© 2023 Elsevier Inc. All rights reserved.
gastro.theclinics.com

suppressor genes for example, TP53.[1] Conventional adenomas are indicative lesions of the chromosomal instability pathway. The serrated pathway accounts for much of the remaining 30% of colorectal carcinogenesis. This pathway is defined by the presence of serrated polyps, and at a molecular level, by mitogen-activated protein kinase (MAP) kinase pathway activation (especially activating *BRAF* mutation) and in many cases, a CpG island methylator phenotype (CIMP).[2–4] Cancers arising via these pathways have distinctive morphologic features and behavior. Furthermore, the precursor polyps in each pathway have different risks for progression to colorectal cancer, which allows for individualized surveillance. **Fig. 1** summarizes the precursor lesions and genetic abnormalities involved in both pathways.

This review will consider only epithelial polyps of the large intestine concentrating mainly on conventional adenomas and serrated lesions. Hamartomatous polyps are discussed in the article on polyposis syndromes.

DISCUSSION
Conventional Adenomatous Polyps

General clinical features
Conventional adenomas are the most common type of neoplastic growth of the colonic epithelium and are precursors of approximately 70% of all colorectal adenocarcinomas through the chromosomal instability pathway.[1,5] Three types of conventional adenomas are recognized based on the predominant architectural pattern of the lesion—tubular adenoma (TA), tubulovillous adenoma (TVA), and villous adenoma(VA), with tubular adenoma being most common, accounting for more than 50%.[6,7] Conventional adenomas always exhibit epithelial dysplasia, which is an unequivocal neoplastic change identified histologically by nuclear enlargement, nuclear hyperchromasia, and crowding of the epithelial cells. Dysplasia is graded based on the degree of these changes (see later). The prevalence of conventional adenomas at colonoscopy is at least 30% to 50%,[8] but increases with age and more rapidly beyond 50 years of age.[9] Most conventional adenomas develop in the left colon as opposed to serrated polyps that develop more often in the right colon.[6,8]

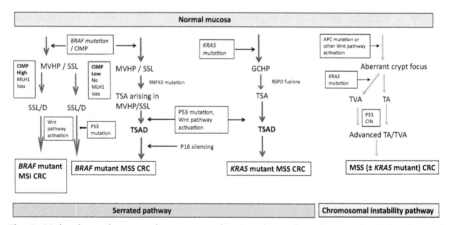

Fig. 1. Molecular pathways and precursor polyps in colorectal carcinogenesis. CRC, colorectal carcinoma; GCHP, goblet cell - rich hyperplastic polyp; MSS, microsatellite stable; MSI, microsatellite instability; MVHP, microvesicular hyperplastic polyp; SSL, sessile serrated lesion; SSLD, sessile serrated lesion with dysplasia; TSA, traditional serrated adenoma; TSAD, traditional serrated adenoma with high grade dysplasia.

Pathogenesis

Most conventional adenomas develop from sporadically acquired DNA mutations. By middle age, about 1% of normal-appearing colonic crypts contain cells with driver mutations for colorectal cancer.[10] Activating mutations of *APC* or other *WNT* family members initiate the development of conventional adenomas while mutations in *TP53* and accelerating chromosomal instability underlie progression to advanced adenoma and colorectal cancer.[1,11] *KRAS* mutation is strongly correlated with the presence of villous architecture in conventional adenomas.[12,13] The earliest appreciable adenoma is a single dysplastic crypt (aberrant crypt focus or microadenoma) that develops from mutations in colonic stem cells located in the crypt bases,[14] with proliferation of cells eventually replacing the entire crypt. Further growth of the adenoma occurs by either the spread of proliferating cells into adjacent crypts or by fission of dysplastic crypts.[15]

In small adenomas, the tubular pattern of the normal colonic crypts is retained. In larger adenomas, the crypts become more convoluted, and finger-like projections (villous structures) are more likely to be found. It remains unclear whether villous architecture always develops from a tubular adenoma or whether it can arise de novo.

Most conventional adenomas are sporadic lesions but they also develop in inherited colon cancer syndromes including familial adenomatous polyposis (FAP), attenuated FAP, Lynch syndrome, MUTYH-associated polyposis (MAP), AXIN2-associated polyposis, POLE/POLD1, NTHL-1 polyposis, and MSH3-Associated Polyposis.[16] Clues to an inherited origin are the development of adenomas at a young age (<30 years), the finding of a polyposis or multiple cumulative adenomas (>10), and neoplasms at other body sites. Lynch syndrome is the commonest inherited colon cancer syndrome, but conventional adenomas are generally not numerous and are more likely to be in the right colon and to harbor high-grade dysplasia and a villous component, even when small.[17,18] Lynch syndrome results in mismatch repair (MMR) deficiency, usually with immunohistochemical loss of expression for any of the DNA MMR proteins, MLH-1, MSH-2, MSH-6, and PMS-2. Three pathways to colorectal cancer may operate in Lynch syndrome patients. The first is by the acquisition of MMR deficiency in a sporadic adenoma. The second is cancer arising directly from colonic crypts showing MMR deficiency without a preceding adenoma, and the third pathway is an adenoma developing due to secondary APC mutations in a background of non-dysplastic colonic crypts showing MMR deficiency.[19] Up to 70% of conventional adenomas in Lynch syndrome patients show a loss of MMR protein staining concordant with the pathogenetic mutation identified in the patient.[20,21] Loss is more likely to be found in older patients and larger adenomas and/or those with high-grade dysplasia.[22] However, the corollary is that retained expression of MMR proteins in a conventional adenoma does not exclude Lynch syndrome.

Pathology

Endoscopic. Conventional adenomas may be either polypoidal or non-polypoidal. Polypoidal adenomas arising from mucosa via a stalk are termed "pedunculated," and those without a stalk are considered sessile. Non-polypoidal lesions may be flat or depressed and those extending more than 10 mm are termed "laterally spreading tumors."[23] Endoscopically, conventional adenoma presents an NBI International Colorectal Endoscopic (NICE) type 2 appearance, with a brown color relative to the background and oval, tubular, or branched white structures surrounded by brown vessels.[24] The brown color is also a feature of the endoscopically resected polyp. **Table 1** outlines the important features of the NICE classification.

Table 1
NBI International Colorectal Endoscopic Classification of polyps

NICE Classification	Color	Vasculature	Surface Pattern
Type 1 (HP or SSA)	Lighter than background mucosa	Few vessels	Dark or light spots (but uniform)
Type 2 (conventional adenoma, SSAD, TSA)	Darker than background mucosa	Many vessels	Irregular (oval or branched) white structures surrounded by vessels

HP, hyperplastic polyp; SSA, sessile serrated adenoma; SSAD, sessile serrated adenoma with dysplasia; TSA, traditional serrated adenoma.

Microscopic. Conventional adenomas are categorized based on the amount of villous change they exhibit. The definition of "villous" is poorly defined. The World Health Organization (WHO) states that a villous should resemble normal small intestinal villi, but acknowledges there is poor reproducibility in subtyping adenomas based on villosity. TAs have less than 25% villous architecture. TVAs have a villous component of between 25% and 75% of the polyp (**Fig. 2**A and B). VA, which is very rare outside of the rectum, has a villous component of greater than 75% of the polyp. These cutoffs are arbitrary, and it has been argued that any degree of villous architecture defines a lesion different from TA.[13] It is well established that villous architecture is more likely to be found in larger adenomas. At least one-third of adenomas ≥10 mm in size have a villous component.[25]

Dysplasia is graded on the degree of nuclear and glandular abnormality into low grade and high grade. In the large intestine, high-grade dysplasia includes carcinoma

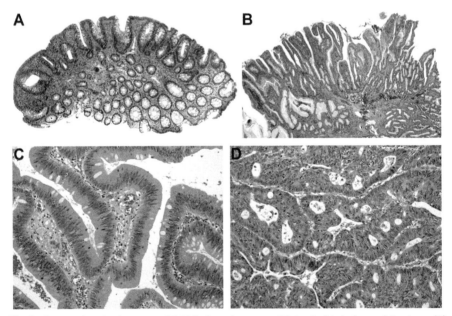

Fig. 2. Conventional adenomas. (*A*) Tubular adenoma with typical tubular architecture; (*B*) Tubulovillous adenoma with villous structures at the surface and tubular architecture at the base; (*C*) Low-grade dysplasia—multilayered epithelium with hyperchromatic, penicillate nuclei; and (*D*) High-grade dysplasia—back-to-back glands with enlarged nuclei and prominent nucleoli.

in situ and intramucosal carcinoma. This two-tier system results in better interobserver concordance and is more clinically relevant since only a minority of adenomas, less than 5% overall,[6,7,26] exhibit high-grade dysplasia, which is predictive of a higher risk of developing invasive adenocarcinoma. As with villous change, the finding of high-grade dysplasia is more common in adenomas ≥10 mm in size.[7,25,27] Low-grade dysplasia has a uniform gland architecture and lining epithelium composed of multilayered cells with hyperchromatic, penicillate nuclei (see **Fig. 2**C). In high-grade dysplasia, the glands are more closely packed with a back-to-back configuration, complex budding, cribriform patterns, and papillary infolding. In general, these architectural features should be identifiable at low-power magnification. The epithelial cells show loss of the normal perpendicular nuclear polarity, nuclear pleomorphism, prominent nucleoli, and a dispersed chromatin pattern (see **Fig. 2**D).

Unfortunately, among pathologists, there may be significant interobserver variation in reporting the presence and degree of villous architecture[28–30] and high-grade dysplasia.[28–33] This variation is more problematic in adenomas less than 10 mm in diameter, potentially affecting subsequent surveillance[29,30] and leading to the suggestion to abandon pathologic reporting of villous architecture and high-grade dysplasia in colorectal adenomas.[34] However, concordance in diagnosis improves in pathologists who are better trained by the use of discrete diagnostic criteria.[28,35] On balance, the benefits of reporting these features outweigh the downside.[36,37]

Differential diagnosis
The histologic diagnosis of conventional adenoma is usually straightforward but secondary changes can cause some difficulty. These changes include ulceration, stromal fibrosis, and mucin extravasation into a polyp stalk secondary to torsion with mucosal displacement, and stromal hemorrhage. This imparts a red appearance when the reaction is acute, and a brown appearance when the reaction is older, due to iron deposition. The cytoplasm of the adenoma cells may show clear cell change and there may be abundant Paneth cells, stromal ossification, squamous metaplasia ("morules"),[38] or neuroendocrine cell proliferation[39] associated with the adenoma. Squamous metaplasia and neuroendocrine cell proliferation can appear infiltrative and give a false impression of high-grade dysplasia or invasive carcinoma.[38,40]

Parts of an adenoma may herniate into the submucosa mimicking invasive carcinoma. This may be the result of torsion of a pedunculated polyp (discussed below) or via extension into normally present lymphoglandular complexes through deficiency in the muscularis mucosae.[41] Epithelial misplacement into the submucosa generally occurs in large pedunculated adenomas, especially in the sigmoid colon. It may be limited to the polyp head or extend into the stalk. The rich stromal reaction to the displaced glands may resemble that seen in invasive cancer, hence the process is alternatively called "pseudo invasion."[42] Distinction from adenocarcinoma is one of the most common reasons for a second opinion referral in gastrointestinal pathology.[43] Some adenomas show both true invasive carcinoma and pseudo invasion further complicating this issue.

The cytologic and/or architectural abnormality of conventional adenomas can be mimicked by epithelial regeneration after ischemic injury (so-called mass-forming ischemia)[44] or other local injury or inflammatory process with polypoidal regeneration, such as occurs in diverticulitis or inflammatory bowel disease. Knowledge of the background history generally helps exclude adenoma. Serrated polyps can be mistaken for a conventional adenoma in 2 situations. The first is an early traditional serrated adenoma lacking well-developed features. This distinction could change the surveillance interval for the patient. The second situation is when the dysplastic component of a sessile serrated lesion is accompanied by either minimal, or none, of the background serrated lesion, or when the dysplastic process overgrows most of the precursor lesion (discussed further later).

Natural history and risk prediction

The overall risk of a conventional adenoma progressing to colorectal carcinoma (CRC) is estimated to be about 5% with a lag time over 10 years.[8] However, patients who have conventional adenomas with at least a 25% villous component and/or high-grade dysplasia and/or size $\geq$10 mm (called "advanced adenomas") are at increased risk of developing colorectal cancer.[45,46] Adenomas with a laterally spreading pattern also exhibit a higher risk for developing cancer.[23] Conversely, a small tubular adenoma has a negligible risk for progression to CRC,[47] and small adenomas are only rarely found to contain invasive adenocarcinoma.[7,48]

Treatment

Standard management of conventional adenomas is resection, which is accomplished endoscopically in most cases. Follow up after resection depends on the nature and number of adenomas resected. National guidelines vary, but in general, patients with fewer than 5 adenomas without advanced features ($\geq$25% villous component, high-grade dysplasia, size $\geq$10) should have a follow-up endoscopy at between 5 and 10 years. Patients with 5 or more adenomas or with an advanced adenoma should undergo follow-up endoscopic surveillance at a shorter interval, typically 3 years or less.[49,50]

Malignant Colorectal Polyp

General clinical features

The diagnosis of adenocarcinoma throughout most of the gastrointestinal tract is defined by invasion of neoplastic cells through the connective tissue basement membrane that normally surrounds the glands. This occurs within the mucosal layer and the term "intramucosal carcinoma" is applied. However, in the large intestine, the term "intramucosal carcinoma" is not recommended because there is no evidence that adenocarcinoma confined to the mucosa can spread beyond the colon.[51,52] This is also true of rare cases of intramucosal carcinoma that show invasion of mucosal lymphatics,[53] although, there is conflicting evidence as to whether poorly differentiated intramucosal carcinoma can be considered potentially capable of metastasis.[54,55] Nevertheless, carcinoma invading the submucosa, often accompanied by a desmoplastic stromal response, is regarded as "malignant colorectal polyp." Using this definition approximately 1% of all polyps in community practice are malignant,[6] and this is largely restricted to polyps that are 10 mm or more in diameter.[7] Malignant polyps are more common in men and over two-thirds are found in the left colon or rectum.[56]

Pathogenesis

Precursor lesions of both the serrated and chromosomal instability pathways can give rise to malignant colorectal polyps. Residual precursor lesion is usually evident at the edge of the carcinoma.[56]

Pathology

Macroscopically, malignant polyps may be polypoid (sessile or pedunculated) or non-polypoid. Endoscopically, these lesions present a NICE 3 pattern with areas of absent vessels and an amorphous or absent surface pattern.[24] Non polypoidal laterally spreading tumors with a non-granular or granular-nodular mixed endoscopic pattern are more likely to contain invasive carcinoma.[23]

Histology

As discussed earlier, the defining feature of malignancy in the large bowel is invasion of the submucosa. Although conceptually simple, many cases of early invasion can be difficult to diagnose with confidence. Problems arise when the polyp is removed piecemeal and the fragments are small, superficial, and/or poorly oriented. The muscularis mucosae can reduplicate itself and in small biopsy fragments it can be very difficult (or impossible) to be certain of submucosal invasion. A desmoplastic stromal response is good evidence of submucosal invasion, but in some cases, the fibrotic stroma of a chronically prolapsed polyp can mimic desmoplasia. A prior biopsy site can also closely mimic a desmoplastic stromal response.

In other cases, there are clearly neoplastic glands in the submucosa, but the distinction between pseudo invasion (dysplastic glands misplaced into the submucosa) and truly malignant glands can be very challenging. Features that can be used to separate the 2 are presented in **Box 1** and **2**.[57]

Natural history

Overall, malignant polyps have a risk of lymph node metastases of approximately 5% and infrequently recur at the polypectomy site if completely excised.[58] So endoscopic resection is curative treatment in most cases.

Risk prediction

Several pathologic features in the removed polyp consistently predict a higher risk for regional lymph node metastases or local recurrence at the polypectomy site that warrants surgical resection. These include large tumor size/invasive tumor depth, poor differentiation (high grade), tumor budding, margin involvement, and lymphatic and/or venous invasion.[58–65] These risk factors are independent of the precursor lesion and the molecular pathway leading to cancer. The approximate risk for lymph node metastasis of each factor in malignant polyps is summarized in **Table 2**. The risk increases as more adverse features are present.[58,66]

Vascular invasion is the pre-eminent risk factor for metastasis in malignant colorectal polyps[59,61,67] and its presence is a recommendation for colectomy in all published management guidelines.[17,60,63,68–72] Direct measurement of the depth of submucosal invasion has effectively replaced Kikuchi and Haggitt levels previously used for sessile and pedunculated polyps, respectively. For sessile polyps, a depth <1 mm (<1000 μm), represents a low-risk lesion,[63] while a depth ≥2 mm, is high risk.[61,73,74] Refinement of the risk between 1 and 2 mm is required. A recent study suggests a cut-off of greater than 1.5 mm should be considered high risk (**Fig. 3**A).[56] For pedunculated polyps, depth of invasion is assessed by referencing 4 anatomic landmarks proposed by Haggitt and colleagues.[75] Level 1 is invasion confined to the head of the polyp, level 2 is invasion to the junction between the head and stalk ('neck of polyp'), level 3 is invasion into the stalk, and level 4 is invasion into the native

---

Box 1
Histologic features favoring pseudo invasion in a colorectal adenoma

1. A mix of neoplastic and non-neoplastic glands in the submucosa

2. Lamina propria accompanying the glands

3. Similar cytology between adenoma and submucosal glands

4. Continuity of glands between mucosa and submucosa

5. Evidence of polyp prolapse/torsion (hemorrhage, hemosiderin, muscular proliferation)

Box 2
Histologic features favoring true invasion in a colorectal adenoma

1. A desmoplastic stromal response

2. Single cells or tumor buds in the submucosa

3. Lymphatic or vascular invasion

4. High-grade adenocarcinoma (poor differentiation)

---

submucosa. Cancers in levels 1 and 2 were considered at low risk for metastasis, however, metastasis occurs in approximately 5% of these cancers if vascular invasion is present.[74] Conversely, if no vascular invasion exists then cancer invading <3 mm into the stalk (level 3) has a low risk for metastasis (see **Fig. 3**B).[74] Poor tumor differentiation reflects either advanced cytoarchitectural abnormality in the carcinoma or a special type of carcinoma known to have aggressive behavior most commonly signet ring cell carcinoma and neuroendocrine carcinoma.[58] More recently, dedifferentiation in the pattern of high-level tumor budding has been identified as a significant risk factor for metastasis in several studies.[56,63,64,76]

There is a consensus that a polypectomy margin of ≥2 mm from cancer is not associated with local recurrence at the resection site. However, several recent studies have concluded that the risk for local recurrence only exists when the true cut edge of the polyp or the adjacent zone of diathermy artifact, usually up to 0.5 mm in thickness, is directly involved by carcinoma or the margin cannot be adequately assessed because of piecemeal resection.[56,58,66,70,77] Currently, only true margin involvement is considered for colectomy in the Japanese Society for Cancer of the Colon and Rectum management guidelines.[63]

Other factors that may increase the risk for a malignant polyp include sessile morphology[62] and location in the distal one-third of the rectum.[78,79] **Box 3** summarizes the recommended features of a histopathology report of a malignant polyp.

Treatment

Malignant polyps that show no high-risk features and that are completely resected can be followed conservatively with a surveillance colonoscopy in 12 months.

Serrated Colorectal Polyps

Serrated colorectal polyps are the precursor lesions involved in the serrated neoplasia pathway. Approximately 20% to 30% of CRC arises via this pathway, with the relative contribution increasing with advancing age.[80] Serrated polyps comprise a wide range of lesions with distinctive morphology and clinical significance. **Tables 3** and **4** describe some of the clinicopathological and molecular features of serrated polyp.

Hyperplastic polyps

As per the fifth edition of Tumors of the Digestive Tract, hyperplastic polyps are now divided into 2 subtypes—microvesicular hyperplastic polyp (MVHP) and goblet cell hyperplastic polyp (GCHP). A former third category of mucin-poor hyperplastic polyp was abandoned in the most recent iteration of the WHO blue book as this is now generally considered to represent a form of MVHP.

Clinical features

Hyperplastic polyps are incidental findings and are not associated with any clinical symptoms. Due to their relative lack of abnormal surface vessels, they are not associated with overt or occult blood loss.[81] Hyperplastic polyps are common and typically

Table 2
Features associated with an increased risk of lymph node metastases in a malignant polyp

Feature	Prevalence of feature	Rate of lymph Node Metastasis when Present	Relative Risk for lymph Node Metastasis	Odds Ratio for lymph Node Metastasis
Sessile Polyp				
Sessile polyp depth ≥2 mm	~60%	~5%	2.5 ×	3 ×
Vascular invasion[a]	~20%	~10%	5 ×	5 ×
Poor differentiation[a]	~5%–10%	~10%	5 ×	5 ×
High tumor budding[a]	~10%–20%	~5%	5 ×	7 ×
Pedunculated Polyp				
Pedunculated polyp with stalk invasion ≥3 mm	Insufficient data	~10%	Insufficient data	Insufficient data
Vascular invasion (irrespective of Haggitt level)	~20%	~5%	Insufficient data	Insufficient data

[a] Data for sessile polyps.
Table compiled from data in references[5]

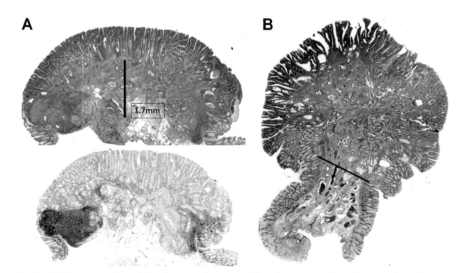

Fig. 3. Malignant polyp. (*A*) Adenocarcinoma arising from a small sessile tubular adenoma in a patient with Lynch syndrome. The carcinoma invades the submucosa for a depth of 1.7 mm. There is loss of expression of MLH-1 in both the adenocarcinoma and the tubular adenoma in this case. (*B*) Adenocarcinoma arising from a pedunculated tubulovillous adenoma. The carcinoma invades the polyp stalk (*arrow*). Depth of invasion is measured from the commencement of the stalk (*horizontal line*).

increase in prevalence with age.[82] They are identified in 10% to 20% of screening colonoscopies, but many diminutive and distal hyperplastic polyps are not resected, and as such, the numbers reported in the literature are likely an underestimate.

Pathogenesis
The initiating molecular event in the development of hyperplastic polyps is not known, but activating *BRAF* (MVHP) or *KRAS* (GCHP) mutation are the most likely candidates.[83] Subsequently, many MVHPs will develop the CpG island methylator phenotype (CIMP).[83] In general, hyperplastic polyps are not considered to have malignant

---

Box 3
Important features of the pathology report of a colorectal malignant polyp:

1. Tumor site
2. Tumor type
3. Differentiation
4. Depth of invasion#
5. Haggitt level (in pedunculated polyps)
6. Tumor budding
7. Vascular invasion
8. Margin status
9. Mismatch repair marker immunohistochemistry

Depth below muscularis mucosae in sessile polyps. Depth into the stalk of pedunculated polyps

Table 3					
Clinicopathological features of serrated colorectal polyps					
Polyp Type	Age	Sex (% Female)	Size (mm)	Location (% including and Distal to Splenic Flexure)	Cancer Risk
Microvesicular hyperplastic polyp	58	47	4.6	84	Negligible
Goblet cell hyperplastic polyp	60	48	4.5	83	Negligible
Sessile serrated adenoma	59	55	8.5	18	Low
Sessile serrated adenoma with dysplasia	69	56	7.8	11	High
Traditional serrated adenoma	62	50	10.6	79	Moderate

potential. It is postulated that oncogene-induced senescence prevents proliferation in these polyps.[84]

Endoscopic features
Endoscopically, hyperplastic polyps present as NICE 1 polyps.[24] Most arise in the distal colon and rectum but they can occur throughout the large bowel. The majority of hyperplastic polyps are diminutive or small.[82,85]

Histology
There are 2 histologic types termed "microvesicular (MVHP)" and "goblet cell–rich hyperplastic polyps" (GCHP) (**Fig. 4**A and B). MVHPs are characterized by their crypt cytoarchitectural features which include crypt elongation, serration in the upper crypt, expanded but symmetric proliferation zone, and a relative lack of mature goblet cells (cells contain microvesicular mucin only).[86] GCHPs are more subtle and can be overlooked as normal mucosa. They are characterized by longer and more crowded crypts than the adjacent normal mucosa, superficial serration, abundance of goblet cells, and occasionally a thick subepithelial collagen layer.[86]

Differential Diagnosis

From a clinical perspective, the major significance of the hyperplastic polyp is in its distinction from the sessile serrated lesion (SSL) (this is particularly an issue for the MVHP subtype) and its contribution to the diagnosis of serrated polyposis syndrome.[86]

Natural History and Treatment

Hyperplastic polyps are generally not considered to harbor malignant potential and as such are of limited clinical significance. Treatment can be by polypectomy but many colonoscopists will choose not to remove typical small and distal hyperplastic polyps.

Sessile Serrated Lesion (Sessile Serrated Adenoma)

Sessile serrated lesion (SSL) is the prototype polyp of the serrated neoplasia pathway and is the major precursor for cancers arising from the serrated neoplasia pathway.[80]

Clinical features
Similar to most other colorectal polyps, SSL is an asymptomatic lesion. Because SSL also does not have a markedly abnormal vasculature, occult blood loss is uncommon from these polyps.[81] As such, they are only identified as incidental polyps during

Table 4
Molecular features of serrated colorectal polyps

Polyp Type	BRAF	KRAS	CIMP	APC Pathway	MLH1 loss	P16 loss	P53	Cancer Subtype
Microvesicular hyperplastic polyp	72	10	10	N/A	N/A	N/A	N/A	N/A
Goblet cell hyperplastic polyp	20	51	7	N/A	N/A	N/A	N/A	N/A
Sessile serrated adenoma	80	9	51	10	0	9	0	As per SSAD below
Sessile serrated adenoma with dysplasia	93	<1	93	55	75	43	14	BRAF mutated; MSI or MSS
Traditional serrated adenoma	67	22	46	15	<1	29	15	BRAF mutated; MSS or KRAS mutated

SSAD, sessile serrated adenoma with dysplasia; MSI, microsatellite instability; MSS, microsatellite stable.

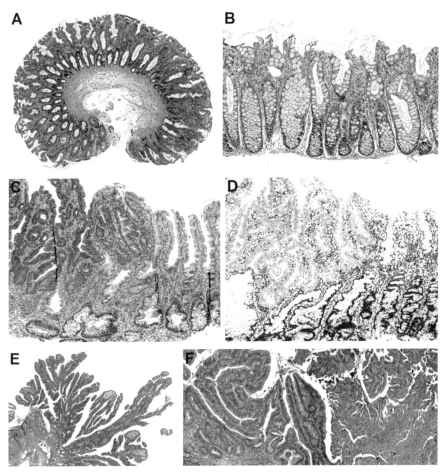

Fig. 4. Serrated polyps. (*A*) Microvesicular hyperplastic polyp; (*B*) Goblet cell hyperplastic polyp; (*C*) Sessile serrated lesion with dysplasia. Loss of staining for MLH1 demonstrated in (*D*); (*E*) Traditional serrated adenoma at low power; and (*F*) a traditional serrated adenoma transitioning to high-grade dysplasia.

endoscopy for investigation of unrelated symptoms or during screening or surveillance endoscopy. Their prevalence is highly variable in the literature, and this is likely due to several factors, including patient factors, endoscopic factors (serrated polyp detection rates), and pathologic factors (histologic criteria for making the diagnosis of SSL).[6,87–89] However, the more recent literature would suggest that SSLs are common, and with expert colonoscopy and pathology, the prevalence can be as high as 20% in a screening population.[90]

Pathogenesis
Risk factors for the development of SSLs are relatively poorly defined but include smoking, diabetes, and obesity.[91] Similar to MVHPs, SSL has frequent activating *BRAF* mutation and high levels of CIMP.[92] Of note, methylation levels are low in younger patients (<50 years of age) and show a sudden increase in the sixth decade,[93] which may be important in driving malignant progression.[94]

Endoscopic features

At colonoscopy, they present as NICE 1 polyps, often with an ill-defined border.[95,96] They range from diminutive to large lesions and often have an adherent mucin covering after bowel preparation. Sometimes a rim of bubbles or fecal debris will collect around the border of the polyp.[95] Most cases are proximal and are identified in older patients. However, some studies have demonstrated that the prevalence can be remarkably consistent across age groups.[90]

Histologic features

Sessile serrated lesions are best defined by their crypt architectural abnormalities[80,86,97] These include uneven crypt spacing, basal crypt dilation, horizontal growth along the muscularis mucosae, crypt branching, deep serration, irregular proliferation centers, and no (or very minimal) cytologic atypia.

Differential diagnosis

As noted earlier, the critical differential diagnosis is with MVHP. These polyps occur on a spectrum, with the final diagnosis dependent on the number of typical SSL-type crypts.[6] Current WHO guidelines recommend that a single, unequivocal SSL-type crypt is sufficient to make a diagnosis of SSL. However, many pathologists argue that there is limited evidence for this recommendation and prefer to see more evidence (in the form of more abnormal crypts) before making a diagnosis of SSL. This difference in pathologic practice can impact SSL detection rates.[6]

Natural history and treatment

Sessile serrated lesions are premalignant polyps. Although the risk of any 1 polyp progressing to cancer is relatively low, complete endoscopic removal is the preferred management option. SSLs can present challenges to the endoscopist, both in detection and complete removal.[88] For these reasons, cancers of the serrated neoplasia pathway tend to be over-represented in series on interval CRC.[98,99]

Sessile Serrated Lesion with Dysplasia

Sessile serrated lesion with dysplasia (SSLD) is the dysplastic form of SSL. Their size and distribution are similar to the SSL, but they tend to occur about 10 years later than SSLs.[100]

Clinical features

Because these polyps have developed overt dysplasia, they develop abnormal vasculature and are potentially more amenable to detection via fecal occult blood tests than ordinary SSLs.

Pathogenesis

The transition to overt dysplasia typically coincides with the development of advanced genetic/epigenetic alterations. The best known is methylation-induced silencing of the *MLH1* gene.[101,102] This can be readily identified by abrupt loss of staining for MLH1 in the dysplastic component of the SSLD (see **Fig. 4**D). This occurs in about 75% of SSLDs.[103] These polyps are, thus, the major precursor of sporadic, MMR- deficient (microsatellite instability — MSI) CRC, which have an overall better prognosis than cancers arising via the chromosomal instability pathway. The remaining 25% progress through a MMR proficient molecular pathway and are a major precursor of the aggressive *BRAF*-mutated microsatellite stable (MMR proficient) form of CRC .[103] Around half of the cases show activation of the *APC* pathway, but this tends to occur via upstream mechanisms rather than via *APC* mutation.[104] *TP53* mutation and *p16/INK4a* pathway abnormalities occur but are relatively uncommon.[100]

Endoscopic features
Colonoscopy may recognize SSLDs as a polyp with a NICE 2 component within a background NICE 1 polyp. A pitfall for the endoscopist is to identify and resect only the NICE 2 component but miss and leave behind the subtle surrounding NICE 1 component.[88,105]

Histology
By histology, there is an abrupt transition from the ordinary SSL component to a cytologically dysplastic component (see **Fig. 4**C). The dysplasia can show a multitude of morphologic patterns.[103] Broadly, these can be divided into conventional and serrated patterns. More than 75% show a conventional pattern and most of the remainder show a serrated pattern.[103] The conventional dysplasia is similar to that seen in conventional adenomas, although the patterns are more variable in serrated polyps. These cases nearly always show loss of staining for MLH1 via gene promoter methylation. The serrated pattern of dysplasia is characterized by tightly packed glands with limited maturation toward the luminal surface. The glands are composed of cells with abundant eosinophilic cytoplasm. There is usually marked nuclear atypia, prominent nucleoli, and frequent and atypical mitoses. These cases are nearly always MMR proficient and are an important precursor of the aggressive BRAF-mutated microsatellite stable form of CRC. As per the WHO, grading of dysplasia in SSLDs is not recommended, as all of these lesions are considered to have a high risk of malignant progression. The concern being that a designation of low-grade dysplasia in this context may inappropriately reassure the colonoscopist that the polyp is of low risk, resulting in inadequate surveillance.

Differential diagnosis
Diagnosis is usually straight-forward but 2 scenarios can cause misdiagnosis. The first instance is with SSLD where either the NICE 1 component has not been resected, and as such the pathologist is presented only with the dysplastic component or the dysplastic component has completely overgrown the SSL component of the polyp. In these cases, rendering a diagnosis of a conventional adenoma is possible and this may lead to under-surveillance of the patient. Avoiding this pitfall is difficult, since the pathologist is required to recognize that the dysplasia is atypical for a conventional adenoma. If the pathologist is suspicious about the diagnosis, the best investigation to confirm the suspicion is *BRAF* mutation testing (either by immunohistochemistry or molecular methods). A *BRAF* mutation clinches the diagnosis.

The second and more common scenario is confusing traditional serrated adenoma (TSA) arising from a precursor SSL as an SSLD with serrated dysplasia. This is quite a common occurrence. TSA can be readily distinguished by identifying the typical histologic features (described later) and recognizing that the serrated histology in TSA is cytologically bland, whereas in SSLD it is highly atypical (as described earlier). Some authors argue that both represent a progressed form of SSL and thus, this distinction is not important. However, SSLD is known to have more molecular abnormalities than a TSA and as such is likely to be a higher risk lesion.[100,106]

Natural history and treatment
From a clinical perspective, these polyps are rare, but if recognized endoscopically, they should be completely removed with a clear margin of normal mucosa. Because the transition from SSLD to invasive carcinoma can be rapid, close surveillance postpolypectomy is recommended. Some authors have referred to the "triple threat" presented by SSL/SSLD; the authors would add a fourth threat, that of pathologic underdiagnosis.[105]

Traditional Serrated Adenoma

Traditional serrated adenoma (TSA) is one of the rarest types of epithelial colorectal polyp, representing less than 1% of all polyps in most series.[6,106,107]

Clinical features

Traditional serrated adenomas are usually asymptomatic, but do have a propensity to arise in the very distal rectum where they can prolapse and cause bleeding. They occur primarily in the distal large bowel and are often large at the time of diagnosis.[106] The mean age at polypectomy is in the seventh decade.

Pathogenesis

Activating *BRAF* and *KRAS* mutations are common in TSAs.[106] The *BRAF-mutated* subtype is more likely to show CIMP and is more likely to have *RNF43* mutations.[108] In contrast, the *KRAS*-mutated cases show frequent *RSPO* fusions.[108]

As for conventional adenomas, occasional TSAs with high-grade dysplasia are identified (see **Fig. 4F**). Similar to the SSLD, this tends to correspond with the development of advanced molecular abnormalities including *TP53* mutation, *WNT* pathway activation, and *p16* inactivation.[106]

Epigenetic silencing of *MLH1* is very rare in TSAs, and as such, *BRAF*-mutated cases are another important precursor of the aggressive *BRAF*-mutated microsatellite stable form of CRC.

Endoscopic features

Macroscopically, they are often pedunculated or protuberant and often have a "pinecone" or "raspberry" appearance.[2] As noted above, TSAs can be separated into 2 major groups, *BRAF* mutated or *KRAS* mutated (double wild-type TSAs tend to segregate best with *KRAS*-mutated cases).[106,107] *BRAF*-mutated cases have frequent origin in other polyp types (MVHP and SSL) and are relatively more common in the proximal colon and can show a sessile growth pattern. *KRAS-mutated* polyps mostly arise de novo in the distal colon and rectum.

Histology

Histologically, the TSA has 3 distinctive features: characteristic cytology, presence of ectopic crypt formation, and slit-like serrations.[106,107,109] The cytologic features are perhaps the most distinctive since the cells show abundant eosinophilic cytoplasm and centrally placed, pencillate nuclei (see **Fig. 4E**). Ectopic crypt formation refers to rounded buds of proliferative epithelium that have lost connection to the muscularis mucosae.[109] Slit-like serrations are indentations in the polyp surface epithelium similar to that seen in the normal small bowel mucosa and often occurring over an ectopic crypt.

Most TSAs display a villous architecture, although this feature is more common in distal compared with proximal polyps. Occasional (usually large and distal) cases will show a "filiform" pattern characterized by an exaggerated villous architecture with bulbous and oedematous villi. Although histologically distinctive, the filiform variant is a subtype of TSA without any distinctive biology. Other rare subtypes include goblet cell rich and mucinous.

Most authors consider the TSA, as described earlier, to be inherently a low-grade dysplastic lesion. Occasional cases show progression to overtly high-grade dysplasia. In the majority of TSAs, this high-grade dysplasia takes a serrated morphology, much the same as for SSLDs with serrated dysplasia as described earlier. That is, the TSA will develop an area with closely packed glands lined by large cells with abundant eosinophilic cytoplasm with large pleomorphic nuclei and a prominent nucleolus.

Mitoses are frequent and atypical. Occasional cases will retain the normal TSA architecture, but the lining epithelium becomes highly atypical, usually with the same cytologic features just described.

Natural history and treatment
The TSA is considered an "advanced" colorectal polyp with a relatively high risk of progression to colon cancer. Treatment is usually achieved by endoscopic polypectomy but some large and distal polyps may require endoscopic submucosal dissection or transanal microscopic surgery. Rare cases require colectomy.

CLINICS CARE POINTS

A. Conventional adenoma and potential misdiagnosis by the pathologist
  1. Overdiagnosis of high-grade dysplasia
  2. Epithelial misplacement misdiagnosed as malignant
  3. Inflammatory or regenerative polyps misinterpreted as conventional adenoma
  4. Squamous metaplasia or benign neuroendocrine proliferation misinterpreted as high-grade dysplasia or malignancy

B. Sessile serrated lesion as a threat to the endoscopist*
  1. Subtle sessile lesions that can be easily overlooked at colonoscopy
  2. Poorly defined borders make incomplete resection a problem
  3. The dysplastic part of an SSLD may distract the endoscopist from the true nature of the lesion—the NICE2 component is resected but the NICE1 component is left in situ
  4. SSL under-diagnosed as MVHP by the pathologist leading to inadequate surveillance

*all of these features can contribute to the risk of interval colorectal carcinoma due to missed lesions or incomplete polypectomy

DISCLOSURE

The authors have no disclosures.

REFERENCES

1. Pino MS, Chung DC. The chromosomal instability pathway in colon cancer. Gastroenterology 2010;138(6):2059–72.
2. Bettington M, Walker N, Clouston A, et al. The serrated pathway to colorectal carcinoma: current concepts and challenges. Histopathology 2013;62(3):367–86.
3. Jass JR. Classification of colorectal cancer based on correlation of clinical, morphological and molecular features. Histopathology 2007;50(1):113–30.
4. Kambara T, Simms LA, Whitehall VLJ, et al. BRAF mutation is associated with DNA methylation in serrated polyps and cancers of the colorectum. Gut 2004; 53(8):1137–44.
5. Burnett-Hartman AN, Passarelli MN, Adams SV, et al. Differences in Epidemiologic Risk Factors for Colorectal Adenomas and Serrated Polyps by Lesion Severity and Anatomical Site. Am J Epidemiol 2013;177(7):625–37.
6. Bettington M, Walker N, Rosty C, et al. Critical appraisal of the diagnosis of the sessile serrated adenoma. Am J Surg Pathol 2014;38(2):158–66.
7. Turner KO, Genta RM, Sonnenberg A. Lesions of All Types Exist in Colon Polyps of All Sizes. Am J Gastroenterol 2018;113(2):303–6.
8. Øines M, Helsingen LM, Bretthauer M, et al. Epidemiology and risk factors of colorectal polyps. Best Pract Res Clin Gastroenterol 2017;31(4):419–24.

9. Pendergrass CJ, Edelstein DL, Hylind LM, et al. Occurrence of colorectal adenomas in younger adults: an epidemiologic necropsy study. Clin Gastroenterol Hepatol 2008;6(9):1011-5.

10. Lee-Six H, Olafsson S, Ellis P, et al. The landscape of somatic mutation in normal colorectal epithelial cells. Nature 2019;574(7779):532-7.

11. Vogelstein B, Kinzler KW. Cancer genes and the pathways they control. Nat Med 2004;10(8):789-99.

12. Maltzman T, Knoll K, Martinez ME, et al. Ki-ras proto-oncogene mutations in sporadic colorectal adenomas: relationship to histologic and clinical characteristics. Gastroenterology 2001;121(2):302-9.

13. Ishii T, Notohara K, Umapathy A, et al. Tubular adenomas with minor villous changes show molecular features characteristic of tubulovillous adenomas. Am J Surg Pathol 2011;35(2):212-20.

14. Barker N, Ridgway RA, van Es JH, et al. Crypt stem cells as the cells-of-origin of intestinal cancer. Nature 2009;457(7229):608-11.

15. Wright NA, Poulsom R. Top down or bottom up? Competing management structures in the morphogenesis of colorectal neoplasms. Gut 2002;51(3):306-8.

16. Rebuzzi F, Ulivi P, Tedaldi G. Genetic Predisposition to Colorectal Cancer: How Many and Which Genes to Test? Int J Mol Sci 2023;24(3).

17. Aarons CB, Shanmugan S, Bleier JI. Management of malignant colon polyps: current status and controversies. World J Gastroenterol 2014;20(43):16178-83.

18. Iino H, Simms L, Young J, et al. DNA microsatellite instability and mismatch repair protein loss in adenomas presenting in hereditary non-polyposis colorectal cancer. Gut 2000;47(1):37-42.

19. Ahadova A, Gallon R, Gebert J, et al. Three molecular pathways model colorectal carcinogenesis in Lynch syndrome. Int J Cancer 2018;143(1):139-50.

20. Dabir PD, Bruggeling CE, van der Post RS, et al. Microsatellite instability screening in colorectal adenomas to detect Lynch syndrome patients? A systematic review and meta-analysis. European journal of human genetics : EJHG (Eur J Hum Genet) 2020;28(3):277-86.

21. Walsh MD, Buchanan DD, Pearson SA, et al. Immunohistochemical testing of conventional adenomas for loss of expression of mismatch repair proteins in Lynch syndrome mutation carriers: a case series from the Australasian site of the colon cancer family registry. Mod Pathol 2012;25(5):722-30.

22. Tanaka M, Nakajima T, Sugano K, et al. Mismatch repair deficiency in Lynch syndrome-associated colorectal adenomas is more prevalent in older patients. Histopathology 2016;69(2):322-8.

23. Bogie RMM, Veldman MHJ, Snijders L, et al. Endoscopic subtypes of colorectal laterally spreading tumors (LSTs) and the risk of submucosal invasion: a meta-analysis. Endoscopy 2018;50(3):263-82.

24. Hewett DG, Kaltenbach T, Sano Y, et al. Validation of a simple classification system for endoscopic diagnosis of small colorectal polyps using narrow-band imaging. Gastroenterology 2012;143(3):599-607 e1.

25. Shinya H, Wolff WI. Morphology, anatomic distribution and cancer potential of colonic polyps - analysis of 7,000 polyps endoscopically removed. Annals of surgery 1979;190(6):679-83.

26. Lieberman DA, Weiss DG, Harford WV, et al. Five-year colon surveillance after screening colonoscopy. Gastroenterology 2007;133(4):1077-85.

27. Gillespie PE, Chambers TJ, Chan KW, et al. Colonic adenomas-a colonoscopy survey. Gut 1979;20(3):240-5.

28. Osmond A, Li-Chang H, Kirsch R, et al. Interobserver variability in assessing dysplasia and architecture in colorectal adenomas: a multicentre Canadian study. Journal of clinical pathology 2014;67(9):781–6.
29. Lasisi F, Mouchli A, Riddell R, et al. Agreement in interpreting villous elements and dysplasia in adenomas less than one centimetre in size. Dig Liver Dis : official journal of the Italian Society of Gastroenterology and the Italian Association for the Study of the Liver 2013;45(12):1049–55.
30. Mahajan D, Downs-Kelly E, Liu X, et al. Reproducibility of the villous component and high-grade dysplasia in colorectal adenomas <1 cm: implications for endoscopic surveillance. Am J Surg Pathol 2013;37(3):427–33.
31. Kuijpers CC, Sluijter CE, von der Thüsen JH, et al. Interlaboratory variability in the grading of dysplasia in a nationwide cohort of colorectal adenomas. Histopathology 2016;69(2):187–97.
32. Foss FA, Milkins S, McGregor AH. Inter-observer variability in the histological assessment of colorectal polyps detected through the NHS Bowel Cancer Screening Programme. Histopathology 2012;61(1):47–52.
33. Turner JK, Williams GT, Morgan M, et al. Interobserver agreement in the reporting of colorectal polyp pathology among bowel cancer screening pathologists in Wales. Histopathology 2013;62(6):916–24.
34. Appelman HD. High-grade dysplasia and villous features should not be part of the routine diagnosis of colorectal adenomas. Am J Gastroenterol 2008;103(6): 1329–31.
35. Madani A, Kuijpers C, Sluijter CE, et al. Decrease of variation in the grading of dysplasia in colorectal adenomas with a national e-learning module. Histopathology 2019;74(6):925–32.
36. Odze R. Pathologist - Clinician interaction is essential. Am J Gastroenterol 2008; 103(6):1331–3.
37. Rex DK, Goldblum JR. Should HGD or degree of villous changes in colon polyps be reported. Am J Gastroenterol 2008;103(6):1327–9.
38. Lee HE, Chandan VS, Lee CT, et al. Squamoid morules in the pseudoinvasive foci of colonic polyp morphologically mimic invasive carcinoma. Hum Pathol 2017;68:54–60.
39. Lin J, Goldblum JR, Bennett AE, et al. Composite intestinal adenoma-microcarcinoid. Am J Surg Pathol 2012;36(2):292–5.
40. Pulitzer M, Xu R, Suriawinata AA, et al. Microcarcinoids in large intestinal adenomas. Am J Surg Pathol 2006;30(12):1531–6.
41. Lee HE, Wu TT, Chandan VS, et al. Colonic Adenomatous Polyps Involving Submucosal Lymphoglandular Complexes: A Diagnostic Pitfall. Am J Surg Pathol 2018;42(8):1083–9.
42. Pascal RR, Hertzler G, Hunter S, et al. Pseudoinvasion with high-grade dysplasia in a colonic adenoma - distinction from adenocarcinoma. Am J Surg Pathol 1990; 14(7):694–7.
43. Panarelli NC, Somarathna T, Samowitz WS, et al. Diagnostic Challenges Caused by Endoscopic Biopsy of Colonic Polyps: A Systematic Evaluation of Epithelial Misplacement With Review of Problematic Polyps From the Bowel Cancer Screening Program, United Kingdom. Am J Surg Pathol 2016;40(8):1075–83.
44. Khor TS, Lauwers GY, Odze RD, et al. "Mass-forming" variant of ischemic colitis is a distinct entity with predilection for the proximal colon. Am J Surg Pathol 2015;39(9):1275–81.
45. Click B, Pinsky PF, Hickey T, et al. Association of Colonoscopy Adenoma Findings With Long-term Colorectal Cancer Incidence. JAMA 2018;319(19):2021–31.

46. He X, Hang D, Wu K, et al. Long-term Risk of Colorectal Cancer After Removal of Conventional Adenomas and Serrated Polyps. Gastroenterology 2020;158(4):852–61.e4.

47. Atkin WS, Morson BC, Cuzick J. Long-term risk of colorectal cancer after excision of rectosigmoid adenomas. N Engl J Med 1992;326(10):658–62.

48. Hassan C, Gimeno-García A, Kalager M, et al. Systematic review with meta-analysis: the incidence of advanced neoplasia after polypectomy in patients with and without low-risk adenomas. Alimentary pharmacology & therapeutics 2014;39(9):905–12.

49. Parker J, Gupta S, Torkington J, et al. Comparison of recommendations for surveillance of advanced colorectal polyps: A systematic review of guidelines. J Gastroenterol Hepatol 2023;38(6):854–64.

50. Gupta S, Lieberman D, Anderson JC, et al. Recommendations for Follow-Up After Colonoscopy and Polypectomy: A Consensus Update by the US Multi-Society Task Force on Colorectal Cancer. Gastroenterology 2020;158(4):1131–53.e5.

51. Kojima M, Shimazaki H, Iwaya K, et al. Intramucosal colorectal carcinoma with invasion of the lamina propria: a study by the Japanese Society for Cancer of the Colon and Rectum. Hum Pathol 2017;66:230–7.

52. Loughrey MB, Webster F, Arends MJ, et al. Dataset for Pathology Reporting of Colorectal Cancer: Recommendations From the International Collaboration on Cancer Reporting (ICCR). Annals of surgery 2022;275(3):e549–61.

53. Hashimoto H, Horiuchi H, Kurata A, et al. Intramucosal colorectal carcinoma with lymphovascular invasion: clinicopathological characteristics of nine cases. Histopathology 2019;74(7):1055–66.

54. Lewin MR, Fenton H, Burkart AL, et al. Poorly differentiated colorectal carcinoma with invasion restricted to lamina propria (intramucosal carcinoma): A follow-up study of 15 cases. Am J Surg Pathol 2007;31(12):1882–6.

55. Shia J, Klimstra DS. Intramucosal poorly differentiated colorectal carcinoma: Can it be managed conservatively? Am J Surg Pathol 2008;32(10):1586–8.

56. Brown I, Zammit AP, Bettington M, et al. Pathological features associated with metastasis in patients with early invasive (pT1) colorectal carcinoma in colorectal polyps. Histopathology 2023. https://doi.org/10.1111/his.14970.

57. Shepherd NA, Griggs RK. Bowel cancer screening-generated diagnostic conundrum of the century: pseudoinvasion in sigmoid colonic polyps. Mod Pathol 2015;28(Suppl 1):S88–94.

58. Brown IS, Bettington ML, Bettington A, et al. Adverse histological features in malignant colorectal polyps: a contemporary series of 239 cases. Journal of clinical pathology 2016;69(4):292–9.

59. Brockmoeller SF, West NP. Predicting systemic spread in early colorectal cancer: Can we do better? World J Gastroenterol 2019;25(23):2887–97.

60. Williams JG, Pullan RD, Hill J, et al. Management of the malignant colorectal polyp: ACPGBI position statement. Colorectal Dis 2013;15(Suppl 2):1–38.

61. Beaton C, Twine CP, Williams GL, et al. Systematic review and meta-analysis of histopathological factors influencing the risk of lymph node metastasis in early colorectal cancer. Colorectal Dis 2013;15(7):788–97.

62. Hassan C, Zullo A, Risio M, et al. Histologic risk factors and clinical outcome in colorectal malignant polyp: a pooled-data analysis. Dis Colon Rectum 2005;48(8):1588–96.

63. Hashiguchi Y, Muro K, Saito Y, et al. Japanese Society for Cancer of the Colon and Rectum (JSCCR) guidelines 2019 for the treatment of colorectal cancer. Int J Clin Oncol 2020;25(1):1–42.

64. Bosch SL, Teerenstra S, de Wilt JH, et al. Predicting lymph node metastasis in pT1 colorectal cancer: a systematic review of risk factors providing rationale for therapy decisions. Endoscopy 2013;45(10):827–34.
65. Zammit AP, Lyons NJ, Chatfield MD, et al. Patient and pathological predictors of management strategy for malignant polyps following polypectomy: a systematic review and meta-analysis. Int J Colorectal Dis 2022;37(5):1035–47.
66. Ueno H, Mochizuki H, Hashiguchi Y, et al. Risk factors for an adverse outcome in early invasive colorectal carcinoma. Gastroenterology 2004;127(2):385–94.
67. Hassan C, Zullo A, Risio M, et al. Histologic risk factors and clinical outcome in colorectal malignant polyp: A pooled-data analysis. Dis Colon Rectum 2005; 48(8):1588–96.
68. Shaukat A, Kaltenbach T, Dominitz JA, et al. Endoscopic Recognition and Management Strategies for Malignant Colorectal Polyps: Recommendations of the US Multi-Society Task Force on Colorectal Cancer. Gastroenterology 2020; 159(5):1916–34.e2.
69. Richards CH, Ventham NT, Mansouri D, et al. An evidence-based treatment algorithm for colorectal polyp cancers: results from the Scottish Screen-detected Polyp Cancer Study (SSPoCS). Gut 2018;67(2):299–306.
70. Richards C, Levic K, Fischer J, et al. International validation of a risk prediction algorithm for patients with malignant colorectal polyps. Colorectal Dis 2020.
71. Pedraza R, Siddharthan R. Management of Malignant Colon Polyps. Dis Colon Rectum 2021;64(3):262–6.
72. Shaukat A, Kaltenbach T, Dominitz JA, et al. Endoscopic Recognition and Management Strategies for Malignant Colorectal Polyps: Recommendations of the US Multi-Society Task Force on Colorectal Cancer. Am J Gastroenterol 2020; 115(11):1751–67.
73. Ueno H, Shirouzu K, Eishi Y, et al. Characterization of perineural invasion as a component of colorectal cancer staging. Am J Surg Pathol 2013;37(10):1542–9.
74. Kitajima K, Fujimori T, Fujii S, et al. Correlations between lymph node metastasis and depth of submucosal invasion in submucosal invasive colorectal carcinoma: a Japanese collaborative study. J Gastroenterol 2004;39(6):534–43.
75. Haggitt RC, Glotzbach RE, Soffer EE, et al. Prognostic factors in colorectal carcinomas arising in adenomas - implications for lesions removed by endoscopic polypectomy. Gastroenterology 1985;89(2):326–36.
76. Koelzer VH, Zlobec I, Lugli A. Tumor budding in colorectal cancer—ready for diagnostic practice? Hum Pathol 2016;47(1):4–19.
77. Berg KB, Telford JJ, Gentile L, et al. Re-examining the 1-mm margin and submucosal depth of invasion: a review of 216 malignant colorectal polyps. Virchows Arch 2020;476(6):863–70.
78. Nascimbeni R, Burgart LJ, Nivatvongs S, et al. Risk of lymph node metastasis in T1 carcinoma of the colon and rectum. Dis Colon Rectum 2002;45(2):200–6.
79. Butte JM, Tang P, Gonen M, et al. Rate of residual disease after complete endoscopic resection of malignant colonic polyp. Dis Colon Rectum 2012;55(2): 122–7.
80. Snover DC, Jass JR, Fenoglio-Preiser C, et al. Serrated polyps of the large intestine - A morphologic and molecular review of an evolving concept. Am J Clin Pathol 2005;124(3):380–91.
81. Chang LC, Shun CT, Hsu WF, et al. Fecal Immunochemical Test Detects Sessile Serrated Adenomas and Polyps With a Low Level of Sensitivity. Clin Gastroenterol Hepatol 2017;15(6):872–879 e1.

82. Fernando WC, Miranda MS, Worthley DL, et al. The CIMP Phenotype in BRAF Mutant Serrated Polyps from a Prospective Colonoscopy Patient Cohort. Gastroenterol Res Pract 2014;2014:374926.

83. Yang S, Farraye FA, Mack C, et al. BRAF and KRAS mutations in hyperplastic polyps and serrated adenomas of the colorectum - Relationship to histology and CpG island methylation status. Am J Surg Pathol 2004;28(11):1452–9.

84. Collado M, Gil J, Efeyan A, et al. Tumour biology: senescence in premalignant tumours. Nature 2005;436(7051):642.

85. Spring KJ, Zhao ZZ, Karamatic R, et al. High prevalence of sessile serrated adenomas with BRAF mutations: A prospective study of patients undergoing colonoscopy. Gastroenterology 2006;131(5):1400–7.

86. Torlakovic E, Skovlund E, Snover DC, et al. Morphologic reappraisal of serrated colorectal polyps. Am J Surg Pathol 2003;27(1):65–81.

87. Abdeljawad K, Vemulapalli KC, Kahi CJ, et al. Sessile serrated polyp prevalence determined by a colonoscopist with a high lesion detection rate and an experienced pathologist. Gastrointest Endosc 2015;81(3):517–24.

88. Pohl H, Srivastava A, Bensen SP, et al. Incomplete polyp resection during colonoscopy-results of the complete adenoma resection (CARE) study. Gastroenterology 2013;144(1):74–80 e1.

89. Kahi CJ, Hewett DG, Norton DL, et al. Prevalence and variable detection of proximal colon serrated polyps during screening colonoscopy. Clin Gastroenterol Hepatol 2011;9(1):42–6.

90. Bettington M, Walker N, Rahman T, et al. High prevalence of sessile serrated adenomas in contemporary outpatient colonoscopy practice. Intern Med J 2017; 47(3):318–23.

91. Anderson JC, Rangasamy P, Rustagi T, et al. Risk factors for sessile serrated adenomas. J Clin Gastroenterol 2011;45(8):694–9.

92. O'Brien MJ, Yang S, Mack C, et al. Comparison of microsatellite instability, CpG island methylation phenotype, BRAF and KRAS status in serrated polyps and traditional adenomas indicates separate pathways to distinct colorectal carcinoma end points. Am J Surg Pathol 2006;30(12):1491–501.

93. Liu C, Bettington ML, Walker NI, et al. CpG Island Methylation in Sessile Serrated Adenomas Increases With Age, Indicating Lower Risk of Malignancy in Young Patients. Gastroenterology 2018;155(5):1362–5.e2.

94. Bettington M, Brown I, Rosty C, et al. Sessile Serrated Adenomas in Young Patients may have Limited Risk of Malignant Progression. J Clin Gastroenterol 2019;53(3):e113–6.

95. Tadepalli US, Feihel D, Miller KM, et al. A morphologic analysis of sessile serrated polyps observed during routine colonoscopy (with video). Gastrointest Endosc 2011;74(6):1360–8.

96. Hazewinkel Y, Lopez-Ceron M, East JE, et al. Endoscopic features of sessile serrated adenomas: validation by international experts using high-resolution white-light endoscopy and narrow-band imaging. Gastrointest Endosc 2013; 77(6):916–24.

97. Torlakovic EE, Gomez JD, Driman DK, et al. Sessile serrated adenorna (SSA) vs. Traditional serrated adenoma (TSA). Am J Surg Pathol 2008;32(1):21–9.

98. Arain MA, Sawhney M, Sheikh S, et al. CIMP status of interval colon cancers: another piece to the puzzle. Am J Gastroenterol 2010;105(5):1189–95.

99. Sawhney MS, Farrar WD, Gudiseva S, et al. Microsatellite instability in interval colon cancers. Gastroenterology 2006;131(6):1700–5.

100. Bettington M, Walker N, Rosty C, et al. Clinicopathological and molecular features of sessile serrated adenomas with dysplasia or carcinoma. Gut 2017; 66(1):97–106.
101. Cunningham JM, Christensen ER, Tester DJ, et al. Hypermethylation of the hMLH1 promoter in colon cancer with microsatellite instability. Cancer Res 1998;58(15):3455–60.
102. Sheridan TB, Fenton H, Lewin MR, et al. Sessile serrated adenomas with low- and high-grade dysplasia and early carcinomas. An immunohistochemical study of serrated lesions "caught in the act". Am J Clin Pathol 2006;126(4):564–71.
103. Liu C, Walker NI, Leggett BA, et al. Sessile serrated adenomas with dysplasia: morphological patterns and correlations with MLH1 immunohistochemistry. Mod Pathol 2017;30(12):1728–38.
104. Borowsky J, Dumenil T, Bettington M, et al. The role of APC in WNT pathway activation in serrated neoplasia. Mod Pathol 2018;31(3):495–504.
105. Burgess NG, Tutticci NJ, Pellise M, et al. Sessile serrated adenomas/polyps with cytologic dysplasia: a triple threat for interval cancer. Gastrointest Endosc 2014; 80(2):307–10.
106. Bettington ML, Walker NI, Rosty C, et al. A clinicopathological and molecular analysis of 200 traditional serrated adenomas. Mod Pathol 2015;28(3):414–27.
107. Tsai JH, Liau JY, Lin YL, et al. Traditional serrated adenoma has two pathways of neoplastic progression that are distinct from the sessile serrated pathway of colorectal carcinogenesis. Mod Pathol 2014;27(10):1375–85.
108. Sekine S, Yamashita S, Tanabe T, et al. Frequent PTPRK-RSPO3 fusions and RNF43 mutations in colorectal traditional serrated adenoma. J Pathol 2016; 239(2):133–8.
109. Torlakovic EE, Gomez JD, Driman DK, et al. Sessile serrated adenoma (SSA) vs. traditional serrated adenoma (TSA). Am J Surg Pathol 2008;32(1):21–9.

Pathology of Gastrointestinal Polyposis Disorders

Christophe Rosty, MD, PhD[a,b,c],*, Lodewijk A.A. Brosens, MD, PhD[d]

KEYWORDS

- Gastrointestinal polyposis • Adenomatous polyposis • Serrated polyposis
- Hamartomatous polyposis • Hereditary cancer

KEY POINTS

- Gastrointestinal polyposis syndromes can be classified based on the predominant histologic type of colorectal polyp and associated gene mutation.
- Most syndromes are associated with polyps in the upper gastrointestinal tract and an increased risk of colorectal cancer.
- Serrated polyposis syndrome is defined by arbitrary clinical criteria and is very rarely associated with a genetic defect.
- Hamartomatous polyposis syndromes are autosomal dominant disorders with an increased risk of cancer in the colon and other organs, and frequent extraintestinal manifestations.

INTRODUCTION

The study of gastrointestinal polyposis syndromes has been instrumental in unraveling the molecular pathways involved in colorectal cancer (CRC) pathogenesis.[1,2] Gastrointestinal polyposis syndromes are generally classified based on the histologic subtype of the colorectal polyps most frequently present in each of these syndromes (**Table 1**).

Familial adenomatous polyposis (FAP) is the prototypical polyposis syndrome. Several other polyposis syndromes with predominantly adenomatous polyps have been recently recognized (see **Table 1**). In addition, there are syndromes with predominantly hamartomatous polyps, serrated colorectal polyps, or a mixture of histologic polyp types. Several of these syndromes are also associated with upper gastrointestinal tract polyps, extraintestinal manifestations, and increased risks of cancer.

[a] Envoi Specialist Pathologists, Brisbane, Queensland 4059, Australia; [b] University of Queensland, Brisbane, Queensland 4072, Australia; [c] Department of Clinical Pathology, Colorectal Oncogenomics Group, Victorian Comprehensive Cancer Centre, The University of Melbourne, Victoria 3051, Australia; [d] Department of Pathology University Medical Center Utrecht, Utrecht University, Postbus 85500, 3508, Utrecht, Galgenwaad, The Netherlands
* Corresponding author. Unit 5/ 38 Bishop Street, Kelvin Grove, Queensland, 4059.
E-mail address: c.rosty@uq.edu.au

Gastroenterol Clin N Am 53 (2024) 179–200
https://doi.org/10.1016/j.gtc.2023.09.006
0889-8553/24/© 2023 Elsevier Inc. All rights reserved.

Table 1
Gastrointestinal polyposis syndromes classified according to histologic subtype of colorectal polyps

Polyp Subtype	Mode of Inheritance	Gene(s)	Pathway
Adenomatous polyps			
FAP	Autosomal dominant	APC	WNT pathway
MAP	Autosomal recessive	MUTYH	DNA base excision repair
PPAP	Autosomal dominant	POLE, POLD1	DNA polymerase proofreading
NTHL1 tumor syndrome	Autosomal recessive	NTHL1	DNA base excision repair
Serrated polyps			
SPS	ND	RNF43 (2%)	WNT pathway
Hamartomatous polyps			
PJS	Autosomal dominant	STK11	-
Juvenile polyposis syndrome	Autosomal dominant	BMPR1A, SMAD4	TGFβ pathway
PTEN hamartoma tumor syndrome/CS	Autosomal dominant	PTEN	PI3K pathway
CCS	NA	NA	

Abbreviations: NA, Not applicable (non-hereditary condition); ND, not determined.

In this review, the clinical genetic and histopathologic aspects of adenomatous polyposis, serrated polyposis, hamartomatous polyposis syndromes, Lynch syndrome (LS), and Cronkhite-Canada syndrome (CCS) are presented.

FAMILIAL ADENOMATOUS POLYPOSIS
Definition

FAP is an autosomal dominant inherited syndrome caused by germline (constitutional) mutations (pathogenic variants) in the *adenomatous polyposis coli* (*APC*) gene, resulting in the upregulation of the WNT signaling pathway. The estimated prevalence is 1 in 8000 to 10,000 affecting both sexes equally.[3]

Clinical Features

The phenotype of the classic form of FAP is the development of more than 100 colonic adenomatous polyps starting in teenage years. Attenuated FAP is characterized by fewer colorectal adenomatous polyps (10–100, average 30). In addition to colorectal adenomas and adenocarcinomas, most patients with FAP develop duodenal and gastric polyps and a variety of benign and malignant extraintestinal tract manifestations. Desmoid tumors, mainly in the small bowel mesentery, abdominal wall, or extremities, are the most frequent extraintestinal tract neoplasia, occurring in about 10% of patients and can cause severe morbidity and mortality.[4,5] Benign extraintestinal features include osteomas, dental abnormalities, and congenital hypertrophy of the retinal pigment epithelium.[3]

A rare subtype of FAP, called gastric adenocarcinoma and proximal polyposis of the stomach (GAPPS) is characterized by carpeting fundic gland polyposis of the proximal stomach sparing the antrum, increased risk of gastric carcinoma and absence or a small number of duodenal and colorectal adenomas.[6,7]

Pathogenesis

A germline mutation in *APC* resulting in a truncated or absent APC protein is identified in most patients. In 20% to 30% of cases, no family history is found; these patients may have de novo variants in *APC* or a recessive polyposis syndrome.[8] Several associations between the location of the *APC* variant and the clinical manifestations have been reported (**Table 2**).[9,10] GAPPS is caused by a mutation in the YY1 binding site of the *APC* exon (promoter) 1B.

Pathologic Condition

Patients with classic FAP have hundreds to thousands of polyps carpeting the entire large bowel, with a predominance for the distal colon. In attenuated FAP, fewer polyps are present and show a proximal colon predominance. Size of polyps varies from barely visible macroscopically to very large polyps measuring several centimeters in diameter. Malignant transformation occurs essentially in larger polyps.

FAP-associated colorectal adenomas show similar tubular, tubulovillous, or villous histologic features that are indistinguishable from sporadic adenomas. Dysplasia can be restricted to a single or a few colonic crypts in otherwise normal mucosa, which is very suggestive of FAP. Invasive adenocarcinomas are also identical morphologically to sporadic colorectal adenocarcinomas.

Duodenal polyps occur in almost all patients with FAP and are conventional intestinal-type adenomas.

Gastric polyps are present in most patients with FAP. Most of these polyps are fundic gland polyps (FGPs), characterized by cystically dilated gastric glands. Although low-grade dysplasia is present in about a third of FGPs, progression to high-grade dysplasia or carcinoma is extremely rare.[11] Other histologic subtypes of gastric polyps are low-grade foveolar adenomas, with a low risk of neoplastic progression,[12] and pyloric gland adenomas (PGAs), which seem to have a higher risk of neoplastic progression (**Fig. 1**). Histologically, PGAs are composed of densely packed glands lined by cuboidal to low columnar epithelium resembling pyloric gland cells. These glands are positive, and the pyloric gland mucin MUC6 and the overlying foveolar epithelium are positive for foveolar mucin MUC5A and often show dysplasia.[13] Of note, the endoscopic assessment and histologic distinction among FGP with dysplasia, foveolar adenoma, and PGA can be difficult in case of extended polyposis carpeting the stomach.[14]

Table 2
Genotype phenotype associations in familial adenomatous polyposis

FAP Phenotype	Location of APC Mutation
Classic FAP	Central part of the gene (between codons 160 and 1393)
Profuse polyposis (>1000 polyps)	Mid-portion of the gene (between codons 1250 and 1464)
Attenuated FAP	Far proximal (5′) end, far distal (3′) end, or certain locations of exon 9 of the APC gene
Desmoid tumors	3′ end of codon 1444
Congenital hypertrophy of the retinal pigment epithelium	Between codons 463 and 1444
Multiplicity of extraintestinal lesions	Codons 1465, 1546, and 2621
GAPPS	Promoter 1B (YY1 binding site)

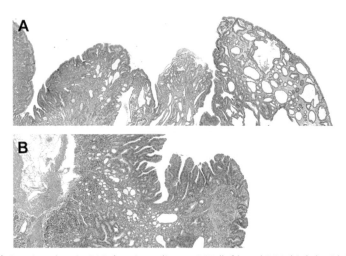

Fig. 1. (*A*) Gastric polyps in FAP showing adjacent FGP (left) and PGA (right) with low-grade foveolar type dysplasia. (*B*) This patient also had multiple foci of high-grade foveolar dysplasia overlying both FGPs (shown) and PGAs.

Risk of Malignancy

If prophylactic colectomy is not performed, virtually all patients with FAP develop CRC at a mean age of 45 years. Attenuated FAP patients have a slightly reduced risk and later onset of CRC (70%–80%) mean age at diagnosis of 56 years.[15,16]

The risk of duodenal adenocarcinoma is 5%.[17] Gastric adenocarcinomas are almost exclusively reported in the proximal stomach and associated with extensive carpeting fundic gland polyposis, a large size (>20 mm) of polyps and dysplasia.[18]

Although less frequent, FAP has also been associated with an increased risk of thyroid carcinoma, hepatobiliary tree tumors, childhood hepatoblastoma, adrenocortical adenomas and carcinomas, and brain tumors particularly medulloblastoma.

Treatment

Treatment strategies of patients with FAP are guided by the severity of polyposis and the clinical presentation. Screening colonoscopy starts early in childhood and followed by surveillance colonoscopy. The age of prophylactic colectomy depends on polyp burden and is followed by surveillance of the ileal pouch. Chemoprevention with nonsteroidal anti-inflammatory drugs may be used to prevent further polyp development. Management of duodenal adenomas in FAP is in most current guidelines guided by the (modified) Spigelman stage of duodenal adenomas, which grades the severity of duodenal polyposis.[19,20] The European FAP consortium recently proposed a novel flowchart for the management of duodenal and gastric adenomas, which will be prospectively evaluated.[21]

MUTYH-ASSOCIATED POLYPOSIS
Definition

MUTYH-associated polyposis (MAP) is an adenomatous polyposis caused by autosomal recessively inherited pathogenic variants in *MUTYH*.[22] The estimated prevalence is 1 in 2000.[23]

Clinical Features

MAP shares many clinical features with attenuated FAP. Most affected patients develop multiple adenomatous polyps throughout the large bowel (usually 10–100, rarely >100 polyps).[24] Duodenal adenomatous polyps are present in 20% of affected patients.[25]

Pathogenesis

MAP is caused by pathogenic variants in the DNA-base excision repair gene *MUTYH*.[22] The biallelic MUTYH loss prevents the removal of incorrectly incorporated adenine residues opposite 8-oxoguanine, resulting in C:G > A:T transversions. The c.34 G > T *KRAS* mutation is frequently observed in MAP-associated tumors.

Pathologic Condition

The colonic phenotype overlaps with that of attenuated FAP although some patients with MAP tend to develop multiple serrated polyps.[26] MAP-associated adenomas and adenocarcinomas do not have any distinctive histologic features.

Risk of Malignancy

The cumulative lifetime of CRC is 63% at the age of 60 years.[27] Other increased tumor risks include duodenal adenocarcinoma, sebaceous skin tumors, and ovarian and bladder cancers.[28] Heterozygous carriers of monoallelic *MUTYH* variants have a mild increased risk of CRC.[28]

Treatment

Patients with MAP are managed by colonoscopy with polypectomy starting at 25 to 30 years and every 1 or 2 years, or colectomy depending on polyp burden. Baseline upper gastrointestinal endoscopy is recommended at the age of 30 to 35 years with surveillance depending on initial findings.

POLYMERASE PROOFREADING–ASSOCIATED POLYPOSIS
Definition

Polymerase proofreading–associated polyposis (PPAP) is an autosomal dominant inherited syndrome caused by germline mutations in the exonuclease (proofreading) domains of *POLD1* and *POLE*.[29]

Clinical Features

Patients with PPAP present with an attenuated or oligoadenomatous colorectal polyposis and duodenal adenomas.[30,31] The phenotype overlaps with LS and attenuated adenomatous polyposis (*APC/MUTYH*).

Pathogenesis

POLE or *POLD1* mutations result in a defect in replication-associated polymerase proofreading, leading to an increased mutation rate in tumors.

Pathologic Condition

Adenomas and adenocarcinomas associated with PPAP are similar to sporadic tumors but are associated with a hypermutant phenotype.

Risk of Malignancy

Affected patients have a high risk of CRC (identified in 60%–64% of *POLE* and *POLD1* carriers) and probably an increased risk of brain tumors.[30,31] *POLD1* female carriers have an increased risk of endometrial and breast cancers.

Treatment

Hypermutant carcinomas associated with PPAP may be responsive to PD1/PDL1 inhibitors.[32] Colonoscopy is recommended every 1 to 2 years. Gastroduodenal endoscopy screening should start at the age of 20 to 25 years with follow-up every 3 years or more depending on the initial findings. Screening for endometrial cancer and breast cancer should also be considered.[30]

NTHL1 TUMOR SYNDROME
Definition

NTHL1 tumor syndrome (also called *NTHL1*-associated polyposis) is an autosomal recessive DNA base excision repair disorder caused by biallelic *NTHL1* pathogenic variants.[33]

Clinical Features

The phenotype of *NTHL1* tumor syndrome is not clearly defined and includes attenuated or oligoadenomatous colorectal polyposis originating in adulthood and duodenal polyps.[33,34]

Pathogenesis

The *NTHL1* gene encodes a base excision repair glycosylase. *NTHL1*-associated CRC are associated with frequent C > T mutations.

Pathologic Condition

Adenomas and adenocarcinomas are similar to sporadic tumors. Colorectal serrated polyps are frequently diagnosed.

Risk of Malignancy

Affected patients have a high risk of CRC. The cumulative lifetime risk of developing extracolonic cancer by age 60 years has been estimated at 35% to 78%. This includes endometrial cancer, breast cancer, urothelial cancer, brain tumors, hematologic malignancies, and various skin tumors.[33,34]

Treatment

The management of *NTHL1* tumor syndrome overlaps with LS and attenuated FAP. Breast cancer screening is recommended.

SERRATED POLYPOSIS SYNDROME
Definition

Serrated polyposis syndrome (SPS) is condition of largely unknown genetic cause, characterized by the development of multiple serrated polyps in the large bowel and an increased risk of CRC for affected individuals and their first-degree relatives.[35–37] The revised World Health Organization (WHO) clinical criteria are presented in **Box 1**.[38] The prevalence is up to 0.1% in primary screening colonoscopies.[39]

Box 1
Clinical diagnostic criteria for serrated polyposis syndrome.

Criterion 1	≥5 serrated lesions/polyps proximal to the rectum, all being ≥5 mm in size, with ≥2 being ≥10 mm in size
Criterion 2	>20 serrated lesions/polyps of any size but distributed throughout the large bowel, with ≥5 proximal to the rectum

The polyp count is cumulative over multiple colonoscopies. Any histologic subtype of serrated polyps is included in the final polyp count. The upper gastrointestinal tract is not affected

Clinical Features

Most patients are diagnosed at 50 to 60 years of age, with some patients diagnosed earlier in their 30s.[40–43] Men and women are equally affected. The phenotype is heterogeneous encompassing patients who barely meet the WHO criteria and those with multiple large polyps fulfilling both criteria. About 25% of patients fulfill only criterion 1, 45% only criterion 2, and the remaining 30% meet both criteria.[41,42]

Some well-characterized genetic syndromes may present with a phenotype overlapping with SPS. This has been documented for MAP, juvenile polyposis syndrome, and Cowden syndrome (CS).[26,44,45] However, serrated polyps are usually not the dominant polyp type and are associated with polyps that are more characteristic of each syndrome. Moreover, testing for germline mutation in *BMPR1A*, *SMAD4*, *PTEN*, *MUTYH*, and *GREM1* did not show any pathogenic variants in a large series of patients with SPS.[46]

Pathogenesis

Pathogenic germline variants in *RNF43* (*Ring Finger Protein 43*), a negative feedback regulator of the WNT signaling pathway, have been reported in less than 2% of affected individuals.[47,48]

Approximately 50% of CRC in patients with SPS have a *BRAF* mutation, less than 5% a *KRAS* mutation, and 40% are *MLH1*-deficient.[49,50] This molecular phenotype suggests that half of CRC develop from serrated polyps via the serrated neoplasia pathway and the other half presumably following the conventional adenoma–carcinoma pathway.

Pathologic Condition

All subtypes of serrated polyps can develop in the large bowel: hyperplastic polyps, sessile serrated lesion (SSL), SSL with dysplasia, and traditional serrated adenoma[51] (**Fig. 2**). Conventional adenomas are also commonly seen and may be associated with

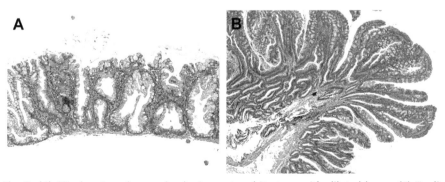

Fig. 2. (*A*) SSL showing abnormal colonic crypt architecture with dilated bases. (*B*) Traditional serrated adenoma with villous projections showing ectopic crypt formations and lined by cells with eosinophilic cytoplasm.

an increased risk of CRC.[50] SPS-associated serrated polyps are identical histological-ly and molecularly to those occurring outside SPS.[52,53] Most nondysplastic serrated polyps in SPS are in the proximal colon and show histologic features of SSL with atyp-ical symmetric dilatation of the crypt bases.[54] The median cumulative polyp number is most commonly 30 to 40, with a range as wide as 6 to 240 polyps and frequent pan-colonic distribution.[37]

Risk of Malignancy

Affected patients have a 15% to 30% risk of CRC.[41,42] Despite serrated polyps being predominant in the proximal colon, nearly 50% of CRC are in the rectosigmoid. Re-ported factors associated with CRC included the fulfillment of both WHO criteria, hav-ing more than 2 SSLs proximal to the splenic flexure, at least one SSLD, and at least one advanced conventional adenoma.

Treatment

The current guidelines recommend initial colonoscopic clearing of all relevant polyps (≥5 mm in size or any size and suspicious for dysplasia) followed by colonoscopy sur-veillance with 1 to 3 years intervals depending on findings from the last procedure.[55–57] Surgery may be required if colonoscopy control of polyps is not feasible. Surgical referral may be as low as 5% when patients with SPS are closely monitored with effec-tive reduction of polyp burden by colonoscopy.[58]

In first-degree relatives, screening colonoscopy is recommended at the age of 40 years or starting 10 years younger than the age at diagnosis of the youngest affected relative. Follow-up colonoscopy should be performed every 5 years or more frequently depending on polyp burden.[59]

HAMARTOMATOUS POLYPOSIS SYNDROMES
Peutz-Jeghers Syndrome

Definition
Peutz-Jeghers Syndrome (PJS) is an autosomal dominant hereditary syndrome char-acterized by hamartomatous gastrointestinal polyps and pigmented cutaneous and mucosal membrane macules. The clinical diagnostic criteria of PJS are summarized in **Box 2**.

Clinical features
Patients with PJS often present in the first 2 decades of life with symptoms of abdom-inal pain, intestinal bleeding, anemia, or intussusception.[60] Although the histologically typical PJS polyps are the main hallmark of PJS, the characteristic mucocutaneous

---

Box 2
Peutz-Jeghers syndrome diagnostic criteria.

Criterion 1	≥3 histologically confirmed Peutz-Jeghers polyps
Criterion 2	Any number of Peutz-Jeghers polyps with a family history of PJS
Criterion 3	Characteristic, prominent* mucocutaneous pigmentation with a family history of PJS
Criterion 4	Any number of Peutz-Jeghers polyps and characteristic, prominent mucocutaneous pigmentation

*Some melanin pigmentation is also regularly seen in unaffected individuals, hence the emphasis on the prominence of the pigmentation. Moreover, the pigmentation in patients with PJS may disappear with time or can, in rare cases, be absent altogether

pigmentations sometimes allows diagnosis of otherwise asymptomatic individuals in affected families.

Pathogenesis
PJS is caused by constitutional pathogenic variants in *STK11* (*Serine Threonine Kinase 11*) gene, which can be found in more than 90% of patients fulfilling the clinical diagnostic criteria. Most variants are point mutations and small intragenic deletions. In some patients, larger deletions of one or more exons have been found.[61]

Pathologic Condition
Patients usually have 10 to 20 gastrointestinal hamartomatous polyps. Polyps are most frequently found in the small intestine (60%–90%), but also in the large bowel (50%–60%), stomach (15%–30%), and rarely in the gallbladder, respiratory, and urinary tract.[62]

Macroscopically, small intestinal and colonic Peutz-Jeghers polyps are usually pedunculated and have a smooth and lobulated surface (**Table 3**). The size varies from several millimeters to centimeters. Microscopically, polyps are characterized by arborizing strands of smooth muscle in the lamina propria (**Fig. 3**). The polyps are lined by nonneoplastic epithelium characteristic for the specific location.[63,64] The differential diagnosis includes other hamartomatous polyps, mucosal prolapse polyps, and hyperplastic polyps. Mucosal prolapse type polyps can closely mimic PJS polyps as both show smooth muscle displacement and proliferation in the lamina propria, which may be related to the role of mucosal prolapse in the pathogenesis of PJS polyps.[65]

Most gastric polyps are found in the antral region and are typically small and asymptomatic. Gastric PJS polyps feature foveolar hyperplasia with cystic change, muscular proliferation, lamina propria edema, and inflammation but the histology of gastric polyps is less distinctive than colonic or small intestinal polyps (see **Fig. 3**). By histology alone, it is often impossible to reliably differentiate gastric PJS polyps from gastric juvenile and hyperplastic polyps, although there may be subtle histologic differences.[66] The diagnosis of hamartomatous gastric polyps remains challenging and, without knowledge of the clinical history, a note about the differential diagnosis that includes other hamartomatous polyps and hyperplastic polyps, may be most appropriate.

Dysplasia is very rare, and it is has been suggested that PJS polyps are in fact an epiphenomenon to the cancer-prone condition instead of the obligate precursor lesions of cancer.[65]

Table 3
Histologic features of polyps in Peutz-Jeghers syndrome and in juvenile polyposis syndrome

	Peutz-Jeghers Syndrome	Juvenile Polyposis Syndrome
Predominant site	Small bowel (jejunum) > large bowel > stomach	Large bowel > stomach > small bowel
Small bowel polyp	Lobulation with arborizing smooth muscle	Rarely seen
Large bowel polyp	Smooth surface Normal lamina propria Smooth muscle proliferation Lobulation with distorted crypts	Red appearance, eroded Inflamed lamina propria Scant smooth muscle Cystic glands with mucin and neutrophils
Gastric polyp	Hyperplastic/inflammatory polyp	Hyperplastic/inflammatory polyp

A

B

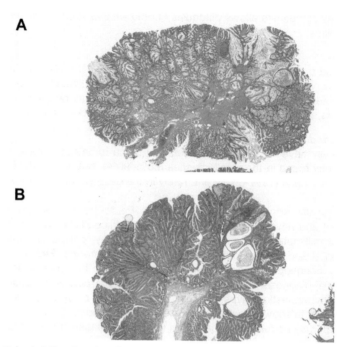

Fig. 3. (A) Colonic PJS polyp showing strands of smooth muscle in the lamina propria and nonneoplastic colonic epithelium with lobulated clusters of colonic crypts. (B) Gastric PJS polyp showing foveolar hyperplasia, some cystic dilatation, and increased inflammatory stroma.

Risk of malignancy

Patients with PJS have a high lifetime risk of a variety of gastrointestinal and extraintestinal malignancies and an overall lifetime risk of any cancer of 81% by the age of 70 years (**Table 4**).[60,67] The main extraintestinal tumors in PJS are breast and pancreatic adenocarcinoma and rare gonadal tumors of the ovary (sex-cord tumors with annular tubules) and testis (Sertoli cell tumors).

Table 4
Peutz-Jeghers syndrome cancer risks for specific site at 65 to 70 y of age[60,67]

Site	Cancer Risk (%)
Colorectum	39
Small intestine	13
Stomach	29
Pancreas	11–36
Breast	32–54
Uterus	9
Ovary	21
Cervix	10
Testes	9
Lung	7–17

Treatment

Management of patients with PJS including upper gastrointestinal endoscopy and colonoscopy should be performed every 2 to 3 years, starting from the late teens.[57] Small bowel visualization is recommended from age 8 to 10 years and repeated every 2 to 3 years. Other screening procedures related to cancer risk of the breast, female genital tract, testis, and pancreas can also be implemented.

JUVENILE POLYPOSIS SYNDROME
Definition

Juvenile polyposis syndrome (JPS) is an autosomal dominant syndrome defined by the presence of multiple colorectal juvenile polyps developing in the first and second decade of life. The clinical diagnosis criteria are presented in **Box 3**.[68,69]

Clinical Features

JPS can present as either colorectal or generalized juvenile polyposis, or as juvenile polyposis of infancy. Gastrointestinal bleeding, anemia, a prolapsed rectal polyp, passage of tissue through the anus, intussusception, and abdominal pain are frequent symptoms. Infant patients with JPS have extensive colorectal and gastric polyposis causing protein losing enteropathy, malabsorption, failure to thrive, and death at a young age. This rare form of JPS is caused by contiguous germline deletion of both the *BMPR1A* and *PTEN* gene.[70]

Pathogenesis

In 50% to 60% of the patients fulfilling these criteria a germline alteration in the TGB-β pathway genes *SMAD4* or *BMPR1A* gene is identified. Patients with *SMAD4* germline defects are more prone to develop gastric polyps, often in a profuse form, and can have hereditary hemorrhagic telangiectasia.[71,72] Immunohistochemistry for SMAD4 can be used as a surrogate marker for genetic *SMAD4* loss in juvenile polyps and as an adjunct in the molecular diagnosis of JPS.[73]

   Although the pathogenesis and neoplastic progression of juvenile polyps is not completely understood, early studies suggested that mechanical mucosal erosion with superimposed inflammatory reaction may lead to the formation of juvenile polyps and stressed the inflammatory basis of these polyps.[74] Recent studies suggest that an exaggerated inflammatory response to mucosal injury due to the inherent transforming growth factor beta (TGFβ) pathway defect in patients with JPS may underlie polyp development and inflammation-driven colon cancer.[75]

Pathologic Condition

Patients with JPS primarily have colorectal polyps but many also have polyps in upper gastrointestinal tract. Gastric polyps are found in 60% to 85% of patients, duodenal polyps in 14% to 33%.[11]

Box 3
Juvenile polyposis syndrome diagnostic criteria.

Criterion 1	>3–5 juvenile polyps of the Colorectum
Criterion 2	Juvenile polyps throughout the gastrointestinal tract
Criterion 3	Any number of juvenile polyps with a family history of juvenile polyposis syndrome
Other syndromes involving hamartomatous gastrointestinal polyps should be ruled out clinically or by pathologic examination	

Colorectal juvenile polyps are 5 to 50 mm in size, spherical and with a smooth surface due to erosion (see **Table 3**). Histologic features are an expanded stroma with edema, a mixed inflammatory infiltrate, and entrapped cystically dilated glands lined by nonneoplastic reactive epithelium (**Fig. 4**). Syndromic juvenile polyps are indistinguishable from sporadic juvenile polyps.[76] Approximately 50% of juvenile polyps show dysplasia but distinction between dysplasia and reactive atypia can be difficult. Inflammatory colorectal polyps form an important differential diagnosis of juvenile polyps.

Gastric juvenile polyps are characterized by abundant edematous stroma lined by hyperplastic and reactive foveolar epithelium[77] (see **Fig. 4**). An "epithelium-rich" variant with varied amount of stroma, tightly packed glands, and hyperplasia of surface epithelium can be seen. As with other hamartomatous polyps, gastric juvenile polyps are virtually indistinguishable from sporadic hyperplastic polyps without knowledge of the correct clinical context. High-grade dysplasia and gastric cancer can develop, particularly in *SMAD4* mutations carriers. The estimated risk of gastric adenocarcinoma is 10% to 30%.[78]

Risk of Malignancy

Affected patients have an increased risk of gastrointestinal cancer, mainly CRC. The risk of CRC is about 40% by the age of 80 years at a mean age of diagnosis of 44 years (range: 15–68 years).[79] Gastric cancer is mainly seen in *SMAD4* germline mutation carriers. The lifetime risk of gastric cancer is estimated between 10% and 30% and the median age of diagnosis is 58 years (range: 21–73 years).[57]

Treatment

Upper gastrointestinal endoscopy and colonoscopy are recommended starting at the age of 15 years or at the time of initial presentation. Depending on endoscopic findings, surveillance every 1 to 3 years should be performed.[57]

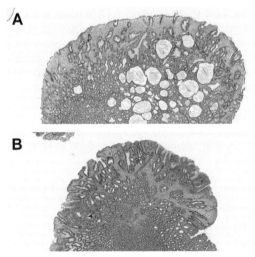

Fig. 4. (*A*) Typical colonic juvenile polyp characterized by eroded surface, expanded stroma with edema and inflammatory infiltrate and cystically dilated glands lined by nonneoplastic epithelium. (*B*) Gastric juvenile polyp showing abundant edematous stroma and hyperplastic and reactive foveolar epithelium.

PHOSPHATASE AND TENSIN HOMOLOG HAMARTOMA TUMOR SYNDROME/ COWDEN SYNDROME

Definition

CS is an autosomal dominant disorder, now part of the phosphatase and tensin homolog (PTEN) hamartoma tumor syndrome that also includes Bannayan-Riley-Ruvalcaba syndrome, PTEN-related Proteus syndrome and Proteus-like syndrome.[80] The reported prevalence of CS is 1 in 200,000 people,[81] a likely underestimate.

Clinical Features

The main features of CS are macrocephaly and multiple benign hamartomatous lesions in various organs, including skin and gastrointestinal tract. Mucocutaneous lesions (trichilemmomas of the face, oral papillomas, and acral and plantar keratosis) are characteristic and nearly always present by the age of 20 years.[82] The National Comprehensive Cancer Network established consensus diagnostic criteria.[82]

Pathogenesis

A constitutional pathogenic variant in *PTEN* is identified in 80% of individuals with a clinical CS diagnosis CS.[80] *PTEN* is a tumor suppressor gene encoding for a phosphatase that regulates cell proliferation, cell migration, and apoptosis through inhibition of the Phosphoinositide 3-kinase/AKT pathway.[83]

Pathologic Condition

Colonic polyps in CS are small sessile lesions that are easily overlooked during colonoscopy.[83] A mixture of hamartomatous and nonhamartomatous benign colonic polyps are typical of CS. Hamartomatous polyps show mildly abnormal crypt architecture and fibrous lamina propria that may contain bland spindle cells with various amount of adipose tissue and lymphoid aggregates (**Fig. 5**). Other histologic types include ganglioneuroma, lipoma, fibrolipoma, and inflammatory pseudopolyps.[84] Conventional adenomas and serrated polyps are also frequently found.[84,85]

In the upper gastrointestinal tract, patients with CS often develop multiple glycogenic acanthosis lesions of the esophagus presenting endoscopically as small white plaques and histologically with hyperplasia of the squamous epithelium showing enlarged cells in the superficial layers caused by glycogen accumulation in the cytoplasm. In the stomach and the duodenum, CS polyps do not have any specific features and often present as small hyperplastic or inflammatory polyps such as in other hamartomatous syndromes.

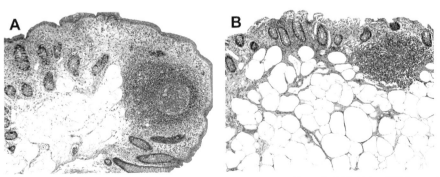

Fig. 5. (*A*) Colonic CS polyp with mixture of adipose tissue and lymphoid follicle. (*B*) Mucosal lipoma of the colon in CS.

Clues for suggesting the diagnosis are a high number of small colonic polyps with various histology identified through multiple colonoscopies and the association with glycogenic acanthosis of the esophagus. Previous history of other CS manifestations may further support the suspicion for the diagnosis and prompt genetic counseling.

Risk of Malignancy

The cumulative lifetime risk for any cancer is 89% by the age of 70 years (**Table 5**).[86] Affected women have an 81% risk of breast carcinoma with 50% penetrance by the age of 50 years.[87] Other cancer risks are 21% for thyroid carcinoma, 19% for endometrial carcinoma, and 15% for renal cell carcinoma. The risk of CRC is 9% to 16%. Benign lesions in the breast and thyroid are also common.

Treatment

The management of patients with CS includes screening for lesions in the breast, thyroid, the endometrium, and kidney.[57] Colonoscopy should start at the age of 35 years and repeated at 5 years interval or more frequently depending on symptoms and polyp findings.

LYNCH SYNDROME
Definition

LS is an autosomal dominant disorder caused by inherited pathogenic variants in one of the DNA mismatch repair (MMR) genes mutL homolog 1 (*MLH1*), mutL homolog 2 (*MLH2*), mutL homolog 6 (*MLH6*), and postmeiotic segregation increased, S. cerevisiae, 2 (*PMS2*) or by deletions in the 3' end of the epithelial cell adhesion molecule (*EPCAM*) gene leading to transcriptional silencing of *MSH2*.[88]

Clinical Features

LS is the most common genetic cause of CRC accounting for approximately 3% of all cases. Affected individuals also develop tumors of the endometrium, ovaries, small intestine, urinary tract, pancreas, hepatobiliary tract, stomach, brain, prostate, and breast.[89] Most individuals do not develop a large number of colorectal polyps.

Pathogenesis

MMR deficiency is the hallmark of LS-associated tumors. This deficiency occurs when the second allele of the same MMR gene that is constitutionally altered is hit by a somatic event. As a result, deficient MMR cells gain a growth advantage and are at risk of acquiring point mutation especially in short DNA repetitive sequences.

Table 5 Cowden syndrome lifetime cancer risks[87,99]	
Site	Lifetime Risk (%)
Breast	25–85
Thyroid	35
Endometrium	19–28
Kidney (Renal cell)	34
Colon	9
Melanoma	6

Immunohistochemistry is used to identify MMR deficiency when the expression of one or more MMR protein(s) is lost in tumor cells. Polymerase chain reaction-based microsatellite instability analysis on tumor tissue is another and sometimes complementary approach to demonstrate MMR deficiency. This phenotype is not specific of LS. Approximately 15% of non-LS associated CRC are MMR deficient caused by somatic hypermethylation of the *MLH1* gene promoter. Most of these sporadic deficient MMR (dMMR) CRC develop from serrated polyps and are associated with a *BRAF* mutation, which can be used to help distinguishing sporadic dMMR CRC from LS-associated CRC. However, most LS-associated CRCs are thought to develop from conventional adenomas.

Pathologic Condition

LS-associated CRC has typical histologic features of MMR deficiency including poor differentiation, mucinous and signet-ring cell features, medullary growth pattern, tumor infiltrating lymphocytes, and Crohn like peritumoral reaction. These characteristics are also present in non-LS dMMR CRC caused by somatic *MLH1* methylation.

Conventional colorectal adenomas in LS can show loss of expression of the MMR protein(s) concordant to the gene that is constitutionally altered in 70% to 80% of cases. Adenomas with high-risk features (large size, with a villous component, with high-grade dysplasia) have the highest rate of dMMR.[90] Testing colorectal adenomas for MMR deficiency by immunohistochemistry may only be warranted if there is a strong family history of CRC suggestive of LS. It is not useful in young patients without a family component.[91] Moreover, a normal MMR protein expression in adenoma does not exclude LS.

Risk of Malignancy

Individuals with a pathogenic variant in *MLH1*, *MSH2*, or *MSH6* have a 20% to 60% cumulative risk of CRC to age 70 years depending on the MMR gene mutated and the sex of the carrier.[92] The risk is lower for *MSH6* carriers and even lower for *PMS2* carriers.

Treatment

Colonoscopy with the removal of all polyps is recommended every 1 to 2 years starting at age 20 to 25 years or 2 to 5 years before earliest CRC diagnosis in the family.

CRONKHITE-CANADA SYNDROME
Definition

CCS is an extremely rare, nonhereditary, protein-losing enteropathy resulting in ectodermal changes and is associated with diffuse gastrointestinal hamartomatous polyposis.

Clinical Features

The clinical presentation is highly variable. Most patients present with diarrhea, weight loss, vomiting, and dysgeusia.[93] In this context, ectodermal changes should raise the suspicion for CCS and include nail dystrophy, alopecia, and diffuse skin pigmentation.

Pathogenesis

The pathogenesis is unknown. However, most studies suggest an autoimmune cause.[94]

Pathologic Condition

Polyps are usually small, broad-based, measuring less than 20 mm and present in the stomach, the duodenum, and the large bowel.[95,96] Endoscopically, these polyps can be described as diffuse mucosal hyperplasia. The gastric mucosa shows an expanded, edematous lamina propria with a moderate mixed inflammatory infiltrate and prominent eosinophils. The architecture is abnormal with cystic dilatation of the glands and foveolar hyperplasia. In the duodenum, there is villus blunting, architectural changes with crypt dilatation, and withering in an inflamed lamina propria. Eosinophilic cryptitis and crypt abscesses are commonly found. The colonic mucosa shows nonspecific inflammatory and architectural changes, resembling inflammatory pseudopolyps.

The most helpful feature that distinguishes CCS from hereditary hamartomatous syndromes is that the mucosa between the polyps is also abnormal with prominent inflammatory changes.

Risk of Malignancy

The risk of malignancy is controversial. However, patients with CCS are at an increased risk of adenoma and adenocarcinoma in the large bowel and the stomach, possibly secondary to the diffuse chronic mucosal inflammation.[97]

Treatment

The prognosis is poor. Correction electrolyte abnormalities and nutritional deficiencies are essential and often associated with immunosuppression.[96]

SUMMARY

The diagnosis of gastrointestinal polyposis syndromes requires a multidisciplinary approach involving pathologists, gastroenterologists, and geneticists.[98] Most hereditary disorders of the gastrointestinal tract present with increased numbers of colorectal polyps of various histologic types and are associated increased risks of cancer. Early diagnosis of these disorders allows appropriate clinical surveillance for the patient and affected relatives.

DISCLOSURE

L.A.A. Brosens: None. C. Rosty: None.

DECLARATION OF INTERESTS

None to declare.

ACKNOWLEDGMENT

None.

REFERENCES

1. Kinzler KW, Vogelstein B. Lessons from hereditary colorectal cancer. Cell. Oct 18 1996;87(2):159–70.
2. Kinzler KW, Vogelstein B. Landscaping the cancer terrain. Science 1998; 280(5366):1036–7.
3. Vasen HF, Moslein G, Alonso A, et al. Guidelines for the clinical management of familial adenomatous polyposis (FAP). Gut 2008;57(5):704–13.

4. Nieuwenhuis MH, De Vos Tot Nederveen Cappel W, Botma A, et al. Desmoid tumors in a dutch cohort of patients with familial adenomatous polyposis. Clin Gastroenterol Hepatol 2008;6(2):215–9.
5. Speake D, Evans DG, Lalloo F, et al. Desmoid tumours in patients with familial adenomatous polyposis and desmoid region adenomatous polyposis coli mutations. Br J Surg 2007;94(8):1009–13.
6. Li J, Woods SL, Healey S, et al. Point Mutations in Exon 1B of APC Reveal Gastric Adenocarcinoma and Proximal Polyposis of the Stomach as a Familial Adenomatous Polyposis Variant. Am J Hum Genet. May 05 2016;98(5):830–42.
7. Worthley DL, Phillips KD, Wayte N, et al. Gastric adenocarcinoma and proximal polyposis of the stomach (GAPPS): a new autosomal dominant syndrome. Gut 2012;61(5):774–9.
8. Gayther SA, Wells D, SenGupta SB, et al. Regionally clustered APC mutations are associated with a severe phenotype and occur at a high frequency in new mutation cases of adenomatous polyposis coli. Hum Mol Genet 1994;3(1):53–6.
9. Lamlum H, Ilyas M, Rowan A, et al. The type of somatic mutation at APC in familial adenomatous polyposis is determined by the site of the germline mutation: a new facet to Knudson's 'two-hit' hypothesis. Nat Med 1999;5(9):1071–5.
10. Nieuwenhuis MH, Mathus-Vliegen LM, Slors FJ, et al. Genotype-phenotype correlations as a guide in the management of familial adenomatous polyposis. Clin Gastroenterol Hepatol 2007;5(3):374–8.
11. Brosens LA, Wood LD, Offerhaus GJ, et al. Pathology and Genetics of Syndromic Gastric Polyps. Int J Surg Pathol 2016;24(3):185–99.
12. Wood LD, Salaria SN, Cruise MW, et al. Upper GI tract lesions in familial adenomatous polyposis (FAP): enrichment of pyloric gland adenomas and other gastric and duodenal neoplasms. Am J Surg Pathol 2014;38(3):389–93.
13. Vieth M, Montgomery EA. Some observations on pyloric gland adenoma: an uncommon and long ignored entity! J Clin Pathol 2014;67(10):883–90.
14. Martin I, Roos VH, Anele C, et al. Gastric adenomas and their management in familial adenomatous polyposis. Endoscopy 2021;53(8):795–801.
15. Sieber OM, Segditsas S, Knudsen AL, et al. Disease severity and genetic pathways in attenuated familial adenomatous polyposis vary greatly but depend on the site of the germline mutation. Gut 2006;55(10):1440–8.
16. Brosens LA, Offerhaus GJ, Giardiello FM. Hereditary Colorectal Cancer: Genetics and Screening. Surg Clin North Am 2015;95(5):1067–80.
17. Brosens LA, Keller JJ, Offerhaus GJ, et al. Prevention and management of duodenal polyps in familial adenomatous polyposis. Gut 2005;54(7):1034–43.
18. Leone PJ, Mankaney G, Sarvapelli S, et al. Endoscopic and histologic features associated with gastric cancer in familial adenomatous polyposis. Gastrointest Endosc 2019;89(5):961–8.
19. van Leerdam ME, Roos VH, van Hooft JE, et al. Endoscopic management of polyposis syndromes: European Society of Gastrointestinal Endoscopy (ESGE) Guideline. Endoscopy 2019;51(9):877–95.
20. Yang J, Gurudu SR, Koptiuch C, et al. American Society for Gastrointestinal Endoscopy guideline on the role of endoscopy in familial adenomatous polyposis syndromes. Gastrointest Endosc 2020;91(5):963–82.
21. Aelvoet AS, Pellise M, Bastiaansen BAJ, et al. Personalized endoscopic surveillance and intervention protocols for patients with familial adenomatous polyposis: the European FAP Consortium strategy. Endosc Int Open 2023;11(4):E386–93.
22. Al-Tassan N, Chmiel NH, Maynard J, et al. Inherited variants of MYH associated with somatic GC–>T: A mutations in colorectal tumors. Nat Genet 2002;30(2):227–32.

23. Win AK, Jenkins MA, Dowty JG, et al. Prevalence and Penetrance of Major Genes and Polygenes for Colorectal Cancer. Cancer Epidemiol Biomarkers Prev 2017; 26(3):404–12.

24. Lipton L, Halford SE, Johnson V, et al. Carcinogenesis in MYH-associated polyposis follows a distinct genetic pathway. Research Support, Non-U.S. Gov't. Cancer Res 2003;63(22):7595–9.

25. Thomas LE, Hurley JJ, Sanchez AA, et al, Collaborative Group on Duodenal Polyposis in MAP. Duodenal Adenomas and Cancer in MUTYH-associated Polyposis: An International Cohort Study. Gastroenterology 2021;160(3):952–4.

26. Boparai KS, Dekker E, Van Eeden S, et al. Hyperplastic polyps and sessile serrated adenomas as a phenotypic expression of MYH-associated polyposis. Gastroenterology 2008;135(6):2014–8.

27. Nieuwenhuis MH, Vogt S, Jones N, et al. Evidence for accelerated colorectal adenoma–carcinoma progression in MUTYH-associated polyposis? Gut 2012; 61(5):734–8.

28. Win AK, Reece JC, Dowty JG, et al. Risk of extracolonic cancers for people with biallelic and monoallelic mutations in MUTYH. Int J Cancer 2016;139(7):1557–63.

29. Palles C, Cazier JB, Howarth KM, et al. Germline mutations affecting the proofreading domains of POLE and POLD1 predispose to colorectal adenomas and carcinomas. Nat Genet. Dec 23 2012;45(2):136–44.

30. Bellido F, Pineda M, Aiza G, et al. POLE and POLD1 mutations in 529 kindred with familial colorectal cancer and/or polyposis: review of reported cases and recommendations for genetic testing and surveillance. Genet Med 2016;18(4):325–32.

31. Buchanan DD, Stewart JR, Clendenning M, et al. Risk of colorectal cancer for carriers of a germ-line mutation in POLE or POLD1. Genet Med 2018;20(8):890–5.

32. Ma X, Dong L, Liu X, et al. POLE/POLD1 mutation and tumor immunotherapy. J Exp Clin Cancer Res. Jul 2 2022;41(1):216.

33. Weren RD, Ligtenberg MJ, Kets CM, et al. A germline homozygous mutation in the base-excision repair gene NTHL1 causes adenomatous polyposis and colorectal cancer. Nat Genet 2015;47(6):668–71.

34. Grolleman JE, de Voer RM, Elsayed FA, et al. Mutational Signature Analysis Reveals NTHL1 Deficiency to Cause a Multi-tumor Phenotype. Cancer Cell. Feb 11 2019;35(2):256–66.

35. Boparai KS, Mathus-Vliegen EM, Koornstra JJ, et al. Increased colorectal cancer risk during follow-up in patients with hyperplastic polyposis syndrome: a multicentre cohort study. Gut 2010;59(8):1094–100.

36. Boparai KS, Reitsma JB, Lemmens V, et al. Increased colorectal cancer risk in first-degree relatives of patients with hyperplastic polyposis syndrome. Gut 2010;59(9):1222–5.

37. Rosty C, Parry S, Young JP. Serrated polyposis: an enigmatic model of colorectal cancer predisposition. Patholog Res Int 2011;2011:157073.

38. Abdulamir AS, Hafidh RR, Abu Bakar F. Abu Bakar F. The association of Streptococcus bovis/gallolyticus with colorectal tumors: the nature and the underlying mechanisms of its etiological role. Review. J Exp Clin Cancer Res 2011;30:11.

39. JEG I, Senore C, et al. Detection rate of serrated polyps and serrated polyposis syndrome in colorectal cancer screening cohorts: a European overview. Gut 2017;66(7):1225–32.

40. Edelstein DL, Axilbund JE, Hylind LM, et al. Serrated polyposis: rapid and relentless development of colorectal neoplasia. Gut 2013;62(3):404–8.

41. Carballal S, Rodriguez-Alcalde D, Moreira L, et al. Colorectal cancer risk factors in patients with serrated polyposis syndrome: a large multicentre study. Gut 2016; 65(11):1829–37.
42. JE I, Atkinson NSS, et al. Clinical risk factors of colorectal cancer in patients with serrated polyposis syndrome: a multicentre cohort analysis. Gut 2017;66(2): 278–84.
43. Win AK, Walters RJ, Buchanan DD, et al. Cancer risks for relatives of patients with serrated polyposis. Am J Gastroenterol 2012;107(5):770–8.
44. Mongin C, Coulet F, Lefevre JH, et al. Unexplained polyposis: a challenge for geneticists, pathologists and gastroenterologists. Clin Genet 2012;81(1):38–46.
45. Heald B, Mester J, Rybicki L, et al. Frequent gastrointestinal polyps and colorectal adenocarcinomas in a prospective series of PTEN mutation carriers. Gastroenterology 2010;139(6):1927–33.
46. Clendenning M, Young JP, Walsh MD, et al. Germline Mutations in the Polyposis-Associated Genes, and Are Not Common in Individuals with Serrated Polyposis Syndrome. PLoS One 2013;8(6):e66705.
47. Buchanan DD, Clendenning M, Zhuoer L, et al. Lack of evidence for germline RNF43 mutations in patients with serrated polyposis syndrome from a large multinational study. Gut 2017;66(6):1170–2.
48. Gala MK, Mizukami Y, Le LP, et al. Germline mutations in oncogene-induced senescence pathways are associated with multiple sessile serrated adenomas. Gastroenterology 2014;146(2):520–9.
49. Boparai KS, Dekker E, Polak MM, et al. A serrated colorectal cancer pathway predominates over the classic WNT pathway in patients with hyperplastic polyposis syndrome. Am J Pathol 2011;178(6):2700–7.
50. Rosty C, Walsh MD, Walters RJ, et al. Multiplicity and molecular heterogeneity of colorectal carcinomas in individuals with serrated polyposis. Am J Surg Pathol 2013;37(3):434–42.
51. Rosty C, Buchanan DD, Walsh MD, et al. Phenotype and Polyp Landscape in Serrated Polyposis Syndrome: A Series of 100 Patients From Genetics Clinics. Am J Surg Pathol 2012;36(6):876–82.
52. Rosty C, Hewett DG, Brown IS, et al. Serrated polyps of the large intestine: current understanding of diagnosis, pathogenesis, and clinical management. J Gastroenterol 2013;48(3):287–302.
53. He EY, Wyld L, Sloane MA, et al. The molecular characteristics of colonic neoplasms in serrated polyposis: a systematic review and meta-analysis. J Pathol Clin Res 2016;2(3):127–37.
54. Pai RK, Bettington M, Srivastava A, et al. An update on the morphology and molecular pathology of serrated colorectal polyps and associated carcinomas. Mod Pathol 2019;32(10):1390–415.
55. Bleijenberg AG, JE IJ van Herwaarden YJ, van Herwaarden YJ, et al. Personalised surveillance for serrated polyposis syndrome: results from a prospective 5-year international cohort study. Gut 2020;69(1):112–21.
56. East JE, Atkin WS, Bateman AC, et al. British Society of Gastroenterology position statement on serrated polyps in the colon and rectum. Gut 2017;66(7):1181–96.
57. Syngal S, Brand RE, Church JM, et al. ACG clinical guideline: Genetic testing and management of hereditary gastrointestinal cancer syndromes. Am J Gastroenterol 2015;110(2):223–62.
58. Parry S, Burt RW, Win AK, et al. Reducing the polyp burden in serrated polyposis by serial colonoscopy: the impact of nationally coordinated community surveillance. N Z Med J 2017;130(1451):57–67.

59. Young JP, Parry S. Risk factors: Hyperplastic polyposis syndrome and risk of colorectal cancer. Nat Rev Gastroenterol Hepatol 2010;7(11):594–5.

60. Boland CR, Idos GE, Durno C, et al. Diagnosis and Management of Cancer Risk in the Gastrointestinal Hamartomatous Polyposis Syndromes: Recommendations From the US Multi-Society Task Force on Colorectal Cancer. Gastroenterology 2022;162(7):2063–85.

61. de Leng WW, Jansen M, Carvalho R, et al. Genetic defects underlying Peutz-Jeghers syndrome (PJS) and exclusion of the polarity-associated MARK/Par1 gene family as potential PJS candidates. Clin Genet 2007;72(6):568–73.

62. Utsunomiya J, Gocho H, Miyanaga T, et al. Peutz-Jeghers syndrome: its natural course and management. Johns Hopkins Med J 1975;136(2):71–82.

63. Tse JY, Wu S, Shinagare SA, et al. Peutz-Jeghers syndrome: a critical look at colonic Peutz-Jeghers polyps. Mod Pathol 2013;26(9):1235–40.

64. Shaco-Levy R, Jasperson KW, Martin K, et al. Morphologic characterization of ha-martomatous gastrointestinal polyps in Cowden syndrome, Peutz-Jeghers syndrome, and juvenile polyposis syndrome. Hum Pathol 2016;49:39–48.

65. Jansen M, de Leng WW, Baas AF, et al. Mucosal prolapse in the pathogenesis of Peutz-Jeghers polyposis. Gut 2006;55(1):1–5.

66. Lam-Himlin D, Park JY, Cornish TC, et al. Morphologic characterization of syn-dromic gastric polyps. Am J Surg Pathol 2010;34(11):1656–62.

67. Giardiello FM, Welsh SB, Hamilton SR, et al. Increased risk of cancer in the Peutz-Jeghers syndrome. N Engl J Med 1987;316(24):1511–4.

68. Giardiello FM, Hamilton SR, Kern SE, et al. Colorectal neoplasia in juvenile polyp-osis or juvenile polyps. Arch Dis Child 1991;66(8):971–5.

69. Jass JR, Williams CB, Bussey HJ, et al. Juvenile polyposis–a precancerous con-dition. Histopathology 1988;13(6):619–30.

70. Delnatte C, Sanlaville D, Mougenot JF, et al. Contiguous gene deletion within chromosome arm 10q is associated with juvenile polyposis of infancy, reflecting cooperation between the BMPR1A and PTEN tumor-suppressor genes. Am J Hum Genet 2006;78(6):1066–74.

71. Blatter R, Tschupp B, Aretz S, et al. Disease expression in juvenile polyposis syn-drome: a retrospective survey on a cohort of 221 European patients and compar-ison with a literature-derived cohort of 473 SMAD4/BMPR1A pathogenic variant carriers. Genet Med 2020;22(9):1524–32.

72. Gallione CJ, Repetto GM, Legius E, et al. A combined syndrome of juvenile pol-yposis and hereditary haemorrhagic telangiectasia associated with mutations in MADH4 (SMAD4). Lancet 2004;363(9412):852–9.

73. Langeveld D, van Hattem WA, de Leng WW, et al. SMAD4 immunohistochemistry reflects genetic status in juvenile polyposis syndrome. Clin Cancer Res 2010; 16(16):4126–34.

74. Lipper S, Kahn LB, Sandler RS, et al. Multiple juvenile polyposis. A study of the pathogenesis of juvenile polyps and their relationship to colonic adenomas. Hum Pathol 1981;12(9):804–13.

75. Kim BG, Li C, Qiao W, et al. Smad4 signalling in T cells is required for suppression of gastrointestinal cancer. Nature 2006;441(7096):1015–9.

76. van Hattem WA, Langeveld D, de Leng WW, et al. Histologic variations in juvenile polyp phenotype correlate with genetic defect underlying juvenile polyposis. Am J Surg Pathol 2011;35(4):530–6.

77. Gonzalez RS, Adsay V, Graham RP, et al. Massive gastric juvenile-type polyposis: a clinicopathological analysis of 22 cases. Histopathology 2017;70(6):918–28.

78. Vos S, van der Post RS, Brosens LAA. Gastric Epithelial Polyps: When to Ponder, When to Panic. Surg Pathol Clin 2020;13(3):431–52.

79. Brosens LA, van Hattem A, Hylind LM, et al. Risk of colorectal cancer in juvenile polyposis. Gut 2007;56(7):965–7.

80. Marsh DJ, Kum JB, Lunetta KL, et al. PTEN mutation spectrum and genotype-phenotype correlations in Bannayan-Riley-Ruvalcaba syndrome suggest a single entity with Cowden syndrome. Hum Mol Genet 1999;8(8):1461–72.

81. Nelen MR, Kremer H, Konings IB, et al. Novel PTEN mutations in patients with Cowden disease: absence of clear genotype-phenotype correlations. Eur J Hum Genet 1999;7(3):267–73.

82. Starink TM, van der Veen JP, Arwert F, et al. The Cowden syndrome: a clinical and genetic study in 21 patients. Clin Genet 1986;29(3):222–33.

83. Blumenthal GM, Dennis PA. PTEN hamartoma tumor syndromes. Eur J Hum Genet 2008;16(11):1289–300.

84. Borowsky J, Setia N, Rosty C, et al. Spectrum of gastrointestinal tract pathology in a multicenter cohort of 43 Cowden syndrome patients. Mod Pathol 2019;32(12): 1814–22.

85. Stanich PP, Pilarski R, Rock J, et al. Colonic manifestations of PTEN hamartoma tumor syndrome: case series and systematic review. World J Gastroenterol 2014; 20(7):1833–88.

86. Riegert-Johnson DL, Gleeson FC, Roberts M, et al. Cancer and Lhermitte-Duclos disease are common in Cowden syndrome patients. Hered Cancer Clin Pract 2010;8(1):6.

87. Tan MH, Mester JL, Ngeow J, et al. Lifetime cancer risks in individuals with germ-line PTEN mutations. Clin Cancer Res 2012;18(2):400–7.

88. Yurgelun MB, Kulke MH, Fuchs CS, et al. Cancer Susceptibility Gene Mutations in Individuals With Colorectal Cancer. J Clin Oncol 2017;35(10):1086–95.

89. Moller P. The Prospective Lynch Syndrome Database reports enable evidence-based personal precision health care. Hered Cancer Clin Pract 2020;18:6.

90. Walsh MD, Buchanan DD, Pearson SA, et al. Immunohistochemical testing of conventional adenomas for loss of expression of mismatch repair proteins in Lynch syndrome mutation carriers: a case series from the Australasian site of the colon cancer family registry. Mod Pathol 2012;25(5):722–30.

91. Ferreira S, Claro I, Lage P, et al. Colorectal adenomas in young patients: micro-satellite instability is not a useful marker to detect new cases of Lynch syndrome. Dis Colon Rectum 2008;51(6):909–15.

92. International Mismatch Repair CVariation in the risk of colorectal cancer in families with Lynch syndrome: a retrospective cohort study. Lancet Oncol 2021; 22(7):1014–22.

93. Cronkhite LW Jr, Canada WJ. Generalized gastrointestinal polyposis; an unusual syndrome of polyposis, pigmentation, alopecia and onychotrophia. N Engl J Med 1955;252(24):1011–5.

94. Sweetser S, Ahlquist DA, Osborn NK, et al. Clinicopathologic features and treatment outcomes in Cronkhite-Canada syndrome: support for autoimmunity. Dig Dis Sci 2012;57(2):496–502.

95. Bettington M, Brown IS, Kumarasinghe MP, et al. The challenging diagnosis of Cronkhite-Canada syndrome in the upper gastrointestinal tract: a series of 7 cases with clinical follow-up. Am J Surg Pathol 2014;38(2):215–23.

96. Slavik T, Montgomery EA. Cronkhite-Canada syndrome six decades on: the many faces of an enigmatic disease. J Clin Pathol 2014;67(10):891–7.

97. Sweetser S, Boardman LA. Cronkhite-Canada syndrome: an acquired condition of gastrointestinal polyposis and dermatologic abnormalities. Gastroenterol Hepatol 2012;8(3):201–3.
98. Rosty C. The Role of the Surgical Pathologist in the Diagnosis of Gastrointestinal Polyposis Syndromes. Adv Anat Pathol 2018;25(1):1–13.
99. Pilarski R, Burt R, Kohlman W, et al. Cowden syndrome and the PTEN hamartoma tumor syndrome: systematic review and revised diagnostic criteria. J Natl Cancer Inst 2013;105(21):1607–16.

Anal and Perianal Preneoplastic Lesions

Maurice B. Loughrey, BSc, MB, MD, MRCP, FRCPath[a],*,
Neil A. Shepherd, DM, FRCPath[b]

KEYWORDS

- Anal cancer • Anal squamous dysplasia • LSIL • HSIL • Paget disease
- Malignant melanoma

KEY POINTS

- Anal squamous cell carcinoma is rare but increasing in prevalence: human papillomavirus (HPV) infection is a major causative factor.
- The 2-tiered Lower Anogenital Squamous Terminology system is preferred, rather than the 3-tiered anal intraepithelial neoplasia classification, for anal squamous dysplasia because it is associated with better interobserver agreement and clear management implications.
- Immunohistochemistry is helpful to corroborate the diagnoses of both squamous dysplasia and Paget disease of the anal region.
- P16 immunohistochemistry is particularly important in the assessment of squamous dysplasia but requires judicious application and careful interpretation.
- Primary Paget disease of the anal region is poorly understood but secondary disease is usually due to spread from a primary rectal adenocarcinoma.

INTRODUCTION

Epithelial tumors of the anal canal and perianal skin are relatively uncommon, with an estimated 9760 new cases in the United States in 2023, in comparison to 153,020 new cases of colorectal cancer.[1] Nevertheless, anal cancer has been steadily increasing in incidence, doubling during the last 30 years. Anal cancer is slightly more common in women, with an incidence in the United States of 2.3 per 100,000 women per year, compared with 1.6 per 100,000 men per year. The median age at diagnosis is 63 years. Anal cancer currently accounts for less than 0.5% of all cancer-related deaths but is associated with significant morbidity for afflicted patients.

[a] Department of Cellular Pathology, Royal Victoria Hospital, Grosvenor Road, Belfast, Northern Ireland BT12 6BA, United Kingdom; [b] Gloucestershire Cellular Pathology Laboratory, Cheltenham General Hospital, Sandford Road, Cheltenham GL53 7AN, United Kingdom
* Corresponding author.
E-mail address: maurice.loughrey@belfasttrust.hscni.net

Gastroenterol Clin N Am 53 (2024) 201–220
https://doi.org/10.1016/j.gtc.2023.09.007
0889-8553/24/© 2023 Elsevier Inc. All rights reserved.
gastro.theclinics.com

Although the vast majority of anal cancers are squamous cell carcinomas, reflecting an origin in the surface mucosal lining of the lower anal canal or perianal skin, other histologic tumor types occur rarely, originating in other cell lineages native to this complex anatomic site. Given their rarity, little is known about precursors to nonsquamous anal neoplasia. In contrast, the precursor to anal squamous cell carcinoma, commonly referred to as anal intraepithelial neoplasia (AIN), is now well understood at morphologic and molecular levels. There have been important developments in nomenclature, with broad acceptance of low-grade and high-grade squamous intraepithelial lesion (SIL) terminology. Current understanding of anal squamous neoplasia represents the focus of this review, including discussions on consensus definitions and nomenclature, pathogenesis, clinical diagnosis, adjunctive diagnostic biomarkers, natural history and treatment, with some additional comments on rarer preneoplastic entities that occur in the anal region.

ANAL SQUAMOUS NEOPLASIA
Definition

Anal squamous neoplasia can originate either in the anal canal or in perianal skin, surrounding the anal verge. The most commonly accepted definition of the anal canal, proposed by the American Joint Committee on Cancer, describes the anal canal extending from the apex of the anal sphincter complex to the palpable intersphincteric groove at the distal edge of the internal sphincter muscle.[2,3] Tumors that originate in the anal canal are significantly different from those originating in perianal skin.[4] The most common tumor of the anal canal is the nonkeratinizing variant of squamous cell carcinoma. In contrast, neoplastic entities of the perianal region emulate their cutaneous counterparts: the most common malignancies are basal cell carcinoma and keratinizing squamous cell carcinoma. Perianal tumors usually require less aggressive treatment. However, squamous dysplasia often occurs at both sites in individual patients.[5]

Nomenclature

The earliest terms introduced to describe anal preinvasive disease used terms from cutaneous pathology practice, such as Bowen disease and carcinoma in situ, and did not distinguish anal canal from perianal skin neoplasia. Awareness of differing biology and clinical behavior of diseases involving these different anatomic sites grew gradually and accelerated after the association between human papillomavirus (HPV) infection and cervical cancer was described, with an HPV link to anal neoplasia following quickly and found to be stronger in anal canal neoplasia than in perianal lesions.[6] In 1986, Fenger and Nielsen described a series of anal canal dysplasia cases and introduced the term anal canal intraepithelial neoplasia, subsequently refined to AIN.[5] Analogous to cervical intraepithelial neoplasia (CIN), AIN was classified by 3 grades according to severity, namely AIN 1, AIN 2, and AIN 3. This terminology became embedded in routine clinical use. Anal squamous intraepithelial lesion (ASIL) was suggested as an alternative in the mid-1990s by Northfelt and colleagues, with a binary subdivision proposed, low-grade ASIL corresponding to AIN 1 and high-grade ASIL to AIN 2 or 3.[7] However, the 3-tier AIN classification remained in common usage, especially in the United Kingdom.

In 2012, representatives from the College of American Pathologists and the American Society for Colposcopy and Cervical Pathology published a set of recommendations to standardize nomenclature applied to HPV-associated noninvasive squamous lesions, under the umbrella term of Lower Anogenital Squamous Terminology (LAST).[8]

The aims were to apply current knowledge of HPV biology, optimize the use of relevant biomarkers and help communication and minimize confusion between anatomic sites. Applying the principle of aligning the number of diagnostic terms with the number of biologically relevant categories, a 2-tier classification was favored across all sites, using the SIL terminology, with an optional additional "-IN" descriptor to specify location for example, AIN or CIN. SIL represents an abnormal cellular proliferation with nuclear atypia in the form of enlargement, pleomorphism, chromatin alterations, and nuclear irregularity. These features become more marked with increasing SIL severity and, in particular, there is a relative loss of maturation in the superficial mucosal layers, associated with an increase in the nuclear to cytoplasmic ratio.

Low-grade SIL (LSIL) demonstrates these atypical nuclear features with loss of maturation and mitotic activity confined to the lower third of the epithelium. Identification of the diagnostic cytopathic effect of HPV infection, known as koilocytosis, and characterized by multinucleation, nuclear enlargement, and/or pleomorphism accompanied by perinuclear halos, also qualifies for the designation of LSIL, provided these appearances are not accompanied by high-grade features. High-grade SIL (HSIL) demonstrates more marked atypical nuclear features as described, with loss of maturation extending into the upper two-thirds of the epithelium. AIN 2, under previous terminology, is therefore included under HSIL but is likely to represent a heterogeneous category. AIN 2 has no unique biological correlate. Its morphologic diagnosis on hematoxylin and eosin (H&E) morphology is poorly reproducible, analogous to cervical intraepithelial neoplasia grade 2.[9,10] For these reasons, the application of biomarkers to assist accurate classification is strongly recommended in this particular setting (see section "Adjunctive Diagnostic Biomarkers" on p16 immunohistochemistry below).

As one would expect, interobserver agreement is greater applying a 2-tier rather than 3-tier system.[10–13] In turn, this implies better diagnostic consistency and more clinically relevant outcome data. LSIL and HSIL terminology is now in widespread use in gynecological and urologic pathologic condition. Importantly with respect to the gastrointestinal (GI) tract, its use for anal neoplasia has been endorsed by the most recent World Health Organization publication.[14]

Pathogenesis

The distinction between LSIL and HSIL is of considerable biological and clinical significance. In the lower anogenital tract, LSIL is much more common than HSIL and is considered to represent a transient, typically self-limited, HPV infection with active replication that is likely to resolve spontaneously. It is most commonly caused by HPV types 6 and 11. In contrast, HSIL is a precancerous lesion that has the potential to progress to invasive carcinoma. It is most commonly caused by HPV types 16 and 18. In these high-risk HPV infections, viral protein products E6 and E7 are expressed initially in the basal squamous layers, enhancing cell proliferation and evasion of host immune surveillance. Persistent high-risk HPV infection over time is associated with decreasing regulation and increasing E6/E7 expression, which is particularly profound if and when the virus becomes integrated into the host genome. This releases the E6/E7 oncogenes from transcriptional control, resulting in a clonal expansion of largely undifferentiated cells and substantially increases the likelihood of malignant transformation.

Clinical Diagnosis

The incidence of anal SIL remains unknown but is likely to be increasing, especially among high-risk groups, given the steadily increasing incidence of anal cancer. It is generally diagnosed in 1 of 2 settings. Most commonly, it is detected on screening of individuals with predisposing risk factors for HPV infection, namely human immuno-deficiency virus (HIV)-positive status, men having sex with men, receptive anal inter-course, and/or HPV infections elsewhere in the lower anogenital tract.[15,16] Less commonly, SIL is found incidentally in anal resection specimens such as hemorrhoi-dectomy or abdominoperineal resection (**Fig. 1**).[17] Smoking is also a risk factor for SIL, although the underlying mechanism for this has not been clearly elucidated.[18,19] Chronic immunosuppression not only predisposes to SIL but also increases the risk of progression to carcinoma, likely due to inefficient viral clearance. Evidence for this comes mainly from the posttransplant population.[20] However, this is likely to apply to other populations and is of considerable clinical importance as a research priority given rapid developments and widespread use of new biologic and other immuno-modulatory therapies, in the settings of oncology and nonneoplastic chronic inflam-matory diseases.

SIL is more likely to develop in the upper anal canal and anal transition zone than in the lower anal canal and perianal region.[4,21] However, many patients show involve-ment of both areas, as well as the perianal skin, and this underscores the importance of widespread sampling to both establish a pathologic diagnosis and assess extent of disease involvement, applying the diagnostic features of LSIL and HSIL as described above. Clinically, SIL may or may not be visible and therefore pathologic assessment is the mainstay of diagnosis. Various macroscopic appearances have been described, including raised erythematous mucosa, white scaling mucosa, pigmented mucosa, or ulceration. A verrucous macroscopic appearance (**Fig. 2** USE **Fig. 1** FROM ANALA-GOUS 2017 PUBLICATION) has been associated with the highest risk of malignant transformation.[22] However, most patients with SIL show no macroscopic changes, which makes early diagnosis and disease management difficult.

Anal cytology demonstrates good sensitivity rates for the detection of SIL. This in-volves the patient or clinician inserting a moist swab into the rectum and then removing it with a twisting motion while applying lateral pressure. This permits sam-pling of the transitional zone and anal canal mucosal lining. The swab is then pro-cessed similar to a cervical smear preparation, using liquid-based cytology and Papanicolaou staining. The stained slide is screened for atypical cells. Some investi-gators have recommended this technique as a method of screening for SIL.[23–25] A lim-itation is that it does not identify the extent and distribution of disease.[26] There is also a

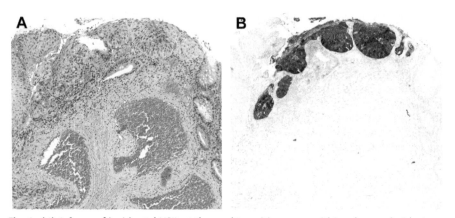

Fig. 1. (*A*) A focus of incidental HSIL at the anal transition zone within a hemorrhoidectomy specimen. (*B*) HSIL is supported by block-positive p16 immunostaining.

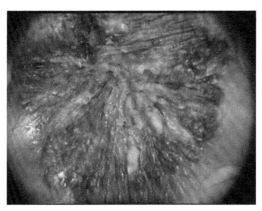

Fig. 2. Macroscopic appearance of verrucous HSIL. The lesion has a papillomatous appearance with marked surface hyperkeratosis.

relatively high rate of atypical but nonspecific findings, so-called atypical squamous cells of undetermined significance, which typically results in the need for further examination and biopsy.[27] Population-based anal cytology screening programs have not been explored, and this approach may have more benefit in selected, high-risk, populations. As in modern cervical screening programs, HPV molecular testing performed on anal cytology specimens may provide improved diagnostic sensitivity but the role of HPV molecular testing in screening for SIL remains unclear.[28]

Anal colposcopy has been advocated as a method to assess the extent of SIL.[18,29,30] Using techniques similar to those applied in the uterine cervix, an operating low-power microscope provides a visual assessment of the anal canal. SIL may be identified as acetowhite epithelium contrasting with iodine-positive (brown) nonneoplastic mucosa. Any suspicious findings are biopsied under direct visualization.[31] In recent years, high-resolution anoscopy (HRA) has been demonstrated to be more effective than standard anoscopy for lesion detection.[32] HRA is usually used in specialist centers after abnormal anal cytology is detected, or for surveillance of established SIL. It also allows the application of localized therapies. HRA is likely an effective approach to the management of SIL but given the relative rarity of HSIL diagnoses in the general population and the significant training time required to be proficient in HRA, this technique is best restricted to specialized centers for best outcomes.

Adjunctive Diagnostic Biomarkers

The diagnosis of SIL relies heavily on standard H&E assessment, and there are few biomarkers of established clinical utility. Ki-67 immunohistochemistry has been extensively investigated but studies reporting its application as an ancillary stain for diagnosing SIL suffer from inconsistent thresholds to define Ki-67 "positivity," hindering comparisons between studies.[31,33] LAST guidelines do not recommend Ki-67 for this purpose, either in isolation or in combination with p16.[8] Ki-67 may however be helpful in distinguishing SIL from benign mimics, such as anal transitional mucosa.[34]

P16 is a 16-kDa protein encoded by *CDKN2A*, which is located within the INK4/ARF tumor suppressor locus on chromosome 9 (9p21.3).[35,36] P16 inhibits cyclin-dependent kinases required to phosphorylate the retinoblastoma protein, pRb. As discussed above, persistent high-risk HPV infection over time results in deregulation of the viral proteins E6/E7, most notably when the virus is integrated and the E6/E7 oncogenes are released from transcriptional control. E6 and E7 can bind and inactivate p53 and pRb, respectively, allowing uncontrolled and rapid progression through the cell cycle. E7-related binding and degradation of pRb releases p16 production from its negative feedback control, resulting in a paradoxic accumulation of p16 protein within the cell, representing an attempt to inhibit the uncontrolled proliferation.[37] In summary, the abnormal p16 overexpression represents a marker of E7-mediated functional inactivation of pRb and can therefore be utilized as a surrogate marker of high-risk transforming HPV infection and HSIL.[38]

P16 is the only biomarker included in the LAST recommendations for the evaluation of lower anogenital squamous lesions.[8] Its use is recommended in specific scenarios, with the overarching aim of ensuring more robust diagnoses of the clinically important precancerous condition HSIL (**Fig. 3**). First, p16 immunohistochemistry should be applied when there is a morphologic differential diagnosis of HSIL versus a benign mimic, specifically immature squamous metaplasia, atrophy, reparative epithelial change, or tangential cutting. Second, if the H&E morphologic features suggest AIN 2, applying old terminology, p16 immunochemistry can help classify this biologically equivocal lesion as either HSIL, a precancer, or LSIL, related to transient HPV infection (or rarely non–HPV-associated pathologic condition). In both scenarios, strong and diffuse block-positive p16 supports classification as HSIL. Weak, patchy, or focal staining patterns are interpreted as negative and do not represent HSIL (**Fig. 4**). Importantly, LAST guidance recommends against the casual use of p16 if the morphologic features are those of LSIL or negative for neoplasia. In a recent study examining p16 immunostaining in 1000 anal biopsies, the 400 cases of LSIL included showed block p16 immunostaining in 151 cases (37%).[39] Furthermore, positive p16 has been reported in 2% of normal anal biopsies (**Fig. 5**).[40] This reinforces the LAST mandate that any block-type p16 positivity must be accompanied by H&E morphologic criteria for HSIL to be interpreted as such. P16 block immunopositivity alone does not define HSIL.

HPV can be identified and classified according to recognized high-risk and low-risk types by applying in situ histochemistry (ISH) for HPV DNA or, more recently, HPV RNA. HPV RNA ISH is much superior to HPV DNA ISH for the detection of high-risk HPV in tissue samples.[41,42] This ancillary test is not within the LAST recommendations, deemed not to offer additional information of clinical value beyond p16 immunohistochemistry, and its routine use is not recommended. However, p16 is not 100%

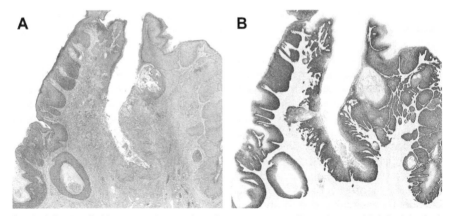

Fig. 3. (*A*) HSIL (left) progressing to invasive squamous cell carcinoma (right). (*B*) Block-positive p16 immunostaining throughout invasive and noninvasive squamous neoplasia.

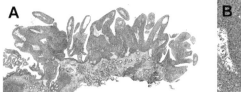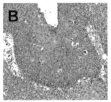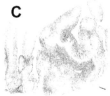

Fig. 4. Papillomatous AIN 2 considered sufficient for HSIL morphologically (*A*, low power; *B*, high power). Nonblock p16 immunostaining (*C*), interpreted as negative, favors downgrading to LSIL applying LAST recommendations, given the rarity of p16-negative HSIL.

sensitive and HPV RNA ISH may offer value in cases that show discordance between H&E morphology and p16 immunostaining.[40,43]

Natural History

Institution of specific guidelines for the management of SIL is difficult because the implications and natural history of SIL remain poorly understood. The concept of HSIL as a precursor of invasive squamous cell carcinoma of the anus is supported by the coexistence of HSIL adjacent to invasive cancer and by the fact that HSIL shows biological and molecular properties that are similar to those of anal cancer, including enhanced angiogenesis, increased proliferation, decreased apoptosis, p53 mutations, and, as discussed, a strong association with high-risk HPV types.

Although LSIL may progress to HSIL and invasive neoplasia, it is also associated with a considerable rate of spontaneous regression, of up to 30%.[30,44–46] This is supported by a pathogenesis related to transient HPV infection. Inconsistent or inaccurate pathology interpretation may also contribute to this finding.[44] Factors associated with LSIL progression have not been well studied but progression seems most common in the setting of immunosuppression, with an LSIL-to-HSIL progression rate of 62% within 2 years reported in HIV-infected men, compared with 36% in HIV-uninfected men.[47,48]

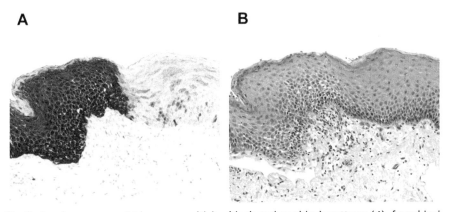

Fig. 5. Focal squamous p16 immunopositivity, block and nonblock patterns (*A*), found incidentally within a hemorrhoidectomy specimen. This is not accompanied by morphologic atypia to suggest HSIL or LSIL, although the abrupt transition line on p16 is also evident, more subtly, on H&E staining (*B*). This is interpreted as negative for neoplasia, despite the positive p16 staining, which can rarely be seen in morphologically normal mucosa and warns against the casual application of p16 immunohistochemistry.

The natural history of HSIL is also poorly understood and has been mainly studied in immunosuppressed populations. In a historic study by Scholefield and colleagues, 35 patients with AIN 3 underwent long-term surveillance after excision.[49] Only 6 patients, all with multifocal disease, were immunosuppressed. Three of the latter developed invasive carcinoma in the follow-up period (maximum 10 years) but none of the immunocompetent patients developed cancer. The investigators concluded that AIN 3 has a relatively low potential for malignant transformation in the immunocompetent patient and that immunosuppression is associated with more extensive AIN 3 and a greater risk of progression to malignancy.

The association of immunosuppression with progression of HSIL to squamous cell carcinoma has been confirmed by larger, more recent studies, which also reported other factors associated with progression, including sex, marital status, smoking, and HIV status.[48,50–52] Burgos and colleagues reported that, within HIV-positive men, treatment with highly active antiretroviral therapy (HAART) or being in a stable personal relationship with another individual protected against progression.[53]

A recent, large, general population-based Danish study reported that having an autoimmune disease, genital warts and living with HIV were all associated with an increased risk of progression from AIN 3 to invasive carcinoma.[54] One US registry-based study estimated that almost 10% of patients in the general population with AIN 3 progressed to invasive carcinoma within 5 years.[50] In general, however, it seems that although LSIL and HSIL can progress to invasive carcinoma, overall progression rates are relatively low, are highest in high-risk populations, and spontaneous regression, particularly of LSIL, can occur in a relatively high proportion of individuals.

Treatment

Given the uncertainty around the natural history of SIL, its management remains uncertain. There is no standard guidance but some recommend treatment of patients with HSIL and observation of those with LSIL.[55] Enhanced surveillance is generally considered appropriate for HSIL and should be augmented in high-risk groups, given higher risk of progression. Surveillance is best undertaken using HRA in specialist centers.

Historically, the treatment of HSIL has been wide local excision after extensive mapping biopsies to assess extent of disease.[26,56] However, this approach is associated with a high rate of recurrence, ranging from 9% to 63%, likely related to multifocal disease.[57] Repeated procedures can result in significant side effects including perianal pain, scarring, stenosis, or fecal incontinence. For these reasons, and given the availability of alternative therapies, a surgical approach to managing HSIL is no longer favored.

Alternative strategies comprise local ablative or topical therapies. Ablative therapeutic options include electrocautery, infrared coagulation, radiofrequency ablation, and photodynamic therapy. These are typically carried out at anoscopy or HRA, with the aim of targeted tissue destruction. Morbidity and side effects are much less than with surgical intervention but all are associated with potential incomplete response and a significant risk of recurrence after treatment.[55] For example, one study examining electrocautery ablation of HSIL in HIV-positive men reported one-third of patients to have a complete response, one-third to have a partial response, and one-third no response.[53] The response was dependent on the number of procedures performed, and the recurrence rate was 25% at 30 months follow-up. A study of infrared coagulation ablation of HSIL reported differential recurrence rates according to HIV status, 61% at 1 year for HIV-positive men compared with 38% for HIV-negative men.[58]

Topical therapies offer a less-invasive option and include trichloroacetic acid (TCA), 5-fluorouracil (5-FU), or imiquimod. These offer good short-term control but are associated with recurrence and local side effects such as hypopigmentation and skin irritation.[59] TCA can clear HSIL in 71% to 79% of patients but may be less effective for extensive or bulky disease.[60] Topical application of the chemotherapeutic agent 5-FU is associated with clearance of HSIL in up to 90% of cases, although with a high-recurrence rate of 50% at 6 months in one study.[61] The synthetic immune modulator imiquimod functions by upregulating the innate immune system to enhance antiviral activity and has been applied with success in gynecological squamous neoplasia.[62] There is some evidence from a double-blind, randomized, controlled trial for its effectiveness in controlling HSIL in HIV-positive men.[63]

In summary, local ablative and topical therapies offer well-tolerated therapeutic options for HSIL that have reasonable efficacy but a substantial portion of patients either do not respond or recur. Best outcomes are likely achieved in combination and within specialist treatment centers. For example, one large US center used serial ablative procedures under HRA, supplemented by office-based surveillance and topical treatments, in 246 patients with HSIL (84% men; 79% immunocompromised) and reported their 10-year experience.[64] They achieved 78% clearance at last follow-up, with complications in 4% and progression to invasive cancer in only 1.2% of patients.

Human Papillomavirus Vaccination

The discovery of the association of HPV infection with cervical neoplasia led to the development of vaccines against this virus. The first vaccine was designed against high-risk HPV types 16 and 18, followed by the "quadrivalent" vaccine targeting HPV types 6, 11, 16, and 18. Given its success in controlling cervical neoplasia, HPV vaccination may also prove a successful tool in preventing and possibly treating anal neoplasia. Potential benefit depends on the timing of vaccination in comparison to HPV exposure, with the greatest benefit for the prevention of anal neoplasia likely stemming from the administration of the vaccine to young people before the onset of sexual activity.[65] A recent multicenter, randomized, placebo-controlled, phase 3 trial of the quadrivalent HPV vaccine in men found that it provided durable protection against anogenital disease.[66] Initial vaccine benefits established in HIV-positive men can be extrapolated to the HIV-negative, immunocompetent population, given the similar pathogenesis related to HPV infection in both settings.[67] Currently, the Center for Disease Control in the United States recommends HPV vaccination for all children aged 11 or 12 years, in addition to older unvaccinated men and women at high risk for HPV-associated anal or cervical neoplasia, up to the age of 26 years.[68]

OTHER SQUAMOUS PROLIFERATIONS OF THE ANAL REGION

A range of other terms is applied to a variety of squamous proliferations of the anal region. Historically, these included Bowen disease and Bowenoid papulosis but both fall under the pathologic definition of HSIL, and these terms are discouraged to avoid confusion, partly because they have been erroneously regarded as specific entities, akin to their cutaneous counterparts.

Condyloma acuminatum is an exophytic lesion that can be encountered in the perianal region. This term is firmly entrenched in clinical practice, and these lesions are commonly described as genital warts. The LAST project considers condyloma acuminatum, by definition, a low-grade papillary proliferation with cytopathic features of HPV infection and is included within the spectrum of LSIL (**Fig. 6**).[8] Most lesions are caused by low-risk HPV types 6 and 11. Accordingly, p16 immuno-expression is

A

B

C

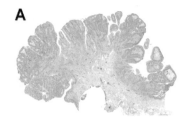
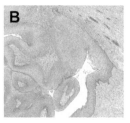
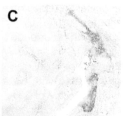

Fig. 6. Condyloma acuminatum with papillomatous growth pattern and acanthosis of maturing squamous epithelium (*A*, low power). Minimal cytologic atypia is evident (*B*, high power). Weak, focal, nonblock p16 immunostaining supports categorization as LSIL (*C*).

typically negative or weak and patchy (nonblock type). Their frond-like growth pattern is readily identified histologically, with papillae lined by thickened squamous epithelium, often with prominent parakeratosis and dyskeratosis. There is minimal cytologic atypia and epithelium often demonstrates characteristic viral cytopathic changes, known as koilocytes. Koilocytes demonstrate nuclear enlargement, hyperchromasia, and irregularity of nuclear membranes. Their nuclei have a shriveled or "raisinoid" appearance and are often surrounded by a zone of cytoplasmic clearing. Rarely, condyloma acuminata may exhibit foci of HSIL, and these can be associated with high-risk oncogenic types, particularly HPV 16 and 18, and corresponding block-positive p16 immunoexpression.[26]

Buschke-Löwenstein tumor, also known as giant condyloma acuminatum, is a rare entity characterized by an exophytic, cauliflower-like squamous proliferation with a locally invasive growth pattern, a high rate of recurrence, and potential for malignant transformation.[69] Its precise incidence is impossible to calculate because there is no agreed minimum size to distinguish it from classic condyloma acuminatum. These lesions share histologic features as described above, including atypia usually in the LSIL range. Accordingly, more than 90% of Buschke-Löwenstein tumors are associated with low-risk HPV types 6 and 11.[70] They differ from squamous cell carcinoma in having an intact basement membrane and lacking features of invasive neoplasia. In one large series of 38 Buschke-Löwenstein tumors, 19 (50%) had an invasive component.[71] Verrucous carcinoma, in particular, represents a difficult differential diagnosis but can be identified by its broad, pushing, invasive margin and absence of koilocytosis because it is not an HPV-associated neoplasm.[72] HPV testing may be diagnostically beneficial if morphologic features are equivocal.

Keratinizing SIL is defined by an abnormal surface keratinizing layer. Dyskeratotic cells are prominent with markedly atypical, pleomorphic nuclei. There is an abnormal basal layer proliferation but this is often accompanied by more cellular maturation and cytoplasmic eosinophilia compared with typical HSIL. Keratinizing SIL is most common in cutaneous sites normally lined by keratinizing epithelium, including the perianal region but it can also be encountered in mucosal epithelium of the anal canal.[8]

GLANDULAR PRENEOPLASTIC LESIONS OF THE ANUS AND PERIANAL REGION

Benign glandular neoplasms of the anal region are well described but are relatively rare. Sweat gland tumors, such as hidradenoma papilliferum, do occur here. Furthermore, primary adenocarcinoma of the anal region is also well recognized but is unusual.[73,74] These often occur as a complication of preexisting pathologic condition such as Crohn disease. Mucinous adenocarcinoma of the anal region is a well-recognized complication of fistulae, within and outwith Crohn disease.[75–77] However, little is known about the precursor glandular lesions before malignancy has intervened. The commonest and most important of the premalignant glandular proliferations in the anal region is Paget disease.

ANAL AND PERIANAL PAGET DISEASE

Paget disease is the clinical manifestation of the intraepidermal proliferation of neoplastic glandular cells within squamous epithelium. Extramammary Paget disease is an enigmatic condition. It is certainly rare with the average pathology department seeing only a handful of cases every year. Ironically, Sir James Paget, the eminent Barts surgeon from London, United Kingdom, and the original describer of the diseases of the breast and bone, to which his name has been appended, did not describe extramammary Paget disease. Instead, two French workers first described this disease in 1893, having noted its similarities to Paget disease of the nipple.[78] Although the latter represents the intraepidermal extension of ductal carcinoma-in situ, extramammary Paget disease, whether of the vulva or anus, has differing pathogenetic mechanisms.[79] Secondary Paget disease, in the anus due to a primary adenocarcinoma of the anus or colorectum, is relatively well understood but primary anal and perianal Paget disease remains poorly understood, particularly with regard to the cell of origin.

Clinical Features

Anal and perianal Paget disease occurs in both genders in almost equal proportions and is mainly a disease of the elderly.[80] It manifests clinically as raised, red, scaling areas in the anal canal or perianal skin[81,82] and clinically resembles other forms of Paget disease, especially that of the breast. There may be subtle clinical and pathologic differences between the 2 main forms of anal and perianal Paget disease. For instance, primary Paget disease is more likely to show an uneven, asymmetrical distribution around the anus, whereas secondary Paget disease has been characterized by fibroepithelioma of Pinkus-like changes and subepidermal mucin deposits histologically.[83] Clinically, the disease is poorly demarcated, and this makes complete excision, if surgery is the chosen option, difficult.[84] This approach requires close co-operation between surgeon and pathologist with either intraoperative frozen sections or Moh's-type surgery, and intraoperative CK7 immunohistochemistry is advocated to ensure that ultimate margins are free of disease.[84,85] As Paget disease can be associated with colorectal, particularly rectal, malignancy, sigmoidoscopy should be performed at the time of diagnosis to rule out an associated malignancy in the rectum or, much more rarely, in the sigmoid colon.[79,86,87]

Pathology and Histogenesis

Histologically, Paget disease demonstrates an intraepidermal proliferation of large vacuolated neoplastic cells, often in clusters but also present discretely (**Fig. 7**). They are typically concentrated in the basal aspect of the epidermis where clustering is more apparent.[88] However, spread of clusters and discrete cells, to the superficial parts of the epidermis, so-called Pagetoid spread, also occurs. The cells have large, irregular nuclei and finely vacuolated cytoplasm. There is intracytoplasmic mucin, which is periodic acid-Schiff-diastase (PAS-D) and alcian blue positive.[89] Thus histochemical stains are often valuable in helping to differentiate Paget disease from its mimics,[88,89] although immunohistochemistry is now the method of choice to corroborate the diagnosis and to determine the type of disease present.[86,89] Among the chief mimics of Paget disease are an entirely benign disease, Pagetoid keratosis, in which intraepidermal vacuolated cells represent a reactive pathology[90] and HPV

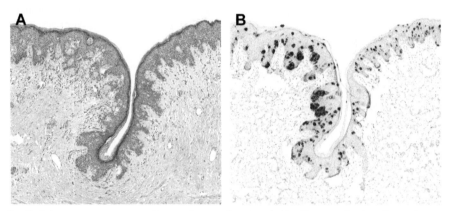

Fig. 7. Primary extramammary Paget disease of perianal skin. The neoplastic cells can be single or nested, have vacuolated cytoplasm, and are predominantly basally orientated (*A*). GCDFP15 immunopositivity highlights the neoplastic cells (*B*).

involvement, described earlier in this article, which can produce similar changes, mimicking Paget disease, and is also characteristically associated with hyperplasia of the squamous epithelium.[88] Premalignant squamous proliferations, especially HSIL, are also potent mimics of Paget disease. Perhaps, the closest mimic of Paget disease is premalignant melanocytic neoplasia because the neoplastic melanocytes can be present and concentrated in the basal region but also show upward extension, as in Paget disease.[88]

The histogenesis of primary or classic anal and perianal Paget disease remains uncertain. However, immunohistochemistry, allied to careful clinical correlation, has provided some evidence for the pathogenesis of this disease.[86,91,92] Classic Paget disease represents an intraepithelial proliferation of neoplastic cells originating either from the ducts of adnexal structures, most notably the apocrine sweat glands of the anal region,[92] the Toker cells, which have been shown to be present at sites of involvement by Paget disease, including the vulva,[93] or hair follicle stem cells.[94] Evidence for an origin in cells of the sweat glands is supported by the presence of apocrine markers, particularly gross cystic fluid protein and this marker is of particular value in differentiating primary perianal Paget disease from secondary disease.[92]

Secondary Paget disease is primarily caused by a primary adenocarcinoma of the rectum although, very unusually, secondary Paget disease has been ascribed to adenomas of the rectum, primary carcinomas of the sigmoid colon, and unusual glandular neoplasms such as goblet cell adenocarcinoma.[87,95–97] Only rarely is classic Paget disease associated with subsequent invasive adenocarcinoma in the anal region.[98,99] When Paget disease is caused by a primary adenocarcinoma of the rectum, the cells demonstrate a characteristic cytokeratin immunophenotype with the expression of cytokeratin 20 (CK20) and only rarely CK7 (**Fig. 8**).[79,100] In contrast, classic or primary Paget disease cells express CK7, gross cystic disease fluid protein 15 (GCDFP15), and only occasionally CK20 (**Table 1**, see **Fig. 8**).[79,86,101] However, primary anal adenocarcinoma usually shows an immunophenotype that closely mimics that of classic apocrine-type Paget disease.[102] In this situation, a panel of antibodies is useful to differentiate the various causes of Paget disease (see **Table 1**).[79,86,89]

Little is known about the molecular changes that occur in primary/classic Paget disease. Various molecular abnormalities and mutations have been described but many of these are different to those that occur in Paget disease of the nipple.[103] Furthermore, the

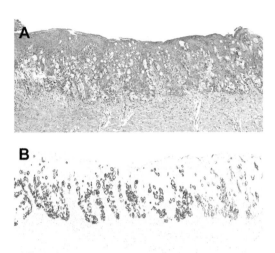

Fig. 8. Secondary Paget disease caused by spread from a primary rectal adenocarcinoma. There is diffuse involvement of the mucosa by neoplastic cells (*A*), highlighted by positive CK20 immunostaining (*B*).

typical absence of microsatellite instability and the lack of PDL-1 expression mean that patients are unlikely to benefit from immunomodulatory treatments that are currently used for more common epithelial malignancies.[103]

Treatment

The treatment of anal and perianal Paget disease entirely depends on the cause of the disease. For Paget disease caused by a primary rectal adenocarcinoma, management is primarily directed at the primary tumor but it may be appropriate to undertake radical abdominoperineal resection to remove the Paget disease at the same operation. For primary or classic Paget disease, various treatment modalities have been described, including radiotherapy, various forms of ablative therapy and drug therapy such as imiquimod.[84,104] Nevertheless, age and comorbidity allowing, relatively radical incisional surgery is the treatment of choice in most cases of primary Paget disease.[84] However, clinically it is difficult to delineate the skin involvement by Paget disease and intraoperative frozen sections or control by CK7 immunohistochemistry can be used to ensure clearance at ultimate margins of excision.[84,85]

MELANOCYTIC PRENEOPLASTIC LESIONS OF THE ANAL REGION

Primary malignant melanoma is a well-recognized, if rare, tumor of the anal region, even if the anus is the commonest site for primary malignant melanoma in the GI tract.[105] It usually presents at a relatively advanced stage with metastatic disease already

Table 1
Immunohistochemical distinction of primary from secondary Paget disease

	Primary Paget Disease	Secondary Paget Disease
GCDFP15	90%	7%
CK7	100%	70%
CK20	12%	95%

demonstrable at presentation in 30% of patients.[105,106] Although it does have a poor prognosis, it has a better prognosis than other primary malignant melanomas in the GI tract, particularly those of the esophagus and stomach.[105] Despite the fact that it originates from melanocytes in the anal canal or perianal skin, it often presents as a lower rectal tumor, and diffuse infiltration of the rectal mucosa is commonly seen histologically.

Melanocytes are present in the upper canal, even above the dentate line, thus accounting for the common presentation of advanced malignant melanoma as an upper anal (or even lower rectal) tumor.[107] Despite this, little is known regarding preneoplastic melanocytic proliferations that presumably occur in the genesis of anal malignant melanoma. There are only isolated reports of an association of premalignant melanocytic proliferations with malignant melanoma.[4]

SUMMARY

In conclusion, anal and perianal preneoplastic lesions comprise a range of entities of which anal squamous dysplasia, the precursor to anal squamous cell carcinoma, is by far the most common and best understood, particularly its relationship to HPV infection and immunosuppression. There is now broad acceptance of LSIL and HSIL terminology from the LAST project. Challenges remain over optimal diagnosis, with judicious use of p16 immunohistochemistry advised, and optimal management. Immunohistochemistry is also helpful to differentiate primary Paget disease, whose pathogenesis remains uncertain, from secondary Paget disease, which is usually due to anal squamous mucosal/epidermal involvement by primary rectal adenocarcinoma. Other forms of premalignant anal neoplasia are rare and poorly understood. A better understanding of the molecular pathology of all these conditions may provide more effective options for managing these diseases.

CLINICS CARE POINTS

- Immunohistochemistry is helpful to corroborate the diagnoses of both squamous dysplasia and Paget disease of the anal region.
- P16 immunohistochemistry is particularly important in the assessment of squamous dysplasia but requires judicious application and careful interpretation.

ACKNOWLEDGMENTS

The authors wish to thank Professor Glenn McCluggage for his helpful comments on the article.

DECLARATION OF INTERESTS

Nothing to declare from either author.

DISCLOSURE

Neither author has any conflicts of interest to disclose.

REFERENCES

1. National Cancer Institute. Surveillance, Epidemiology, and End Results Program. https://seer.cancer.gov/statfacts/html/anus.html. Accessed July, 2023.

2. Bilimoria KY, Bentrem DJ, Rock CE, et al. Outcomes and prognostic factors for squamous-cell carcinoma of the anal canal: analysis of patients from the National Cancer Data Base. Dis Colon Rectum 2009;52(4):624–31.

3. Edge SBBD, Compton CC, Fritz AG, et al. AJCC Cancer staging manual. 7th edition. New York, NY: Springer; 2010.

4. Fenger C, Nielsen VT. Precancerous changes in the anal canal epithelium in resection specimens. Acta Pathol Microbiol Immunol Scand A 1986;94(1):63–9.

5. Fenger C, Nielsen VT. Intraepithelial neoplasia in the anal canal. The appearance and relation to genital neoplasia. Acta Pathol Microbiol Immunol Scand A 1986;94(5):343–9.

6. Frisch MG B, van den Brule AJ, van den Brule AJ, et al. Sexually transmitted infection as a cause of anal cancer. NEJM 1997;337:1350–8.

7. Northfelt DW, Swift PS, Palefsky JM. Anal neoplasia. Pathogenesis, diagnosis, and management. Hematol Oncol Clin N Am 1996;10(5):1177–87.

8. Darragh TM, Colgan TJ, Cox JT, et al, Members of LAST Project Work Groups. The Lower Anogenital Squamous Terminology standardization project for HPV-associated lesions: background and consensus recommendations from the College of American Pathologists and the American Society for Colposcopy and Cervical Pathology. Arch Pathol Lab Med 2012;136(10):1266–97.

9. Castle PE, Stoler MH, Solomon D, et al. The relationship of community biopsy-diagnosed cervical intraepithelial neoplasia grade 2 to the quality control pathology-reviewed diagnoses: an ALTS report. Am J Clin Pathol 2007;127(5):805–15.

10. Stoler MH, Schiffman M, Atypical Squamous Cells of Undetermined Significance-Low-grade Squamous Intraepithelial Lesion Triage Study ALTS Group. Atypical squamous cells of undetermined significance-low-grade squamous intraepithelial lesion triage study group. Interobserver reproducibility of cervical cytologic and histologic interpretations: realistic estimates from the ASCUS-LSIL Triage Study. JAMA 2001;285(11):1500–5.

11. Lytwyn A, Salit IE, Raboud J, et al. Interobserver agreement in the interpretation of anal intraepithelial neoplasia. Cancer 2005;103(7):1447–56.

12. Preti MM M, Robertson C, Sideri M, et al. Inter-observer variation in histopathological diagnosis and grading of vulvar intraepithelial neoplasia: results of an European collaborative study. Br J Obstet Gynaecol 2000;107:594–9.

13. Roma AA, Liu X, Patil DT, et al. Proposed terminology for anal squamous lesions: its application and interobserver agreement among pathologists in academic and community hospitals. Am J Clin Pathol 2017;148(1):81–90.

14. Graham RP. Anal squamous dysplasia (intraepithelial neoplasia). In: Nagtegaal ID, Arends MJ, Odze RD, editors. WHO classification of tumours: Digestive system tumours. Lyon: IARC; 2019.

15. Colon-Lopez V, Shiels MS, Machin M, et al. Anal cancer risk among people with HIV infection in the United States. J Clin Oncol 2018;36(1):68–75.

16. Siddharthan RV, Lanciault C, Tsikitis VL. Anal intraepithelial neoplasia: diagnosis, screening, and treatment. Ann Gastroenterol 2019;32(3):257–63.

17. Navale P, Gonzalez RS, Vyas M. Incidental secondary findings in hemorrhoidectomy specimens: a 16-year experience from a single academic center. Hum Pathol 2021;109:12–20.

18. Palefsky JM, Holly EA, Ralston ML, et al. Anal cytological abnormalities and anal HPV infection in men with Centers for Disease Control group IV HIV disease. Genitourin Med 1997;73(3):174–80.

19. Slama J, Sehnal B, Dusek L, et al. Impact of risk factors on prevalence of anal HPV infection in women with simultaneous cervical lesion. Neoplasma 2015; 62(2):308–14.

20. Ogunbiyi OA, Scholefield JH, Raftery AT, et al. Prevalence of anal human papillomavirus infection and intraepithelial neoplasia in renal allograft recipients. Br J Surg 1994;81(3):365–7.

21. Foust RL, Dean PJ, Stoler MH, et al. Intraepithelial neoplasia of the anal canal in hemorrhoidal tissue: a study of 19 cases. Hum Pathol 1991;22(6):528–34.

22. Kreuter A, Brockmeyer NH, Hochdorfer B, et al. Clinical spectrum and virologic characteristics of anal intraepithelial neoplasia in HIV infection. J Am Acad Dermatol 2005;52(4):603–8.

23. Arain S, Walts AE, Thomas P, et al. The Anal Pap Smear: Cytomorphology of squamous intraepithelial lesions. CytoJournal 2005;2(1):4.

24. Friedlander MA, Stier E, Lin O. Anorectal cytology as a screening tool for anal squamous lesions: cytologic, anoscopic, and histologic correlation. Cancer 2004;102(1):19–26.

25. Mathews WC, Sitapati A, Caperna JC, et al. Measurement characteristics of anal cytology, histopathology, and high-resolution anoscopic visual impression in an anal dysplasia screening program. J Acquir Immune Defic Syndr 2004;37(5): 1610–5.

26. Papaconstantinou HT, Lee AJ, Simmang CL, et al. Screening methods for high-grade dysplasia in patients with anal condyloma. J Surg Res 2005;127(1):8–13.

27. Panther LA, Wagner K, Proper J, et al. High resolution anoscopy findings for men who have sex with men: inaccuracy of anal cytology as a predictor of histologic high-grade anal intraepithelial neoplasia and the impact of HIV serostatus. Clin Infect Dis 2004;38(10):1490–2.

28. Padilla-Espana L, Repiso-Jimenez JB, Fernandez-Sanchez F, et al. [Effectiveness of human papillomavirus genotyping for detection of high-grade anal intraepithelial neoplasia compared to anal cytology]. Enferm Infecc Microbiol Clín 2016;34(7):400–5.

29. Scholefield JH. Anal intraepithelial neoplasia. Br J Surg 1999;86(11):1363–4.

30. Scholefield JH, Ogunbiyi OA, Smith JH, et al. Anal colposcopy and the diagnosis of anal intraepithelial neoplasia in high-risk gynecologic patients. Int J Gynecol Cancer 1994;4(2):119–26.

31. Bean SM, Eltoum I, Horton DK, et al. Immunohistochemical expression of p16 and Ki-67 correlates with degree of anal intraepithelial neoplasia. Am J Surg Pathol 2007;31(4):555–61.

32. Camus M, Lesage AC, Flejou JF, et al. Which lesions should be biopsied during high-resolution anoscopy? Prospective descriptive study of simple morphological criteria. J Low Genit Tract Dis 2015;19(2):156–60.

33. Walts AE, Lechago J, Bose S. P16 and Ki67 immunostaining is a useful adjunct in the assessment of biopsies for HPV-associated anal intraepithelial neoplasia. Am J Surg Pathol 2006;30(7):795–801.

34. Pirog EC, Quint KD, Yantiss RK. P16/CDKN2A and Ki-67 enhance the detection of anal intraepithelial neoplasia and condyloma and correlate with human papillomavirus detection by polymerase chain reaction. Am J Surg Pathol 2010; 34(10):1449–55.

35. Li J, Poi MJ, Tsai MD. Regulatory mechanisms of tumor suppressor P16(INK4A) and their relevance to cancer. Biochemistry 2011;50(25):5566–82.

36. Romagosa C, Simonetti S, Lopez-Vicente L, et al. p16(Ink4a) overexpression in cancer: a tumor suppressor gene associated with senescence and high-grade tumors. Oncogene 2011;30(18):2087–97.

37. Reuschenbach M, Waterboer T, Wallin KL, et al. Characterization of humoral immune responses against p16, p53, HPV16 E6 and HPV16 E7 in patients with HPV-associated cancers. Int J Cancer 2008;123(11):2626–31.

38. Stoler MH, Wright TC Jr, Ferenczy A, et al. Routine use of adjunctive p16 immunohistochemistry improves diagnostic agreement of cervical biopsy interpretation: results from the CERTAIN study. Am J Surg Pathol 2018;42(8):1001–9.

39. Liu Y, McCluggage WG, Darragh TM, et al. p16 immunoreactivity correlates with morphologic diagnosis of hpv-associated anal intraepithelial neoplasia: a study of 1000 biopsies. Am J Surg Pathol 2021;45(11):1573–8.

40. Albuquerque A, Rios E, Dias CC, et al. p16 immunostaining in histological grading of anal squamous intraepithelial lesions: a systematic review and meta-analysis. Mod Pathol 2018;31(7):1026–35.

41. Keung ES, Souers RJ, Bridge JA, et al. Comparative performance of high-risk human papillomavirus RNA and DNA in situ hybridization on College of American Pathologists proficiency tests. Arch Pathol Lab Med 2020;144(3):344–9.

42. Mills AM, Dirks DC, Poulter MD, et al. HR-HPV E6/E7 mRNA in situ hybridization: validation against PCR, DNA in situ hybridization, and p16 immunohistochemistry in 102 samples of cervical, vulvar, anal, and head and neck neoplasia. Am J Surg Pathol 2017;41(5):607–15.

43. Kong CS, Balzer BL, Troxell ML, et al. p16INK4A immunohistochemistry is superior to HPV in situ hybridization for the detection of high-risk HPV in atypical squamous metaplasia. Am J Surg Pathol 2007;31(1):33–43.

44. Colquhoun P, Nogueras JJ, Dipasquale B, et al. Interobserver and intraobserver bias exists in the interpretation of anal dysplasia. Dis Colon Rectum 2003; 46(10):1332–6, discussion 6-8.

45. Scholefield JH, Hickson WG, Smith JH, et al. Anal intraepithelial neoplasia: part of a multifocal disease process. Lancet 1992;340(8830):1271–3.

46. Watson AJ, Smith BB, Whitehead MR, et al. Malignant progression of anal intraepithelial neoplasia. ANZ J Surg 2006;76(8):715–7.

47. Palefsky JM, Holly EA, Hogeboom CJ, et al. Virologic, immunologic, and clinical parameters in the incidence and progression of anal squamous intraepithelial lesions in HIV-positive and HIV-negative homosexual men. J Acquir Immune Defic Syndr Hum Retrovirol 1998;17(4):314–9.

48. Tong WW, Jin F, McHugh LC, et al. Progression to and spontaneous regression of high-grade anal squamous intraepithelial lesions in HIV-infected and uninfected men. AIDS 2013;27(14):2233–43.

49. Scholefield JH, Castle MT, Watson NF. Malignant transformation of high-grade anal intraepithelial neoplasia. Br J Surg 2005;92(9):1133–6.

50. Lee GC, Kunitake H, Milch H, et al. What Is the risk of anal carcinoma in patients with anal intraepithelial neoplasia III? Dis Colon Rectum 2018;61(12):1350–6.

51. Mathews WC, Agmas W, Cachay ER, et al. Natural history of anal dysplasia in an HIV-infected clinical care cohort: estimates using multi-state Markov modeling. PLoS One 2014;9(8):e104116.

52. Tinmouth J, Peeva V, Amare H, et al. Progression From Perianal High-Grade Anal Intraepithelial Neoplasia to Anal Cancer in HIV-Positive Men Who Have Sex With Men. Dis Colon Rectum 2016;59(9):836–42.

53. Burgos J, Curran A, Tallada N, et al. Risk of progression to high-grade anal intraepithelial neoplasia in HIV-infected MSM. AIDS 2015;29(6):695–702.

54. Faber MT, Frederiksen K, Palefsky JM, et al. A nationwide longitudinal study on risk factors for progression of anal intraepithelial neoplasia grade 3 to anal cancer. Int J Cancer 2022;151(8):1240–7.
55. Brogden DRL, Lupi MEE, Warren OJ, et al. Comparing and contrasting clinical consensus and guidelines for anal intraepithelial neoplasia in different geographical regions. Updates Surg 2021;73(6):2047–58.
56. Abbasakoor F, Boulos PB. Anal intraepithelial neoplasia. Br J Surg 2005;92(3): 277–90.
57. Steele SR, Varma MG, Melton GB, et al, Standards Practice Task Force of the American Society of Colon and Rectal Surgeons. Practice parameters for anal squamous neoplasms. Dis Colon Rectum 2012;55(7):735–49.
58. Goldstone RN, Goldstone AB, Russ J, et al. Long-term follow-up of infrared co-agulator ablation of anal high-grade dysplasia in men who have sex with men. Dis Colon Rectum 2011;54(10):1284–92.
59. Brogden DRL, Walsh U, Pellino G, et al. Evaluating the efficacy of treatment options for anal intraepithelial neoplasia: a systematic review. Int J Colorectal Dis 2021;36(2):213–26.
60. Megill C, Wilkin T. Topical therapies for the treatment of anal high-grade squamous intraepithelial lesions. Semin Colon Rectal Surg 2017;28(2):86–90.
61. Richel O, Wieland U, de Vries HJ, et al. Topical 5-fluorouracil treatment of anal intraepithelial neoplasia in human immunodeficiency virus-positive men. Br J Dermatol 2010;163(6):1301–7.
62. de Witte CJ, van de Sande AJ, van Beekhuizen HJ, et al. Imiquimod in cervical, vaginal and vulvar intraepithelial neoplasia: a review. Gynecol Oncol 2015; 139(2):377–84.
63. Fox PA, Nathan M, Francis N, et al. A double-blind, randomized controlled trial of the use of imiquimod cream for the treatment of anal canal high-grade anal intraepithelial neoplasia in HIV-positive MSM on HAART, with long-term follow-up data including the use of open-label imiquimod. AIDS 2010;24(15):2331–5.
64. Pineda CE, Berry JM, Jay N, et al. High-resolution anoscopy targeted surgical destruction of anal high-grade squamous intraepithelial lesions: a ten-year experience. Dis Colon Rectum 2008;51(6):829–35, discussion 35-7.
65. Stier EA, Chigurupati NL, Fung L. Prophylactic HPV vaccination and anal cancer. Hum Vaccin Immunother 2016;12(6):1348–51.
66. Goldstone SE, Giuliano AR, Palefsky JM, et al. Efficacy, immunogenicity, and safety of a quadrivalent HPV vaccine in men: results of an open-label, long-term extension of a randomised, placebo-controlled, phase 3 trial. Lancet Infect Dis 2022;22(3):413–25.
67. Palefsky JM, Giuliano AR, Goldstone S, et al. HPV vaccine against anal HPV infection and anal intraepithelial neoplasia. N Engl J Med 2011;365(17):1576–85.
68. Petrosky E, Bocchini JA Jr, Hariri S, et al, Centers for Disease Control and Prevention CDC. Use of 9-valent human papillomavirus (HPV) vaccine: updated HPV vaccination recommendations of the advisory committee on immunization practices. MMWR Morb Mortal Wkly Rep 2015;64(11):300–4.
69. Nieves-Condoy JF, Acuna-Pinzon CL, Chavarria-Chavira JL, et al. Giant condyloma acuminata (Buschke-Lowenstein tumor): review of an unusual disease and difficult to manage. Infect Dis Obstet Gynecol 2021;2021:9919446.
70. Rydzewska-Rosolowska A, Kakareko K, Kowalik M, et al. An unexpected giant problem - giant condyloma (Buschke-Lowenstein tumor). Int J Infect Dis 2021; 103:280–1.

71. Zhang D, Gonzalez RS, Feely M, et al. Clinicopathologic features of Buschke-Lowenstein tumor: a multi-institutional analysis of 38 cases. Virchows Arch 2020;476(4):543–50.

72. Zidar N, Langner C, Odar K, et al. Anal verrucous carcinoma is not related to infection with human papillomaviruses and should be distinguished from giant condyloma (Buschke-Lowenstein tumour). Histopathology 2017;70(6):938–45.

73. Basik M, Rodriguez-Bigas MA, Penetrante R, et al. Prognosis and recurrence patterns of anal adenocarcinoma. Am J Surg 1995;169(2):233–7.

74. Tarazi R, Nelson RL. Anal adenocarcinoma: a comprehensive review. Semin Surg Oncol 1994;10(3):235–40.

75. Connell WR, Sheffield JP, Kamm MA, et al. Lower gastrointestinal malignancy in Crohn's disease. Gut 1994;35(3):347–52.

76. Jones EA, Morson BC. Mucinous adenocarcinoma in anorectal fistulae. Histopathology 1984;8(2):279–92.

77. Ky A, Sohn N, Weinstein MA, et al. Carcinoma arising in anorectal fistulas of Crohn's disease. Dis Colon Rectum 1998;41(8):992–6.

78. Classic articles in colonic and rectal surgery: Sir James Paget, 1814-1899, on disease of the mammary areola preceeding cancer of the mammary gland. Dis Colon Rectum 1980;23(4):280–1.

79. Goldblum JR, Hart WR. Perianal Paget's disease: a histologic and immunohistochemical study of 11 cases with and without associated rectal adenocarcinoma. Am J Surg Pathol 1998;22(2):170–9.

80. Simonds RM, Segal RJ, Sharma A. Extramammary Paget's disease: a review of the literature. Int J Dermatol 2019;58(8):871–9.

81. Armitage NC, Jass JR, Richman PI, et al. Paget's disease of the anus: a clinicopathological study. Br J Surg 1989;76(1):60–3.

82. Goldman S, Ihre T, Lagerstedt U, et al. Perianal Paget's disease: report of five cases. Int J Colorectal Dis 1992;7(3):167–9.

83. Sasaki Y, Goto K, Sugino T, et al. Characteristic clinicopathological features of secondary extramammary Paget disease with underlying anorectal adenocarcinoma: evenly circumferential perianal distribution, fibroepithelioma of Pinkus-like changes, and subepidermal mucin deposits without invasive tumor cells. Am J Dermatopathol 2021;43(10):721–6.

84. Kibbi N, Owen JL, Worley B, et al. Evidence-based clinical practice guidelines for extramammary Paget disease. JAMA Oncol 2022;8(4):618–28.

85. Brough K, Carley SK, Vidal NY. The treatment of anogenital extramammary Paget's disease as part of a multidisciplinary approach: The use of Mohs surgery moat method with CK7. Int J Dermatol 2022;61(2):238–45.

86. Nowak MA, Guerriere-Kovach P, Pathan A, et al. Perianal Paget's disease: distinguishing primary and secondary lesions using immunohistochemical studies including gross cystic disease fluid protein-15 and cytokeratin 20 expression. Arch Pathol Lab Med 1998;122(12):1077–81.

87. Umemoto S, Inoue S, Amemiya T, et al. A case of perianal Paget's disease associated with a sigmoid colon carcinoma. Gastroenterol Jpn 1993;28(5):719–24.

88. Guenther T. Tumours and tumour-like conditions of the anorectal region. In: Shepherd NA, Warren BF, Williams GT, et al, editors. Morson & Dawson's gastrointestinal pathology. Oxford: Wiley-Blackwell; 2013.

89. Battles OE, Page DL, Johnson JE. Cytokeratins, CEA, and mucin histochemistry in the diagnosis and characterization of extramammary Paget's disease. Am J Clin Pathol 1997;108(1):6–12.

90. Val-Bernal JF, Pinto J. Pagetoid dyskeratosis is a frequent incidental finding in hemorrhoidal disease. Arch Pathol Lab Med 2001;125(8):1058–62.
91. Bussolati G, Pich A. Mammary and extramammary Paget's disease. An immuno-cytochemical study. Am J Pathol 1975;80(1):117–28.
92. Mazoujian G, Pinkus GS, Haagensen DE Jr. Extramammary Paget's disease - evidence for an apocrine origin. An immunoperoxidase study of gross cystic disease fluid protein-15, carcinoembryonic antigen, and keratin proteins. Am J Surg Pathol 1984;8(1):43–50.
93. Belousova IE, Kazakov DV, Michal M, et al. Vulvar toker cells: the long-awaited missing link: a proposal for an origin-based histogenetic classification of extra-mammary Paget disease. Am J Dermatopathol 2006;28(1):84–6.
94. Regauer S. Extramammary Paget's disease - a proliferation of adnexal origin? Histopathology 2006;48(6):723–9.
95. Chumbalkar V, Jennings TA, Ainechi S, et al. Extramammary Paget's disease of anal canal associated with rectal adenoma without invasive carcinoma. Gastro-enterology Res 2016;9(6):99–102.
96. Hutchings D, Windon A, Assarzadegan N, et al. Perianal Paget's disease as spread from non-invasive colorectal adenomas. Histopathology 2021;78(2):276–80.
97. Li M, Yao X. Goblet cell adenocarcinoma of the anal canal with perianal Paget dis-ease: A rare case report with literature review. Medicine (Baltim) 2023;102(16):e33598.
98. Marchesa P, Fazio VW, Oliart S, et al. Long-term outcome of patients with peri-anal Paget's disease. Ann Surg Oncol 1997;4(6):475–80.
99. McCarter MD, Quan SH, Busam K, et al. Long-term outcome of perianal Paget's disease. Dis Colon Rectum 2003;46(5):612–6.
100. Ramalingam P, Hart WR, Goldblum JR. Cytokeratin subset immunostaining in rectal adenocarcinoma and normal anal glands. Arch Pathol Lab Med 2001;125(8):1074–7.
101. Ohnishi T, Watanabe S. The use of cytokeratins 7 and 20 in the diagnosis of pri-mary and secondary extramammary Paget's disease. Br J Dermatol 2000;142(2):243–7.
102. Sasaki M, Terada T, Nakanuma Y, et al. Anorectal mucinous adenocarcinoma associated with latent perianal Paget's disease. Am J Gastroenterol 1990;85(2):199–202.
103. Tse J, Elvin J-A, Vergilo J, et al. Extra-mammary Paget's disease of the skin: a comprehensive genomic profiling study. J Clin Oncol 2019;37:A9591.
104. Rudnicki Y, Stapleton SM, Batra R, et al. Perianal Paget's-an aggressive dis-ease. Colorectal Dis 2023;25(6):1213–21.
105. Zheng Y, Cong C, Su C, et al. Epidemiology and survival outcomes of primary gastrointestinal melanoma: a SEER-based population study. Int J Clin Oncol 2020;25(11):1951–9.
106. Brady MS, Kavolius JP, Quan SH. Anorectal melanoma. A 64-year experience at Memorial Sloan-Kettering Cancer Center. Dis Colon Rectum 1995;38(2):146–51.
107. Clemmensen OJ, Fenger C. Melanocytes in the anal canal epithelium. Histopa-thology 1991;18(3):237–41.

Printed and bound by CPI Group (UK) Ltd, Croydon, CR0 4YY

03/10/2024

01040474-0004